Cognitive and Neuropsychological Approaches to Mental Imagery

NATO ASI Series

Advanced Science Institutes Series

A Series presenting the results of activities sponsored by the NATO Science Committee, which aims at the dissemination of advanced scientific and technological knowledge, with a view to strengthening links between scientific communities.

The Series is published by an international board of publishers in conjunction with the NATO Scientific Affairs Division

A	Life Sciences	Plenum Publishing Corporation
B	Physics	London and New York
C	Mathematical and Physical Sciences	D. Reidel Publishing Company Dordrecht, Boston, Lancaster and Tokyo
D	Behavioural and Social Sciences	Martinus Nijhoff Publishers
E	Applied Sciences	Dordrecht, Boston and Lancaster
F	Computer and Systems Sciences	Springer-Verlag
G	Ecological Sciences	Berlin, Heidelberg, New York, London,
H	Cell Biology	Paris and Tokyo

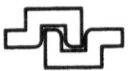

Series D: Behavioural and Social Sciences - No. 42

Cognitive and Neuropsychological Approaches to Mental Imagery

edited by

Michel Denis

Centre d'Etudes de Psychologie Cognitive,
Université de Paris-Sud,
Orsay, France

Johannes Engelkamp

Fachrichtung Psychologie,
Universität des Saarlandes,
Saarbrücken, F.R.G.

and

John T.E. Richardson

Department of Human Sciences,
Brunel University,
Uxbridge, U.K.

1988 **Martinus Nijhoff Publishers**
Dordrecht / Boston / Lancaster
Published in cooperation with NATO Scientific Affairs Division

Proceedings of the NATO Advanced Research Workshop on
"Imagery and Cognition",
Orsay, France,
September 24–26, 1986

Library of Congress Cataloging-in-Publication Data

European Workshop on Imagery and Cognition (1986 :
   Orsay, France)
   Cognitive and neuropsychological approaches to
mental imagery.

   (NATO ASI series. Series D, Behavioural and social
sciences ; no. 42)
   "Proceedings of the European Workshop on Imagery
and Cognition, NATO Advanced Research Workshop, Orsay,
France, September 24-26, 1986"--T.p. verso.
   "Published in cooperation with NATO Scientific
Affairs Division."
   1. Imagery (Psychology)--Congresses. 2. Cognition--
Congresses. 3. Neuropsychology--Congresses. I. Denis,
Michel. II. Engelkamp, Johannes. III. Richardson,
John T. E. IV. North Atlantic Treaty Organisation.
Scientific Affairs Division. V. Title. VI. Series.
[DNLM: 1. Cognition--physiology--congresses.
2. Imagination--physiology--congresses. 3. Mental
Processes--physiology--congresses. BF 367 E89c 1986]
BF367.E95 1986 153.3'2   88-1525

ISBN-13:978-94-010-7121-5   e-ISBN-13:978-94-009-1391-2
DOI: 10.1007/978-94-009-1391-2

Distributors for the United States and Canada: Kluwer Academic Publishers, 101
Philip Drive, Norwell, MA 02061, USA

Distributors for the UK and Ireland: Kluwer Academic Publishers, MTP Press Ltd,
Falcon House, Queen Square, Lancaster LA1 1RN, UK

Distributors for all other countries: Kluwer Academic Publishers Group, Distribution
Center, P.O. Box 322, 3300 AH Dordrecht, The Netherlands

The European Workshop on Imagery and Cognition

The volume "Cognitive and Neuropsychological Approaches to Mental Imagery" presents selected proceedings from the European Workshop on Imagery and Cognition (EWIC), which was held at the Université de Paris-Sud, Orsay, France, 24-26 September 1986.

The decision to organize the EWIC initially came out of discussions among European imagery researchers, who agreed upon the importance of enhancing their level of scientific exchange. It was felt that an appropriate way of doing so would be to set up a workshop which would allow European researchers who had little or no opportunities to meet their counterparts in other countries to become acquainted with the research domains and findings of their colleagues in the imagery field.

The objectives of the EWIC were to extend existing efforts aimed at augmenting scientific exchange among European cognitive psychologists and neuropsychologists involved in imagery research ; to provide a setting where researchers could mutually inform one another of their recent as well as future lines of research ; to provide an opportunity for initiating collaboration in the field of imagery ; to discuss possible new forms of scientific interaction among imagery researchers.

In order for the meeting to be efficient and fruitful, the organizers agreed that the workshop should be restricted to topics on imagery in experimental cognitive-oriented work. The meeting was thus open to papers on theoretical and empirical issues in imagery and cognition, as well as papers dealing with applied fields employing the same conceptual and methodological approaches as those used in cognitive research, in particular, cognitive psychology and neuropsychology.

In order to maintain ties with the wider scientific community, the organizers thought it appropriate to solicit the participation of North American colleagues who have been involved in projects with European researchers, and could contribute to discussions during the EWIC, and the dissemination of ideas emerging from the workshop. The EWIC was pleased to welcome Alain Desrochers, Marc Marschark, and Mark McDaniel, who acted as efficient Invited Discussants.

In addition, the organizers felt that the EWIC would benefit from the participation of internationally recognized contributors in the field of imagery. The organizers are thus especially grateful to Allan Paivio and Steven Pinker, who kindly accepted to participate as Keynote Invited Speakers.

Besides the regular participants, the EWIC organizers opened the workshop to a limited number of observers. The workshop brought together 80 participants, from a total of 11 European countries, in addition to the United States and Canada.

Two Committees were responsible for the preparation of the EWIC :

- The Organizing Committee was in charge of the local organization of the meeting. It was made up of Michel Denis and Marguerite Cocude, both members of the Centre d'Etudes de Psychologie Cognitive, Université de Paris-Sud, Orsay, with the assistance of Maryvonne Carfantan, François Faure, and Constance Greenbaum ;

- The Scientific Committee coordinated the scientific organization of the workshop. It was made up of Michel Denis, Université de Paris-Sud, Orsay, France ; Johannes Engelkamp, Universität des Saarlandes, Saarbrücken, F.R.G. ; and John T.E. Richardson, Brunel University, Uxbridge, England, U.K.

The Committees gratefully acknowledge the support provided to the EWIC by the following institutions : the NATO Scientific Affairs Division, who designated the EWIC as NATO Advanced Research Workshop #86-272 ; the Université de Paris-Sud, Centre d'Orsay, who hosted the workshop and facilitated the preparation of the meeting ; the French Ministère de la Recherche et de l'Enseignement Supérieur, for its support to the Réseau Européen de Laboratoires "Recherche Cognitive en Imagerie" (#411/203/2/4) ; the Centre National de la Recherche Scientifique, for its support provided through the Action Incitative "Europe" (#990023).

The Committees extend their special thanks to the following people for their efforts during the preparatory phases of the workshop : Mme Legendre and Mme Vigny, Université de Paris-Sud, Bureau des Relations Internationales ; Mme Joffrin, Ministère de la Recherche et de l'Enseignement Supérieur, Service International de la Recherche ; Mme Trouillet, Centre National de la Recherche Scientifique, Direction des Relations et de la Coopération Internationales.

Michel Denis

Organization of the Volume

The EWIC was designed to be a forum for the exploration of current issues in imagery research. It is fitting that Part 1 of this volume presents views on these issues by the two Keynote Speakers at the workshop, Allan Paivio and Steven Pinker.

The organization of the rest of the volume reflects to a great extent the way the EWIC was conceived. Parts 2, 3, and 4 correspond to the three days of the workshop. Clearly the fact that a chapter has been assigned to one part does not imply that it is unrelated to the issues dealt with in other parts. Each of the three parts is closed by a concluding chapter written by the Invited Discussant whose role was to highlight the major issues of the session.

Part 2 is devoted to papers dealing with contributions on the nature of imaginal coding, its connections with the representation of visual information in long-term memory, and in particular the ties between this form of coding and the processing of linguistic information. On a lexical level, the main issues are the definition of word imagery value, and the relationships between imagery and the processing of conceptual information. At higher levels of linguistic complexity, the papers presented here deal with the role of imagery in the processing and memorization of sentences and of texts.

Part 3 focuses more directly on imagery as a process. Imagery is first discussed for its role in the functioning of working memory, both as concerns the formation and the manipulation of visuo-spatial representations. Visual imagery is also examined in terms of its structural and functional components and its capacity to handle certain features of temporal information. This part of the volume also includes papers discussing the contribution of imagery-based strategies to problem solving, as well as the role of imagery in the acquisition of motor skills based on mental practice.

Part 4 first presents papers exploring the relationships between imaginal and motor representations in memory systems, and papers on emotional imagery in the framework of a cognitive approach. The second section of part 4 is devoted to neuropsychological approaches to mental imagery, with papers oriented towards detailed characterizations of the neural substrate and mechanisms of visual imagery, and articles examining the incidence of brain damage and sensory handicaps on the elaboration and mnemonic use of visual imagery.

The Editors' Concluding Chapter (part 5 of the volume) summarizes the final remarks presented at the closing session of the workshop.

Michel Denis
Johannes Engelkamp
John T.E. Richardson

The Editors would like to acknowledge the assistance of Maryvonne Carfantan and Constance Greenbaum in the preparation of this volume.

Table of Contents

2.3. Sentence and Text Processing

2.4. Discussion of Part 2

Part 3
Imagery Processes in Adaptive Behavior

3.1. Imagery Processes and Working Memory

Contributors

Alberto Acosta
Seccion de Psicología, Campus Universitario de Cartuja, Universidad de Granada, 18011 Granada, Spain

Ornella Andreani
Istituto di Psicologia, Facoltà di Lettere e Filosofia, Università degli Studi di Pavia, Piazza Botta 6 (Palazzo San Felice), 27100 Pavia, Italy

John Annett
Department of Psychology, University of Warwick, Coventry CV4 7AL, England, United Kingdom

Susan Aylwin
Department of Applied Psychology, University College, Cork, Ireland

Alan Baddeley
MRC Applied Psychology Unit, 15 Chaucer Road, Cambridge CB2 2EF, England, United Kingdom

Anna Berti
Istituto di Clinica Neurologica, Università di Milano, Via Francesco Sforza, 35, 20122 Milano, Italy

Klaus Bischof
Institut für Psychologie, Universität Basel, Bernouillistrasse 14, 4056 Basel, Switzerland

Edoardo Bisiach
Istituto di Clinica Neurologica, Università di Milano, Via Francesco Sforza, 35, 20122 Milano, Italy

Marguerite Cocude
Centre d'Etudes de Psychologie Cognitive, Université de Paris-Sud, Centre scientifique d'Orsay, Bâtiment 335, 91405 Orsay Cedex, France

Martin A. Conway
MRC Applied Psychology Unit, 15 Chaucer Road, Cambridge CB2 2EF, England, United Kingdom

Cesare Cornoldi
Dipartimento di Psicologia Generale, Università degli Studi di Padova, Piazza Capitaniato, 3, 35139 Padova, Italy

Rossana De Beni
Dipartimento di Psicologia Generale, Università degli

Studi di Padova, Piazza Capitaniato, 3, 35139 Padova, Italy

Lüder Deecke
Neurologische Universitätsklinik, Lazarettgasse 14, 1090 Wien, Austria

Michel Denis
Centre d'Etudes de Psychologie Cognitive, Université de Paris-Sud, Centre scientifique d'Orsay, Bâtiment 335, 91405 Orsay Cedex, France

Alain Desrochers
Ecole de Psychologie, Université d'Ottawa, 651 Cumberland, Ottawa, Ontario, K1N 6N5, Canada

Emanuel Donchin
Department of Psychology, University of Illinois at Urbana-Champaign, 603 East Daniel Street, Champaign, IL 61820, U.S.A.

Johannes Engelkamp
Fachrichtung 6.4 - Psychologie, Universität des Saarlandes, 6600 Saarbrücken, F.R.G.

Martha J. Farah
Department of Psychology, Carnegie-Mellon University, Pittsburgh, PA 15213-3890, U.S.A.

Pilar Ferrándiz
Departamento de Psicología General, Facultad de Psicología, Universidad Complutense, Campus de Somosaguas, 28023 Madrid, Spain

Georg Goldenberg
Neurologische Universitätsklinik, Lazarettgasse 14, 1090 Wien, Austria

Marie-Anne Gonon
INSERM Unité 280, 151, cours Albert-Thomas, 69003 Lyon, France

Javier Gonzalez-Marques
Departamento de Psicología General, Facultad de Psicología, Universidad Complutense, Campus de Somosaguas, 28023 Madrid, Spain

Miep van der Ham-van Koppen
Rijksuniversiteit Utrecht, Vakgroep Psychonomie, Sectie Theoretische Psychologie en Functieleer, Postbus 80.140, 3508 TC Utrecht, The Netherlands

Tore Helstrup
Department of Cognitive Psychology, University of Bergen, Sydneshaugen 2, 5000 Bergen Univ., Norway

Gregory V. Jones
Department of Psychology, University of Warwick, Coventry CV4 7AL, England, United Kingdom

Geir Kaufmann
Department of Cognitive Psychology, University of Bergen, Sydneshaugen 2, 5000 Bergen Univ., Norway

Alain Lieury
Laboratoire de Psychologie Expérimentale, Université de Haute-Bretagne, 6, avenue Gaston-Berger, 35043 Rennes Cedex, France

Robert H. Logie
Department of Psychology, University of Aberdeen, King's College, Old Aberdeen AB9 2UB, Scotland, United Kingdom

Anita van Loon-Vervoorn
Rijksuniversiteit Utrecht, Vakgroep Psychonomie, Sectie Theoretische Psychologie en Functieleer, Postbus 80.140, 3508 TC Utrecht, The Netherlands

Amir Mane
Department of Psychology, University of Illinois at Urbana-Champaign, 603 East Daniel Street, Champaign, IL 61820, U.S.A.

Marc Marschark
Department of Psychology, University of North Carolina at Greensboro, Greensboro, NC 27412-5001, U.S.A.

Maryanne Martin
Department of Experimental Psychology, University of Oxford, South Parks Road, Oxford OX1 3UD, England, United Kingdom

Juan Mayor
Departamento de Psicología General, Facultad de Psicología, Universidad Complutense, Campus de Somosaguas, 28023 Madrid, Spain

Mark A. McDaniel
Department of Psychological Sciences, Purdue University, West Lafayette, IN 47907, U.S.A.

Silvia Mecklenbräuker
Universität Trier, Fachbereich I, Psychologie, Postfach 3825, 5500 Trier, F.R.G.

F. Alfonso Medina
Universidad Nacional de Educación a Distancia, C. Embajadores, 7, 28012 Madrid, Spain

Allan Paivio
Department of Psychology, University of Western Ontario,

London, Ontario, N6A 5C2, Canada

Alfonso Palma
Seccion de Psicología, Campus Universitario de Cartuja,
Universidad de Granada, 18011 Granada, Spain

Herminia Peraita
Universidad Nacional de Educación a Distancia, Facultad
de Psicología, Departamento de Psicologia General,
Ciudad Universitaria, 28040 Madrid, Spain

Franck Péronnet
INSERM Unité 280, 151, cours Albert-Thomas, 69003 Lyon,
France

Walter J. Perrig
Institut für Psychologie, Universität Basel,
Bernouillistrasse 14, 4056 Basel, Switzerland

Steven Pinker
Department of Brain and Cognitive Sciences (E10-018),
Massachusetts Institute of Technology, Cambridge, MA
02139, U.S.A.

Ivo Podreka
Neurologische Universitätsklinik, Lazarettgasse 14, 1090
Wien, Austria

Gerard Quinn
Department of Psychology, University of St. Andrews, St.
Andrews, Fife, KY16 9JU, Scotland, United Kingdom

John T. E. Richardson
Department of Human Sciences, Brunel University,
Uxbridge, Middlesex, UB8 3PH, England, United Kingdom

Javier Sainz
Departamento de Psicología General, Facultad de
Psicología, Universidad Complutense, Campus de
Somosaguas, 28023 Madrid, Spain

Alain Savoyant
U.A. Cognition et Mouvement, C.N.R.S. - IBHOP, 5, rue
des Géraniums, 13014 Marseille, France

Russel Sheptak
Department of Psychology, University of Illinois at
Urbana-Champaign, 603 East Daniel Street, Champaign, IL
61820, U.S.A.

John Michael Slack
Department of Psychology, Open University, Walton Hall,
Milton Keynes MK7 6AA, England, United Kingdom

Margarete Steiner
Neurologische Universitätsklinik, Lazarettgasse 14, 1090 Wien, Austria

Erhard Suess
Neurologische Universitätsklinik, Lazarettgasse 14, 1090 Wien, Austria

Manuel de Vega
Departamento de Psicología Básica, Universidad de La Laguna, Tenerife, Islas Canarias, Spain

Jaime Vila
Seccion de Psicología, Campus Universitario de Cartuja, Universidad de Granada, 18011 Granada, Spain

Harold T. A. Whiting
Vakgroep Psychologie IFLO, Vrije Universiteit, De Boelelaan 1081, Amsterdam, The Netherlands

Klaus Willmes
Neurologische Abteilung der RWTH Aachen, Pauwelstrasse, 5100 Aachen, F.R.G.

Barbara Wilson
University Department of Rehabilitation, Southampton General Hospital, Southampton SO9 4XY, England, United Kingdom

Werner Wippich
Universität Trier, Fachbereich I, Psychologie, Postfach 3825, 5500 Trier, F.R.G.

PART 1

KEY ISSUES IN IMAGERY RESEARCH

BASIC PUZZLES IN IMAGERY RESEARCH

ALLAN PAIVIO
UNIVERSITY OF WESTERN ONTARIO

ABSTRACT

Modern research has generated much positive information on the structure and functions of imagery. Unexpectedly, it has also exposed methodological and conceptual obstacles that impede our progress toward a deeper scientific understanding of imagery and are challenging problems in their own right. An overriding methodological problem is the relative difficulty of providing an unambiguous external criterion for the internal process of imagery. Also unsolved are such specific problems as: vividness versus ease of imagery as determinants (or correlates) of image-mediated performance, interpretation of imagery integration and its effects; the complex nature and predictive uncertainty of individual differences; and neural mechanisms of imagery. Using research examples, I discuss the implications of such puzzles and describe attempts that have been made to solve them.

1. INTRODUCTION

The title of this chapter refers to issues that we have encountered in our research and appear often enough in the literature to be considered basic. I exclude the so-called imagery-proposition controversy, although I have strong views on that issue and have presented them elsewhere (Paivio, 1986). I concentrate instead on other conceptual and methodological problems that are challenging to imagery researchers regardless of their theoretical preferences. Discussed in turn are, (a) the problem of specifying an unambiguous criterion for imagery, (b) vividness versus ease of imagery as determinants of image-mediated performance, (c) the functional integration of images, (d) the complexity and predictive uncertainty of individual differences in imagery, and (e) the neural mechanisms of imagery. The first three are specific problems and could be viewed as pieces of the imagery puzzle. Individual differences and neural mechanisms are more general and entail the problem of putting together pieces of the puzzle into an organizing framework.

2. EXTERNAL CRITERIA FOR IMAGERY

The criterion puzzle is an overriding issue with implications for the other four topics that follow. The study of imagery has always been plagued by the difficulty of finding a relatively direct and unambiguous observational criterion for imagery activity. This problem of operational definition is common to all inferential or mentalistic concepts and its consequences have ranged from the outright rejection of such concepts in the behaviorist program to a variety of specific complications in the investigation of imagery. The general problem also

3

M. Denis et al. (eds.), Cognitive and Neuropsychological Approaches to Mental Imagery, 3–16.
© *1988 by Martinus Nijhoff Publishers.*

has a positive side in that it has motivated research designed to show that imagery has unique functional properties. Familiar examples include research on modality specific interference, mental rotation, image scanning, and mental comparisons as ways of testing parallels between imagery and perceptual mechanisms.

On the negative side, however, the subjective nature of imagery makes it difficult to come up with a simple measure of the extent to which imagery is involved in specific tasks, a measure comparable, say, to verbal responses as indicators of language involvement. We encountered the problem most recently when we set out to compare the time required for the reciprocal referential reactions of naming pictures of objects and imaging to the names of the objects. Naming speed is usually measured by means of a voice key that is activated by the spoken name, but imagery cannot be expressed in such a direct way.

Our solution was to have subjects press a key as soon as the name or image occurred to them, and then to externalize the internal reactions in different ways. Thus, in the naming condition, they wrote the name they had thought of and, in the image condition, they drew a rough sketch of the object they had imaged. We hoped thereby to induce sets for verbal and nonverbal internal processing while at the same time having a common neutral response for measuring reaction time. The procedure succeeded in that subjects easily carried out the tasks and the results were interpretable. For example, measures of name uncertainty and image uncertainty were the best predictors of naming and imaging latencies. The results may not generalize to different procedures, however, because even subtle variations in the external criteria affect reaction times and their correlations with other variables. In the case of imagery, drawing is not overlearned and conventionalized to the same degree as writing. Thus, subjects are likely to delay their key press until they are sure they can draw an acceptable fascimile, and the delay would be expected to increase with such variables as the complexity of the drawn object more than if drawing is not required.

We lack direct evidence on the effect of a drawing criterion on image latency, but we do have some on a comparable criterion task. As part of a study of pupillary dilation during an imagery task, Simpson and I (Simpson & Paivio, 1968) obtained keypress latencies for imaging to concrete and abstract words. Half the subjects were required to describe their images after pressing the key and half were not. The pertinent result, illustrated in Figure 1, was that the requirement to describe the images substantially increased the latency of the keypress. A similar delaying effect would be expected with a drawing criterion.

Despite the conventional nature of language, even naming latency is affected by the response criteria used. We have data on average naming latency for items using both keypress and voicekey reactions. Although the two measures are highly correlated, they apparently tap somewhat different processes. For example, word frequency and pronounceability correlated more highly with voicekey naming latency than with keypress latency. The differences are theoretically appropriate because vocal responses presumably are mediated more directly than manual responses by properties of the verbal system that also are the basis of frequency and pronounceability judgments. Nevertheless, such results complicate the measurement problem, though to a lesser extent than in the case of imagery.

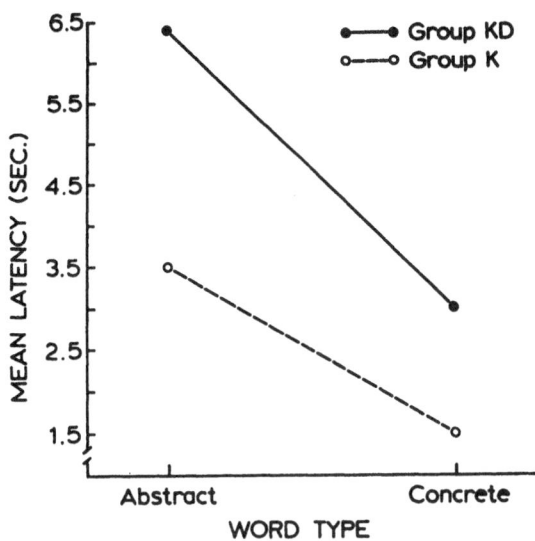

FIGURE 1. Effect of requiring a description of the image (group K versus KD) on key press latencies to abstract and concrete words. Based on Simpson and Paivio (1968).

3. VIVIDNESS VERSUS EASE OF IMAGERY

Galton introduced the empirical study of imagery with an emphasis on vividness as its main functional attribute. This emphasis was reflected in his breakfast table questionnaire, which asked the respondent to judge the vividness of his or her memory images along different sensory dimensions. The emphasis continued in all subsequent versions of the questionnaire (e.g. Betts, 1909; Sheehan, 1967; Marks, 1973). Vividness is turning out to be a good predictor of performance in certain tasks (e.g., see Denis in the present volume) but this had not been the case in earlier research and even today the results are variable (e.g., see the paradoxical negative relations reported recently by Heuer, Fischman, & Reisberg, 1986). Partly because of the doubtful empirical status of vividness, I decided instead to put my money on ease or speed of image arousal in my research on imagery and memory in the early 1960s. The other reason was that I wanted to compare the role of imagery with that of verbal mediators in standard verbal memory tasks in which items were typically presented at rates as rapid as two seconds per item. Thus, imagery had to be aroused quickly if it were to be effective as a mediator, which implied further that ease of image arousal should be an important correlate of the memorability of items. This turned out to be the case and rated ease of imagery continues to be a powerful predictor of memory performance.

However, ease and vividness of item imagery have not been systematically compared as predictors. To my knowledge, both were included only in a correlational study of item attributes and memory that I reported in 1968. Rated ease and vividness were highly correlated but ease nonetheless turned out to be the better predictor of memory. Since

6

I was interested in other theoretical issues at that time, I didn't
pursue the problem more systematically, although sometimes I was tempted
to do so when others published studies in which they incorrectly referred
to our word imagery norms as measures of vividness.

A study by Day and Bellezza (1983) finally prompted us to focus on
the problem. The subjects in their study were shown pairs of
semantically related and unrelated concrete nouns or abstract nouns, to
which they were to generate interactive images. They rated the images on
vividness and were then asked to recall one member of each pair given the
other member as a retrieval cue. The crucial finding was that the
subjects rated abstract related pairs higher in vividness than concrete
unrelated pairs, but they nonetheless recalled more of the concrete
unrelated pairs. This dissociation between vividness and recall led Day
and Bellezza to conclude that Paivio's dual coding and imagery theory of
verbal memory was wrong inasmuch as less vivid images were remembered
better than more vivid images.

Their theoretical analysis was incomplete in various ways that
rendered their conclusion inappropriate (see Paivio, 1986, p. 170) but
the relevant point here is that Day and Bellezza emphasized vividness
rather than ease of imagery in their instructions. Given that the pairs
were presented in an unpaced manner, subjects had unlimited time to
generate vivid images even for abstract pairs. The results might differ
if their attention were drawn to the ease or speed with which items
arouse imagery. That is, abstract related pairs might now be rated lower
in imagery value than concrete unrelated pairs. Jim Clark, Mustaq Kahn,
and I tested that idea in a series of experiments in which we used rating
and other procedures designed to distinguish between vividness and ease.
The result was that we essentially failed to do so. As shown in Figure
2, abstract related pairs were consistently rated higher than concrete
unrelated pairs on both ease and vividness of imagery, but concrete
unrelated pairs were remembered better.

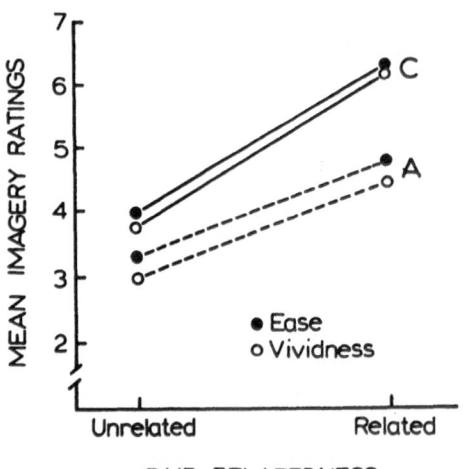

FIGURE 2. Mean ratings of ease and vividness of imagery for semantically
related and unrelated pairs of concrete (c) nouns and abstract (A) nouns.

I point out in passing that pair relatedness and concreteness had partly independent and additive effects on imagery ratings. This observation is quite consistent with the dual coding assumption that imaginal and verbal associative structures result from associative experiences with objects and words, so that stimulus relatedness would be expected to facilitate access to both kinds of structures. The crucial point for present purposes, however, is that ratings of vividness and ease were indistinguishable. Note how different this seems from the analogous perceptual situation: if we orthogonally varied the clarity of a picture and the delay between its presentation and a preceding signal, people should be able to judge clarity and time interval independently and verdically. If my thought experiment is correct, it means that vividness and speed of mental images are much less discriminable than comparable perceptual dimensions, or that the two are actually correlated attributes of imagery, derived from correlated perceptual experiences; or it could simply mean that we haven't yet developed effective procedures that would enable subjects to distinguish similarly between the imaged attributes. The alternatives remain to be investigated.

4. IMAGERY INTEGRATION

One of the most common generalizations about imagery mnemonics is that relationally organized images are more effective than separated images in cued recall tasks. The effect is generally attributed to the spatially integrated properties of such images and their redintegration by the word that serves as the retrieval cue. The question here is whether such integrative properties are unique to imagery.

The dual coding position is that effects suggestive of integration could be produced by strong pre-experimental verbal associative connections between items when the direction of retrieval is congruent with the associative sequence. Such ideas were tested and to some extent supported at the time that associative symmetry was a popular issue. But what if verbal associative relations seemingly are equated whereas imagery varies? Shouldn't the integrative power of imagery still show its effect? Marc Marschark and I (1977) failed to obtain such an effect in a series of experiments on memory for concrete and abstract sentences. The sentences clearly differed in rated imagery value and the subjects reported using imagery to remember concrete but not abstract sentences. Despite these differences, cued recall effects that are presumed to tap integration showed that abstract and concrete sentences were recalled in an equally integrative or holistic manner. At the same time, overall recall was higher for concrete than for abstract sentences. Thus, we had support for the additive effects of dual coding but not for differences in integrative organization of the memory trace.

Marschark (e.g., 1985) has subsequently replicated and extended these findings to show some of the boundary conditions for concrete item superiority in recall and trace integration. Concrete-abstract differences are reduced and even eliminated when rich contextual factors can operate, as in memory for paragraphs. Such observations go part way toward clarifying the issues, although I don't think they resolve them completely. In particular, they don't tell us why integrative imagery effects that appear with simple materials, such as paired associates, should be eliminated or at least obscured in the case of more complex verbal material such as paragraphs. That is, why shouldn't verbal contextual relations and imagery still be additive in their effects?

The empirical issue itself has not yet been fully resolved, judging from Wippich's finding (reported in the present volume) of greater integration effects for concrete than abstract sentences. I remain hopeful that the pieces of the puzzle can be put together within the framework of dual coding theory using a combination of imagery and verbal associative processes, and assuming some tradeoff between facilitative and interfering effects that can result from associative relations and other factors in the memory tasks.

5. INDIVIDUAL DIFFERENCES

I turn now to the first of two general problem areas in which our task at the outset not only is to find missing pieces of a puzzle, but also to organize them into a broader picture. This is the problem of individual differences, which was the first imagery puzzle to be approached quantitatively. Despite its venerable history, however, the individual difference approach has not shown the same degree of systematic empirical and theoretical progress as approaches based on experimental procedures and manipulation of stimulus materials. I base this conclusion partly on the observation that most of the individual difference research has not been designed to explore systematically the nature of imagery differences as a problem in its own right, with the aim of identifying various dimensions of imagery abilities and habits or preferences. Instead, the research has consisted mainly of piecemeal attempts to predict memory or some other cognitive skill using scores on a single test that is assumed to measure imagery ability. The most popular tests include (a) imagery vividness, especially Marks's (1973) VVIQ, (b) space relations or some other measure of spatial ability, (c) imagery controllability as measured by Gordon's (1949) questionnaire, and (d) imagery preference as measured by our Individual Difference Questionnaire (IDQ; Paivio & Harshman, 1983) or some version of it.

Imagery researchers are aware that imagery is multidimensional and complex, but the problem is relatively unexplored and the few attempts to identify imagery dimensions have generally focussed on some specific contrasts, such as factorial distinctions between subjective and objective tests or between imaginal and verbal abilities. The relative narrowness of scope characterized our own early research on the problem. Although I had discussed various dimensions of imagery and verbal habits and skills in my 1971 book, we did not initiate a truly systematic research program on the problem at that time.

Systematic research needs a general theory to guide it and to provide an organizing framework for the individual pieces of the puzzle that the research uncovers. We now have at least the beginnings of such programs. Kosslyn and Jolicoeur (1980) approached the study of individual differences in imagery using the various processes specified in Kosslyn's computational theory. Recently, we began a program of research on individual differences based on an updated version of dual coding theory (Paivio, 1986, Ch. 6). I will outline the framework and the approach to illustrate my general point. The categories and distinctions used in the approach to individual differences all derive from the general theory.

Symbolic habits versus abilities

This distinction refers to the difference between how often and how skilfully we use different modes of thinking. Our IDQ was intended to measure habits or preferences for using imagery as compared to language in various situations, although it also measures independent ability dimensions (Paivio & Harshman, 1983). Spatial manipulation tests tap imagery abilities more directly and scores on such tests also are generally independent of imagery preferences.

Nonverbal (imaginal) versus verbal processes

Dual coding theory would be in deep trouble if the verbal-nonverbal distinction did not show up in the individual difference research. Fortunately, various studies show that scores on tests that depend on nonverbal processes, including those that have been traditionally viewed as imagery tests, are generally uncorrelated with scores on tests that depend primarily on verbal processes. This is consistent with the independence assumption of the general theory.

Symbolic versus sensorimotor modalities

The contrast here is between the verbal-nonverbal symbolic dimension and specific sensory modalities. The two dimensions are assumed to be orthogonal in that both verbal and nonverbal information can be visual (e.g., printed words versus pictures), auditory (spoken words versus environmental sounds), or haptic (writing activity versus tactual exploration of objects). Such modalities as taste and smell are not used as linguistic media, so the orthogonal model is necessarily incomplete, but the general point is that we must have cognitive representational systems for dealing with different modalities of verbal and nonverbal information. Some evidence is available on modality specific abilities (Paivio, 1986, p. 101-102), but the facts are sparse and, accordingly, this area is ripe for systematic research.

Structural interconnections and processing levels

Dual coding theory distinguishes between representational, referential, and associative interconnections and different levels of processing involving those interconnections. The representational level refers to relatively direct activation of cognitive representations corresponding to verbal or nonverbal stimulus units; the referential level refers to cross-system activation via the interconnections between verbal and nonverbal representations; and the associative level, to spreading activation among representations within each system. Individuals presumably differ in the availability of representations and functional interconnections between them, as well as the processing skills involved in making use of the structures.

Representational abilities would be tapped by tests that measure some aspect of an individual's ability to recognize objects and words, without also requiring referential and associative processing of such stimuli. This could be achieved using stimulus recognition or matching tests, but most standard cognitive ability tests do not meet that ideal. For example, although picture recognition tests and figural completion tests entail access to object representations, they usually require a spoken or written naming response to the stimuli, thereby implicating referential processing. Purer test paradigms are available in the experimental literature and could be systematically applied to the study of individual differences in this level of processing.

The available tests of referential ability are generally incomplete from the dual coding perspective because they measure processing in only one direction, from nonverbal to verbal. Picture naming is a familiar example. The opposite, verbal to nonverbal direction is crucial to the study of imagery because most imagery tasks make use of verbal stimuli. Imagery reaction time to words is an appropriate measure that has been used in experimental and some individual difference studies. However, systematic comparisons of the two directions has only begun.

Wilma Bucci and her colleagues (e.g., Bucci, 1984) developed a referential ability test using speed of color naming. They found that scores on the test correlated with other aspects of cognition that directly implicate imagery. Thus, though unidirectional, Bucci's naming test appears to tap referential access to, and processing in, the imagery system as well. This would be expected on the basis of dual coding theory because experiences involving nonverbal stimuli and their descriptive labels are usually bidirectional, although unidirectional experiences could be consistent enough in some cases to produce asymmetries in referential processing efficiency over items and people.

Jim Clark, Nancy Digdon, and I have begun studying individual and item differences in speed of referential processing in both directions, using object naming and word imaging tests. Among other things, we found that reaction times for these reciprocal responses are substantially but not perfectly correlated over individuals (r=.74) as well as items (r=.57). The research needs to be expanded to include such nonverbal referential reactions as imaged environmental sounds, movement patterns, and emotions in response to the relevant descriptive language. Motor referential reactions are implicated in the research reported by Engelkamp and Perrig in this volume, and they could easily extend their research to include relevant individual difference measures.

Associative abilities have been measured by a variety of standard verbal association tests. Once again, however, comparable tests are generally lacking on the imagery side, perhaps because the measurement problem is especially acute. Ideally, we would want measures of the ease, distribution, and quality of the nonverbal images that are associatively aroused by objects, environmental sounds, and so on. We find some approximations in Guilford's tests that tap divergent production of figural systems, but most of the potentially-relevant tests are contaminated by referential processing and verbal associative processing demands. It appears that the necessary tests will have to be developed essentially from scratch.

Transformational processing abilities

According to the dual coding approach, cognitive transformations are constrained and determined by the structure of the information in the two symbolic sytems. The constraints are primarily sequential in the case of language, so that transformations occur on a sequential frame. Conversely, the constraints are spatial and sensory in the case of nonverbal information, so that transformations entail changes on such spatial dimensions as size, shape, and orientation, or changes in the sensory modality of representational information. Spatial manipulation tests of imagery measure an individual's ability to recognize or produce spatial transformations or to re-organize spatial components in some way. Some of the items in Gordon's (1949) imagery control questionnaire appear to tap spatial transformational skills. For example, subjects are asked if they can "see" a car and then image it upside down. However, the scores on such items correlate only slightly if at all with scores on standard spatial manipulation tests (Ernest, 1977). Other items in her questionnaire deal with control of colour, implicating sensory transformational skills that have not yet been studied systematically by more objective procedures.

Thus, despite the many tests that have been developed to tap transformational abilities involving imagery, we are far from having a complete picture of the potential range and limits of such abilities and the degree to which they are correlated or independent. Here, too, dual coding theory provides a framework that draws attention to empirical gaps that might otherwise go unnoticed.

Functional abilities

Other theoretically motivated categories of individual differences pertain to complex adaptive functions served by imaginal and verbal systems. These include evaluative, mnemonic, and motivational functions, which are more general than the categories discussed up to this point because the functions incorporate many of the specific processing abilities in various combinations. For example, a complete inventory of mnemonic abilities would have to include whatever processes are entailed in encoding, storage, and retrieval of information. Most tests of memory ability, however, are designed only to measure storage capacity. Guilford (1967) has used a variety of tests that tap memory for items, sequences, associations, and so on, but these do not tease apart the contributions of such component processes as encoding and retrieval.

From the dual coding perspective, speed of referential processing should be related to performance on tasks that require the use of imagery mnemonics for remembering verbal material or verbal coding for remembering pictures, but such relations have been studied only rarely and incompletely. Transformational abilities have been investigated more often in studies that have correlated memory performance with scores on spatial imagery tests, but even that research has been relatively unsystematic and unanalytic. A systematic analysis suggests, for example, that spatial organizational and transformational skills should be more related to the efficiency with which individuals can generate and use interactive images than separate images because the latter do not require transformations. Numerous problems of that kind merit study if we are to increase our systematic understanding of the role of imaginal representations and processing skills in memory performance.

Motivational functions refer to the role played by imaginal and verbal processes in goal directed activity and affect. The papers by Conway and Bekerian, Martin, and Acosta et al in this volume deal with such functions. Relevant examples from the psychological literature include achievement imagery as studied by McClelland (e.g., 1961) in connection with the measurement of need achievement and by Jerome Singer (1966) in his analysis of daydreams. Both approaches implicate goal directed activity as reflected in the content of mental imagery and language. Affective imagery has been a central focus in psychoanalysis and in cognitive approaches to psychotherapy. Sports psychologists have used relaxation techniques based on imagery to help athletes reduce maladaptive tension. Despite this theoretical and practical attention to the role of imagery in motivation and emotion, researchers have only touched on relevant individual difference variables. Singer and Antrobus (1972) incorporated affective dimensions in their daydream questionnaire and other specific approaches can be found in the literature, but these do not represent systematic empirical and theoretical attempts to study the motivational functions of imagery from an individual difference perspective.

I have not undertaken such research although I studied motivational and affective factors in social behavior before I began programmatic research on imagery. The relation between verbal processes, imagery, and affect were implicit in a study (Paivio & Lambert, 1959) in which we adapted McClelland's thematic story procedure to measure individual differences in audience sensitivity (susceptibility to stage fright in the broad sense). It would be interesting now to study the relation between cognition and motivation more generally from a dual coding perspective, and with an emphasis on individual differences.

6. NEURAL MECHANISMS OF IMAGERY

Like individual differences, the neuropsychology of imagery begs for a conceptual scheme that would organize the available and sought-after pieces of a puzzle. I will point to some salient pieces and provide a sketch of the larger pattern into which they might fit, drawing on general reviews (Paivio, 1986; Paivio & te Linde, 1983) in which I organized the available empirical pieces of the puzzle within the framework of dual coding theory. The fit looks pretty good to me but others will want to judge for themselves and perhaps come up with a different partial sketch.

The question most often asked is, What brain structures are responsible for imagery? The most popular hypothesis is that they are preferentially located in the right hemisphere (e.g., see Ley, 1983), perhaps especially in the parietal or parieto-occipital region of that hemisphere. Another view is that posterior regions in both hemispheres are crucial sites for imagery (e.g., Bisiach, Capitani, Luzzatti, & Perani, 1981). Recently, Farah (1984) and Kosslyn, Holtzman, Farah, and Gazzaniga (1985) have focused on left hemisphere structures in the generation of multipart mental images. My own reading of the data is that all of these interpretations are partly correct. Different regions in both cerebral hemispheres and probably subcortical regions as well carry out different imagery functions, depending on the criteria that are used to define imagery and the kind of task that is used to tap those functions.

Both hemispheres must contain the representational information necessary for generating images of objects, since normal subjects can identify pictures of familiar objects just as easily when they are presented to the right visual field as when they are presented to the left field. Split brain patients also have the ability to identify objects presented to either hemisphere provided that the same hemisphere is used in the test phase. For example, the patient can correctly identify with the right hand an object that had been presented only in the right field, so that the seen and felt objects are processed by the left hemisphere.

Carole Ernest and I (Paivio & Ernest, 1971) obtained evidence that the hemispheric equivalence in object identification implicates spatial imagery. The pertinent results are shown in Figure 3. Note that subjects with high spatial imagery ability were far superior to low ability subjects in tachistoscopic recognition of pictures presented to either field. Field had no effect either alone or in interaction with ability. The results differed for letters and geometric forms; for example, letters were recognized better in the right field by both high and low imagery subjects, which is consistent with the accepted view that the left hemisphere is specialized for processing verbal stimuli. The different pattern for pictures suggests that both hemispheres must have representations for familiar objects and that imagery ability facilitates access to those representations in either hemisphere. The research by Farah and her colleagues suggests further that the left hemisphere can actually surpass the right hemisphere in the generation of mental images of letters and parts of familiar objects to verbal cues.

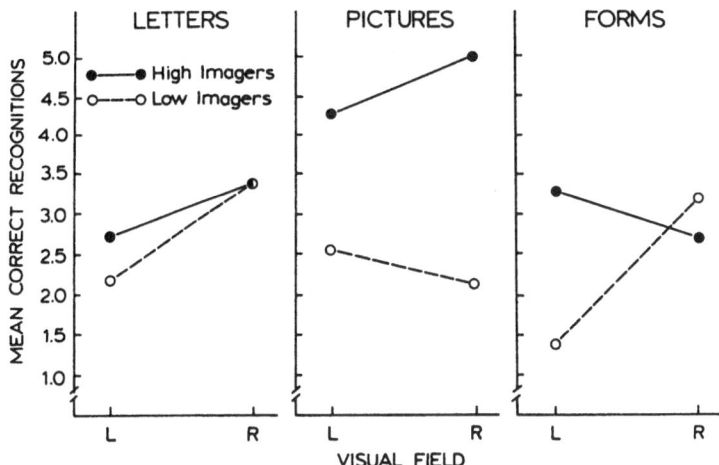

FIGURE 3. Recognition accuracy scores as a function of imagery ability, stimulus attribute, and visual field. From Paivio and Ernest (1971).

Conversely, however, many studies have produced evidence that certain nonverbal spatial processing tasks that implicate imagery are carried out more efficiently by the right hemisphere than by the left. Examples include performance on standard spatial manipulation tests, visual recognition of holistic properties of faces, perceptual closure, and memory for geometric forms, to mention just a few of the better-known findings.

A straightforward interpretation of such contrasting observations is that nonverbal representations in the left hemisphere are especially likely to be activated and used when the task entails referential activity, as in object identification by naming, imaging to words, and describing images verbally. The right hemisphere imagery functions are revealed by tasks that require nonverbal associative processing or transformation of nonverbal information with minimal verbal involvement.

The functional lateralization of referential imagery to the left may be a neuroanatomical consequence of the left hemisphere specialization for speech. This general view is an extension of the classical interpretation of the anomias as involving damage to pathways that connect anterior language processing centers and more posterior object processing systems in the left hemisphere. I stress the relation to speech production in particular because receptive language functions have been demonstrated for the right hemisphere as well. It follows that language-evoked imagery should also be possible in the right hemisphere. This view is supported by such evidence as more efficient right hemisphere processing of concrete than abstract words and, as we shall see later, the possible superiority of the right over the left hemisphere in verbal memory tasks that implicate imagery.

The right hemisphere predominance in certain nonverbal and image-related tasks may be partly a default consequence of the left hemisphere dominance in language functions generally. In any case, the dual coding interpretation is that the right hemisphere tasks entail associative, organizational, and transformational processing of nonverbal representational units and structures. The arousal of a visual image of an object, such as a telephone, by a corresponding environmental sound, such as a telephone ring, would be an example of nonverbal associative processing in the imagery system. The finding that certain environmental sounds (e.g., of a car starting) are better recognized by the left ear than by the right ear (Curry, 1976) suggests that the right hemisphere may predominate in such processing. The construction of integrated images of pairs of objects illustrates imagery organization, and here we are uncertain about which hemisphere dominates in that task. As mentioned above, the evidence is stronger that the right hemisphere dominates in tasks that require transformation of images, such as mental rotation, or in tasks that require mental organization of complex visual patterns, as in the case of closure tests.

Interpretations are further complicated by the distinction, implicit in the discussion up to this point, between episodic and semantic memory tasks. Episodic memory tasks have provided some of the strongest evidence that the two cerebral hemispheres are differentially specialized for verbal and nonverbal processing. Thus, Brenda Milner and her colleagues (e.g., Milner, 1980) have repeatedly observed a double functional dissociation in which memory for verbal material is depressed among patients with lesions in the left temporal lobe but not among those with lesions in the right temporal lobe, whereas memory for nonverbal materials such as faces suffers more from right temporal lobe lesions. Jones-Gotman and Milner (1978) also provided direct experimental evidence that right temporal lobe patients performed more poorly than controls on a verbal memory task in which they were required to use imagery but not on a task in which they used sentences as mnemonic aids. The asymmetry does not show up in tasks that depend on the availability of nonverbal semantic memory representations, such as perceptual identification of familiar pictures and symbolic size comparisons.

A complete dual coding account would include anterior-posterior distinctions in regard to sequential and synchronous processing of verbal and nonverbal materials, hemispheric distinctions in the representation of emotion, as well as other functions covered by dual coding theory. However, my examples suffice to illustrate the approach.

I conclude that systematic neuropsychological studies have provided enough positive evidence to support a number of important generalizations concerning brain structures for different imagery functions, but the evidence is still very fragmentary. In this area as in the others I have discussed, dual coding theory provides one way of organizing and interpreting the known facts and guiding research required to fill in some of the missing pieces.

REFERENCES

1. Betts, G. H. (1909). The distribution and functions of mental imagery. New York: Teacher's College, Columbia University.
2. Bisiach, E., Capitani, E., Luzzatti, C., & Perani, D. (1981). Brain and conscious representation of outside reality. Neuropsychologia, 19, 543-551.
3. Bucci, W. (1984). Linking words and things: Basic processes and individual variation. Cognition, 17, 137-153.
4. Curry, F. K. W. (1967). A comparison of left-handed and right-handed subjects on verbal and non-verbal dichotic listening tasks. Cortex, 3, 343-352.

5. Day J. C., & Bellezza, F. S. (1983). The relation between visual imagery mediators and recall. Memory & Cognition, 11, 251-257.
6. Ernest, C. H. (1977). Imagery ability and cognition: A critical review. Journal of Mental Imagery, 1, 181-216.
7. Farah, M. J. (1984). The neurological basis of mental imagery: A componential analysis. Cognition, 18, 245-272.
8. Gordon, R. (1949). An investigation into some of the factors that favour the formation of stereotyped images. British Journal of Psychology, 39, 156-167.
9. Guilford, J. P. (1967). The nature of human intelligence. New York: McGraw-Hill.
10. Heuer, F., Fischman, D., & Reisberg, D. (1986). Why does vivid imagery hurt colour memory? Canadian Journal of Psychology, 40, 161-175.
11. Jones-Gotman, M., & Milner, B. (1978). Right temporal lobe contribution to image-mediated memory. Neuropsychologia, 16, 61-71.
12. Kosslyn, S. M., Holtzman, J. D., Farah, M. J., & Gazzaniga, M. S. (1985). A computational analysis of mental image generation: Evidence from functional dissociations in split-brain patients. Journal of Experimental Psychology: General, 114, 311-341.
13. Kosslyn, S. M., & Jolicoeur, P. (1980). A theory-based approach to the study of individual differences in mental imagery. In R. E. Snow, P. A. Federico and W. E. Montague (eds.) Aptitude, Learning and Instruction: Cognitive Processes Analysis of Aptitude, Vol. 1. Hillsdale, NJ. Erlbaum.
14. Ley, R. G. (1983). Cerebral laterality and imagery. In A. A. Sheikh (Ed.), Imagery: Current theory, research, and application. New York: Wiley.
15. Marks, D. F. (1973). Visual imagery differences in the recall of pictures. British Journal of Psychology, 64, 17-24.
16. Marschark, M. (1985). Imagery and organization in the recall of prose. Journal of Memory and Language, 24, 734-745.
17. Marschark, M., & Paivio, A. (1977). Integrative processing of concrete and abstract sentences. Journal of Verbal Learning and Verbal Behavior, 16, 217-231.
18. McClelland, D. C. (1961). The achieving society. Princeton, NJ: D. Van Nostrand.
19. Milner, B. (1980). Complementary functional specializations of the human cerebral hemispheres. In R. Levi-Montalcini (Ed.) Nerve cells, transmitters, and behavior. Vatican City: Pontificia Academia Scientiarum.
20. Paivio, A. (1968). A factor-analytic study of word attributes and verbal learning. Journal of Verbal Learning and Verbal Behavior, 7, 41-49.
21. Paivio, A. (1971). Imagery and verbal processes. New York: Holt, Rinehart, & Winston. (Reprinted 1979, Hillsdale, NJ: Lawrence Erlbaum Associates)
22. Paivio, A. (1986). Mental representations: A dual-coding approach. New York: Oxford University Press.
23. Paivio, A., & Ernest, C. (1971). Imagery ability and visual perception of verbal and nonverbal stimuli. Perception & Psychophysics, 10, 429-432.
24. Paivio, A., & Harshman, R. (1983). Factor analysis of a questionnaire on imagery and verbal habits and skills. Canadian Journal of Psychology, 37, 461-483.

25. Paivio, A., & Lambert, W. E. (1959). Measures and correlates of audience anxiety ("stage fright"). Journal of Personality, 27, 1-17.
26. Paivio, A., & te Linde, J. (1982). Imagery, memory, and the brain. Canadian Journal of Psychology, 36, 243-272.
27. Sheehan, P. W. (1967). A shortened form of Betts' questionnaire upon mental imagery. Journal of Clinical Psychology, 23, 386-389.
28. Simpson, H. M., & Paivio, A. (1968). Effects on pupil size of manual and verbal indicators of cognitive task fulfillment. Perception & Psychophysics, 3, 185-190.
29. Singer, J. (1966). Daydreaming: An introduction to the experimental study of inner experience. New York: Random House.
30. Singer, J., & Antrobus, J. S. (1972). Daydreaming, imaginal processes, and personality: A normative study. In P. W. Sheehan (Ed.), The function and nature of imagery. New York: Academic Press.

A COMPUTATIONAL THEORY OF THE MENTAL IMAGERY MEDIUM

STEVEN PINKER

MASSACHUSETTS INSTITUTE OF TECHNOLOGY, CAMBRIDGE, MA, U.S.A.

ABSTRACT

Does it make sense to think of a mental image as a picture in the head? And if it does, how are three-dimensional objects and scenes represented in mental "pictures"? I suggest that these questions can be answered using the theoretical principles of computational cognitive science, analyzing the imagery system in terms of the data structures and processes that manipulate information during imaginal thinking. In particular, I outline a theory in which images are patterns of activation in a 3D array of cells, accessed via two overlayed coordinate systems: a fixed viewer-centered spherical coordinate system, and a movable object-centered or world-centered coordinate system. By inserting information into the array using one system, and accessing it using the other, a variety of 3D spatial information processes, such as generating, inspecting, and transforming images, recognizing shapes, and attending to locations, can be handled within a single framework.

1. INTRODUCTION

As a recent book title has put it (Gardner, 1985), the mind has a new science. Over the past 25 years, the field called "Cognitive Science" has revolutionized our understanding of mental processes. At the heart of this discipline is a central dogma, which plays a role analogous to the doctrine of atomism in physics, the germ theory of disease in medicine, or plate tectonics in geology. This central dogma is the "Computational Theory of Mind": that mental processes are formal manipulations of symbols, or programs, consisting of sequences of elementary processes made available by the information-processing capabilities of neural tissue. The computational theory of mind has led to rapid progress because it has given a precise mechanistic sense to formerly vague terms such as "memory", "meaning", "goal", "perception", and the like, which are indispensable to explaining intelligence. It has also fostered the experimental investigation of mental processes in the laboratory, because computational theories allow one to predict the relative ease or difficulty people will have in performing various tasks by assessing the number and type of computational steps and the amount of memory required by the mechanisms of the theory as it simulates the task in question. (Fodor (1968, 1975), Newell and Simon (1973), and the papers in Haugeland (1981), outline the logic of cognitive science in detail.)

Mental imagery is one of the topics that has benefited the most from this new approach to the mind. Through much of this century philosophers and psychologists have argued that the common sense notion of a mental image is scientifically useless at best and incoherent or misleading at worst (see Kosslyn, 1980; Block, 1981). But the formulation of computational models of imagery has clarified the issues to such an extent that debates over imagery have now shifted to empirical discussions about which theory is correct,

17

M. Denis et al. (eds.), Cognitive and Neuropsychological Approaches to Mental Imagery, 17–32.
© *1988 by Martinus Nijhoff Publishers.*

18

rather than logical discussions about which concepts are coherent. In this
paper, I discuss how one apparent paradox in imagery — that "mental pictures"
imply a two-dimensional medium, whereas people's images can contain 3D
objects — can be resolved by thinking in computational terms. In particular,
I propose a theory of the brain mechanism in which images "occur" and how 3D
spatial information is put into it and read out of it. I also show how the
theory is compatible with the computational demands of other spatial abilities
such as pattern recognition, perceptual stability, attention, and intersensory
coordination.

2. BACKGROUND: THE ARRAY THEORY OF IMAGERY

At least since Plato's time, visual memories have been likened to physical
pictures. Though a literal reading of this "picture metaphor" leads to absurd
consequences (see Pylyshyn, 1973), Stephen Kosslyn (Kosslyn, 1980; Kosslyn,
Pinker, Smith, and Shwartz, 1979; Pinker and Kosslyn, 1983) has shown that
there is a sensible interpretation of the metaphor that is compatible with the
principles of modern computational psychology. Briefly, this "array theory"
is based on the following tenets. The structure underlying our experience of
visual perception and imagery can best be characterized by a two-dimensional
array of cells, each mapping onto a local region of the visual field. Objects
and scenes are depicted in the array by patterns of filled cells isomorphic in
shape to the object or scene. The array cells are filled with information
arriving from the eyes during perception, and from labelled, hierarchically
structured long-term memory files, corresponding to objects and their parts
during imagination. Information from memory placed in the array fades quickly
unless refreshed periodically. The elements filling the cells can be thought
of as primitive elements representing the lightness, color, texture, and
presence and orientation of edges in small local regions of the visual field.
Pattern-matching procedures can operate on the array patterns to construct
symbolic descriptions of the objects and scenes depicted therein, and
transformation procedures can alter the patterns by moving elements from cell
to cell, simulating translations, rotations, size scalings, and so forth.
Figure 1 shows the overall organization of the imagery system according to the
array theory. For a more detailed account, see Kosslyn, Pinker, Smith, &
Shwartz, 1979).

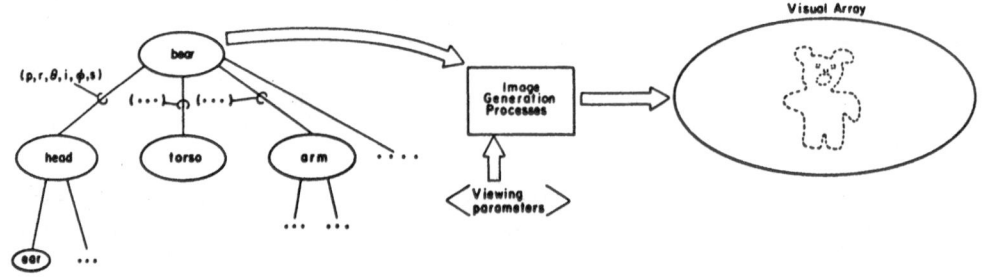

Figure 1. The array theory of imagery. The LTM representation of a shape is on
the left; the information in parentheses specifies the position of a part
relative to the whole.

Evidence for the Array Theory

The Array Theory is supported by four categories of experimental data.

2.1.   First, if there really exists a fixed medium supporting spatial
patterns in imagery and perception, one should be able to obtain stable
measures of the intrinsic spatial properties of the array, such as its shape,
size, grain, isotropy, homogeneity, dimensionality, and brain locus. Since the
theory posits a single array used in imagery and perception, estimates of the
array properties derived when subjects imagine patterns should be similar to
analogous estimates made when subjects perceive those patterns, and it should
be possible to obtain evidence that some of the visual areas of the brain are
used in visual imagery. As predicted, Kosslyn (1978) and Weber and Malmstrom
(1979) were able to estimate the maximum size of images; Finke & Kosslyn
(1980) and Finke and Kurtzman (1981) estimated the fall-off of resolution with
eccentricity in the visual field for images and percepts; and Kosslyn, Brunn,
Cave, and Wallach (1984) measured the resolution of imagined and perceived
patterns of different orientations and spatial frequencies, observing an
"oblique effect" for imagery as well as for perception. Recent studies in
human neuropsychology have supported the idea that there are neural structures
that represent and manipulate information in imagery, which are often shared
by perceptual processes. Farah (1984) reviewed literature showing that an
inability to generate visual images, with preserved abilities to process
visual information, can result from damage to certain areas of the left
hemisphere. She also cited cases of an inability to imagine particular
classes of objects (e.g. animals) accompanied by an inability to recognize
those classes when they are presented visually. Bisiach and Luzatti (1978)
documented neglect patients that not only failed to report the contents of the
left half of their visual field, but failed to report objects that were in the
left sides of scenes imagined from specific vantage points. Peronnet, Farah,
and Gonon (this volume) showed altered event-related potentials from early
stages of visual processing resulting from exact matches between images and
visual stimuli.
2.2.   The second body of evidence is useful in attempting to distinguish
the array theory from theories that hold that abstract propositions are the
only form of internal representation. When a visual pattern is represented as
a set of propositions, its size, shape, location, and orientation are factored
apart into separate propositions, one per attribute. For example, a slightly
tilted square might be represented as follows: SHAPE(x,square); SIZE(x,27);
LOCATION(x,50,75); ORIENTATION(x,75) (e.g., Anderson, 1978; Miller & Johnson-
Laird, 1976).   In contrast, an array representation of a pattern conflates
these four attributes into one and the same collection of dots or elements in
the array.   Thus if the representation underlying imagery is an array, when
one of these attributes of an image must be compared with a remembered
attribute value, the others can be expected to interfere. This prediction has
been borne out many times. For example, Shepard & Metzler (1971) found that
subjects could not decide whether two depicted 3D objects had the same shape
until they mentally rotated one object into the orientation of the other,
taking proportionally more time to perform the rotation when the objects were
separated by greater angles (see also Cooper & Shepard, 1973). This shows that
orientation can interfere with shape judgments.   Kosslyn (1975) found that
subjects took longer to verify the presence of parts of imagined animals when
either the part was intrinsically small or the animal was imagined at a small
size. This shows that size can interacts with shape judgments.   Shwartz
(1979) has shown that when subjects prepare for a visual stimulus whose shape
must be discriminated from a remembered pattern, they rotate an image of the
remembered pattern into the anticipated orientation of the stimulus, doing so
at a faster rate when the image is smaller. I have replicated this effect in
two unpublished experiments, one using 3D shapes, another using a Cooper-
Shepard paradigm with 2D shapes. The dependence of mental rotation rate on

size shows that size, orientation, and shape mutually interact in visual imagery, as one would expect if normalizing orientation was an operation performed iteratively on a bounded region of array cells, with smaller regions of cells requiring fewer operations per iteration. Finke & Pinker (1982, 1983) and Pinker, Choate, and Finke (1984; see also Spoehr & Williams, 1978) showed that when subjects are asked to determine whether a visible arrow points to the position of an imagined dot, the time they require is a linear function of how far the arrow is from the dot position (as if subjects were mentally extrapolating the arrow until it hit or missed the image of the dot). All of these findings can be explained under the theory that images are two-dimensional distributions of local elements that can be matched against templates constructed from memory, but only after being transformed so as to normalize the irrelevant attributes (e.g., differences in size, orientation, or location) that would otherwise vitiate the template match. In contrast, a propositions-only model would lead one to expect that each spatial attribute could be interrogated directly, without displaying effects of the values of other attributes, since each attribute is defined in a separate, modular proposition.

2.3. The third body of evidence concerns the facilitation of perception by imagery in a way that is sensitive to the precise spatial distribution of the imagined and physical patterns in the visual field. Brooks (1967) and Segal & Fusella (1970) showed that mental images and perceptual processing mutually interfere if both are in the same sensory modality. Cooper & Shepard (1973), Metzler (1973), Shwartz (1979), and many others (see Kosslyn et al, 1979) have shown that classification latencies for visual stimuli are greatly reduced, and the need to normalize irrelevant attributes is eliminated, if subjects form an image of the stimulus in advance for use as a template against the stimulus when it appears. But if image and stimulus differ in orientation, size, or location, or if the information given the subject in advance does not allow an image of a determinate shape, size, orientation, and location to be formed (e.g., information about orientation but not shape, as in Cooper & Shepard (1973), or information about shape but not location, as in Posner, Snyder & Davidson, 1980), the benefits are reduced or nonexistent. The most dramatic illustration of the template-like properties of images come from Farah (1985), who found that forming an image facilitated the sensitivity of detecting near-threshold visual stimuli but only if they were of the same shape and location as the image. A different kind of facilitation was demonstrated by Freyd and Finke (1984), who showed that imagining a context frame around a set of line segments facilitated discriminating the lengths of those segments, in the same way that a visually presented frame would have led to such facilitation. All this implies that preparation for a stimulus is maximally effective only if one can "prime" or fill in the set of cells that will be occupied by the stimulus when it appears. Again, this argues against a representation factoring visual attributes apart, since in that case, any attribute, spatially localizable or not, should be primable. Together with the rest of the evidence cited here, it also argues for a single array structure representing specifically visual information in imagery and perception.

2.4. Finally, there is evidence related to the function of imagery. People report using images to "see" patterns that they had not encoded explicitly when they originally inspected a scene, such as the shape of a beagle's ears (Kosslyn, 1980), how many windows are in one's living room (Shepard and Cooper, 1982), or the emergent properties that objects would display when juxtaposed or positioned in various ways (Pinker & Finke, 1980; Shepard, 1978). Many of these properties could only be detected if images represented the basic geometric properties of local parts of a shape in a single frame of reference, as opposed to descriptions of the parts in terms of their function or identity with respect to the object as a whole. For example, Finke, Pinker, and Farah (1987) read descriptions of arrangements of objects to people, such as "Imagine a capital letter 'D'. Rotate the figure 90 degrees to the left. Now place a capital letter 'J' at the bottom". Most subjects could "see" that the result was a depiction of an umbrella, a symbolic description that was not in the original instructions. This ability required "undoing" the mental description of the curved segment of the 'D' as being to the right of its spine with concave region pointing left, the description of the top of the 'J' as being part of the same object as the hooked segment and distinct from the spine of the 'D', and so on. It required "seeing" a pattern that cut across the original description of each part as belonging to a whole, and representing each part neutrally in terms of its overall position and orientation in the visual field (technically, in a global, viewer-centered coordinate system, rather than in a set of distributed object-centered coordinate systems; see Hinton, 1979a; Pinker, 1984). An array, in which parts are represented in terms of a single frame of reference, makes the detection of parts that cut across the description or "parse" of an object easy to do; a conceptual description of parts relative to the objects that they are parts of does not. See Hollins (1985), Pinker and Finke (1980), Slee (1980), and Shepard and Feng (reported in Shepard & Cooper, 1982) for other demonstrations of the ability to detect novel geometric patterns in images, and Kosslyn (1980), Kosslyn et al (1979), Pinker and Kosslyn (1983), Pinker (1984), Shepard (1978), Finke (1980), and Finke and Shepard (1986), for extensive general reviews of the experimental literature on the properties of images.

3. PROBLEMS FOR THE ARRAY THEORY

The evidence outlined above suggest that the array theory is a plausible account of the short-term mental representation of visuospatial information. The theory, however, remains controversial. For example, Pylyshyn (1981) argues that the theory as a whole has too many free parameters to be explanatory, and that the supporting experiments can be given alternative explanations in terms of subjects' tacit knowledge about the physical world and their perceptual systems. Hinton (1979a, b) and Chambers and Reisberg (1985) point out that certain image inspection processes seem to operate on the interpretation of an object as a whole, or upon the role that a part plays in a reference frame aligned with the object, rather than being able to access arbitrary local regions of a pattern. Though these counterarguments are important, I will focus here upon a different and equally serious class of criticisms: that the array theory is ill-suited to represent information about three-dimensional objects and scenes. In particular, there are two problems with the two-dimensional array. The first is that mental rotation in depth, which yields just as precise a linear relation between reaction time and angular disparity as rotation in the frontal plane (Shepard & Metzler, 1971), is difficult to model within a 2D array, for three reasons: a) 2D depictions of 3D objects are ambiguous—an ellipse in a 2D array could represent an ellipse viewed head-on or a circle tilted about its vertical axis. Rotating it in depth would yield very different results on the different interpretations (e.g., a narrowing in one case and a widening in the other), so the rotation operator could not proceed correctly if all it accessed was the array. b) One can formulate accounts of the incremental nature of mental rotation for picture-plane rotations (e.g., perhaps because of a constraint that cell contents can only be shifted to neighboring cells in a given iteration, or because small increments of rotation minimize shape distortion introduced by noise in the rotation operation), but not for depth rotations, since for each increment of rotation, different points in the rotated pattern shift by very different amounts across the array. c) As an object rotates in depth, new surfaces come into view. This information was not in the array to begin with, and so the rotation cannot be accomplished solely by operations on array cells.

The second problem with the 2D array (e.g., Neisser, 1979) is that of perceptual stability: If the experience of imagery is analogous to perceptual experience, as introspection as well as much of the empirical imagery literature suggests, both experiences should be of a world of meaningful solid objects, available to all sensory modalities, and stable despite changes in eye position, head position, or body movement in any direction. But these properties are difficult, if not impossible, to simulate on an internal two-dimensional "screen" or array.

Clearly, the array theory (and the age-old picture metaphor that preceded it) will stand or fall depending on its ability to account for the representation of the three-dimensional world in perception and imagery. I will first present, and reject, a series of simple extensions of the array theory that might give it an ability to deal with the representation of 3D information. Then I will propose a new theory, which I believe solves the problems inherent in the earlier approaches.

4. SIMPLE EXTENSIONS OF THE ARRAY THEORY TO HANDLE THE THIRD DIMENSION
4.1. 3D array

The most natural way to extend the array theory to handle the three-dimensional case is to build the third dimension right into the array, giving it the equivalent of rows, columns, and layers instead of just rows and columns. In contrast to the 2D array, this allows one to model rotation in depth as a set of uniform displacements of elements from cell to cell, and allows one to explain the incremental nature of the rotation by a putative constraint on how far (i.e., across how many intervening cells) an element can be displaced in a single computational step (see also Attneave & Block, 1973; Shepard & Judd, 1976). Similarly, it can account for people's ability to scan mentally along a straight trajectory in any direction in an imagined 3D scene, a performance that requires proportionally more time for greater 3D Euclidean distances between the source and destination of scanning (Pinker & Kosslyn, 1978; Pinker, 1980b; see also Attneave and Pierce, 1978).

Despite the intuitive appeal of the "sandbox in the head" theory (Attneave, 1972), it faces several major problems (Pinker and Kosslyn, 1978; Pinker, 1980a, b). The introspective experience of imagery is of a perspective glimpse of a scene from a particular vantage point (Pinker, 1979b; Hinton, 1979a). Furthermore, experimental evidence supports this introspection: imagined objects are reported by subjects to "loom large" as one imagines moving toward them (Kosslyn, 1978); and objects that are imagined as concealed, out of view, distant, or foreshortened are recalled less frequently in an incidental memory test than objects imagined to be visible (Abelson, 1976; Fiske, Taylor, Etcoff, & Laufer, 1979; Keenan & Moore, 1979; Pinker, Nimgade, and Wiesenfeld, 1982). Perspective information is easily accessed in scenes imagined "from a vantage point": for example, when subjects are asked to scan mentally across an image of a 3D scene by imagining a rifle sight sweeping from one object to another, their scan times are proportional to the separation between the objects in the 2D projection of the scene orthogonal to the "line of sight" (Pinker, 1980b; Pinker & Finke, 1980), showing the accuracy of the representation of projective interpoint distances in images. Other experiments, involving psychophysical and pattern-matching tasks, reported in Pinker and Finke (1980), confirm the availability of accurate perspective information. Barring the absurd interpretation that the "mind's eye" has a lens and a retina onto which "images of images" are projected, data on perspective effects in imagery are hard to reconcile with the 3D array theory, for perspective effects arise when a 3D scene is accessed via its projection onto a 2D surface, not when the scene or a 3D representation thereof is accessed directly.

4.2. 2D array + memory files

This hypothesis, suggested by results in Pinker (1980b) and Pinker and Finke (1980), keeps the array two-dimensional, but puts information about the three-dimensional shapes of objects and scenes in the long-term memory files from which array patterns are generated. The process that "paints in" the array would accept as input not just a memory file containing information about the intrinsic 3D shape of the object (say, in the form of a list of object-centered 3D coordinates defining the object's surface), but also a vector specifying the intended "viewing" angle and distance. The process would then use a perspective transformation to compute the coordinates of the cells that would have to be filled in to depict the object accurately with respect to that "vantage point". Mental transformations would consist of successively repainting the array pattern, feeding in a slightly different value for the vantage point each time.

Unfortunately, this account has its own problems. First, it posits that the image painting process can immediately generate a depiction of a pattern at any orientation. Empirical evidence suggests otherwise. Pinker, Stromswold, and Beck (1984) found that subjects were unable to generate images of remembered 3D objects at arbitrary orientations given an orientation cue; rather, they first imagined the object in the orientation at which they had studied it, or in its canonical orientation, and then mentally rotated it into the target orientation. In any case, if humans <u>could</u> generate images at prespecified orientations, we would not be able to explain the incremental nature of mental rotation: if subjects can generate an image at a desired orientation immediately, why do they take proportionally longer to match stimulus pairs separated by greater disparities? In addition, if objects are mentally transformed by altering the viewer's vantage point relative to the scene, these transformations would resemble movements of the observer relative to the entire scene, as opposed to movements of parts of the scene relative to the rest. This is contrary both to subjects' introspections, and to data showing that subjects can imagine parts of an image moving with respect to a perceived (hence stationary) display (Pinker, 1980b; Pinker & Finke, 1980).

4.3. 2 1/2D array

In Pinker (1980), I proposed that the 2D array be enriched along the lines of Marr and Nishihara's (1978) "2 1/2D sketch", a structure sometimes used in computer vision systems at an intermediate stage of the shape recognition process. This would involve filling each cell in the array not just with elements representing the lightness, color, texture, or edge-orientation of the corresponding local region of the depicted surface, but with quantities specifying its depth and surface orientation with respect to the viewer as well. In the simple 2D array theory of Kosslyn (1980), the rotation operator computed the trajectories of elements by sweeping across the array, and using the address of each filled cell (specifying its 2D position) to compute the address of the cell to which its contents must be moved in that iteration. In the 2 1/2D array theory, the rotation operator would access not just the cell address, but also the contents of the cell (specifying its depth from the vantage point). This additional piece of information is all that is needed mathematically for the rotation operator to compute the address and depth value of the destination cell for that element. Thus this account satisfies the three conditions that in combination strained the earlier approximations:

it represents perspective effects (since the array cells are isomorphic to the two-dimensional layout of the visual field as experienced from a particular vantage point); it contains information about the third dimension (making 3D transformations such as rotation or translation in depth possible); and it allows such transformations to be performed by operating on the information displayed in the array, rather than by constructing the array pattern from scratch repeatedly.

Still, the theory is not wholly satisfactory. First, there is no simple mechanism for bringing new material into the array at the trailing edge of an object rotating in depth. But another problem is more fundamental. Since the addresses and depth values in the array are specified relative to the viewer (that is, in a viewer-centered coordinate system), the perspective appearance of objects are represented explicitly: a given visual angle corresponds to a precise number of adjacent array cells. On the other hand, objects' intrinsic sizes and shapes, and their locations in the world, are represented implicitly and must be computed indirectly from the cell addresses and contents using a set of coordinate transforms (that is, a given real world size corresponds to a large number of adjacent cells with "near" depth values or a small number of adjacent cells with "far" depth values). This predicts that tasks accessing perspective information about objects in immediate visual memory should be easier and less consuming of mental effort than those accessing objective information about intrinsic size and shape. Though both perspective ("visual field") and objective ("visual world") percepts are possible (see Gibson, 1950, 1952; Boring, 1952; Pinker, 1980a), contrary to the prediction of the 2 1/2D array theory, the latter are clearly more primary in several ways. Children see objects as three-dimensional long before they can use perspective information, say, in drawings (Spelke, in press; Phillip, Hobbs & Pratt, 1978); our primary phenomenal experience is of a world of solid objects laid out in a fixed 3D framework despite the wildly fluctuating retinal images, the properties of which we are usually unaware of (Gibson, 1950; Neisser, 1976, 1979); and judgments about shape and size seem to be chronometrically sensitive to three-dimensional properties of objects such as intrinsic shape and intrinsic size, and relatively insensitive to factors such as depth and occlusion that affect perspective properties (Metzler & Shepard, 1974; Uhlarik, Pringle, Jordan & Misceo, 1980; Pringle & Uhlarik, 1979). Though the primacy of objective over perspective judgments can be handled by making certain assumptions about the temporal properties of the processes that operate on the information in the 2 1/2D array (i.e., that accessing a cell address is as time-consuming as accessing its contents, or that deriving object-centered from viewer-centered coordinates is a computationally primitive step invariably invoked while transforming images), the resulting theory becomes unparsimonious and counterintuitive.

5. A NEW THEORY: DUAL-ADDRESS ARRAY

The chief problem for each of the theories outlined above is an inability to deal parsimoniously with the dual nature of visual experience: The visual field, such as when railroad tracks stretching to the horizon are seen to converge, and the visual world, such as when those same tracks are seen as parallel (Gibson, 1950, 1952; Boring, 1952; Pinker, 1980a). Each of these mental sets plays a role in perception and in imagery. The theory to be outlined in this section tries to capture this duality within the confines of a single array structure.

In a 2 1/2D array as described here, the depth of a local region of a surface is specified by filling an array cell with a number representing that depth. Say we took the array and replaced each cell by a string of cells, so that each cell in the string would represent a specific depth from the viewer when filled with a primitive element or mark. The mapping between physical depth and the cells in the string could be nonlinear, like the focusing scale on a camera lens barrel, so that objects at apparently infinite distances (e.g., heavenly bodies) would be represented by elements in the last cell of each string. Furthermore, one could stipulate that only one cell in a string can be filled at one time, so that only visible, not occluded surfaces, would be represented (though the fact that we can perceive transparency might call for a weaker assumption than this). If we consider cells representing the same depth in adjacent strings to be adjacent to one another, then this array is half-way between a 2 1/2D array and a 3D array (though I will resist the temptation to christen it a "2 3/4D array"). The array cells map topographically onto distinct regions of visible three-dimensional space, as in the 3D or sandbox theory. But unlike that theory, the mapping from array cell to physical region is nonlinear and nonhomogeneous; only visible surfaces are represented; and the cell addresses are in viewer-centered coordinates (i.e., horizontal visual angle, vertical visual angle, and depth, all relative to the "Cyclopean" fovea), therefore displaying the perspective, not intrinsic, sizes and shapes of objects. In fact, Downing and Pinker (1985) showed that the accessing of visual space by focal attention seems to be determined by this type of coordinate system: when people attend to a location, they detect a stimulus presented at that location more quickly; for stimuli presented at various distances from the attended locus, this enhancement falls off as a function of distance in terms of visual angle and distance in depth.

So far the theory is barely different from the 2 1/2D model. But say we now gave each cell in the array a second address, reflecting its coordinates in a 3D, world-centered, homogeneous, isotropic coordinate system mapping linearly into physical space. Such an array is represented schematically in Figure 2. It should be apparent from the figure that the mapping from world-centered to viewer-centered addresses is nonlinear and nonhomogeneous, so that a given number of adjacent array cells are assigned a small range of horizontal world-centered addresses in the "front" of the array and a large range in the "rear". Let us posit, as a final assumption, that the world-

(Depth from the vantage point)	∞	$-\infty,0$	$-\infty,\infty$	$-\infty,\infty$	$0,\infty$	∞,∞	∞,∞	$\infty,0$
	1000	−1000,0	−900,500	−500,900	0,1000	500,900	900,500	1000,0
	100	−100,0	−90,50	−50,90	0,100	50,90	90,50	100,0
	10	−10,0	−9,5	−5,9	0,10	5,9	9,5	10,0
	1	−1,0	−.9,.5	−.5,.9	0,1	.5,.9	.9,.5	1,0
	.1	−.1,0	−.09,.05	−.05,.09	0,.1	.05,.09	.09,.05	.1,0
		−90°	−60°	−30°	0°	30°	60°	90°

Visual angle from the fixation point

Figure 2. Schematic diagram of the dual-address array. The Y- or height dimension is collapsed, yielding a "top-view" so to speak, of the array. The grain is vastly enlarged, and the known physiological characteristics of the visual field like anisotropy and nonhomogeneity with eccentricity are ignored. Viewer-centered addresses are listed in the margins, world-centered addresses are listed in each cell (no theoretical difference is implied by this notational difference). The origin of the world-centered system has been placed on the origin of the viewer-centered system.

centered addresses can be specified in "base + index" format, like modern computer memories, which is equivalent to being able to move the origin of the coordinate system to lie on any cell of the array. (Thus what I am calling a "world-centered" coordinate system can be centered on or aligned with salient environmental surfaces such as walls and floors, or upon an object being attended to). Since "mental arrays" of any sort owe many of their functional properties to their addressing or coordinate system (Pylyshyn, 1984), providing each cell with two addresses, one perspective-specific, and one world-centered, provides the advantages of separate 2D and 3D arrays without having to posit an additional structure plus processes linking it to all the others.

Marr and Nishihara (1978) and Hinton (1979b) point out that a variety of visual and inferential processes require a transformation from retinal or viewer-centered coordinates to object- or world-centered coordinates or vice-versa. The substantive hypothesis submitted here is that these translations are accomplished in effect as simple lookup operations on array cells, each cell pairing a viewer-centered coordinate triple with an object-centered coordinate triple for a distinct local region of the visual field. In the following sections I show how the theory provides succinct and plausible prima facie accounts of each of these processes, at the same time raising testable empirical hypotheses about various aspects of the mechanisms involved.

How the Dual-Address Theory Handles Spatial Information Processing

5.1. The visual field and the visual world. In the dual-address theory, the processing of visual patterns via the world-centered addresses of the cells they fill yields visual world percepts (and hence is used in judgments about objects' real world shapes, sizes, and locations); processing the viewer-centered addresses yields visual field percepts. The current theory allows both mental sets to operate in imagery as well as perception, consistent with demonstrations that imagery transformations can obey either set (see Pinker, 1980a, for a review). For example, while driving on the highway, when I mentally place five cars between my car and the one up ahead to maintain the proper following distance, I can be confident that the judged distance really is five times one car length in the world though I can "see" each car as smaller than the one behind it.

5.2. Mental transformations. In performing transformations like rotation in depth, the world-centered coordinate system is first centered upon the object to be rotated. The rotation operator sweeps through cells in a bounded region of the array encompassing the object, and looks up the world-centered or object-centered address. Assuming that the object-centered coordinate system can be either cylindrical or spherical (see Marr, 1982; Pinker, 1984), the operator subtracts a constant from the angular coordinate of the address, fetches the contents of the cell with that new world/object-centered address, and deposits them into the cell being worked upon. A constraint that the fetched-from and deposited-into cells must be in close proximity within the array is one way to guarantee the incremental nature of the rotation. Sometimes the desired "source" cell is blocked because another cell in its string, representing an occluding surface at a nearer distance, is filled (i.e., at the trailing edge of a rotating object). In that case, the object-centered coordinates of the blocked cell are passed to the long-term memory file for the object's shape, which is assumed to be specified with respect to an object-centered coordinate system (e.g., as in Marr & Nishihara, 1978; Kosslyn & Shwartz, 1977). The desired surface element can now be retrieved from the LTM file by subtracting the angle through which the object has been rotated so far from the angular coordinate of the blocked cell. In contrast, the 2 1/2D array theory outlined earlier is far more complex, involving viewer-to-object-centered translations at every step, and the theory fails to provide concise accounts of the incremental nature of the rotation or of the approximately equal rates for depth- and picture-plane rotations. And unlike the 3D array theory, the current theory correctly implies that new 2D perspective patterns will emerge as an object rotates in depth (Pinker & Finke, 1980), since these patterns will be accessible via the viewer-centered coordinates of the rotated pattern.

5.3. Mental image generation. In the Kosslyn & Shwartz (1977) version of the array theory, images are generated from LTM files hierarchically organized in terms of (a) the skeletal shape of the object, and (b) the details or parts attached to it, with additional information specifying the spatial relations of parts to the skeleton. Say the skeletal image is generated by first aligning the world-centered coordinate system with the desired position of the object, then by using these coordinate addresses to fill in the cells as specified by the skeletal file (this is a simple identity mapping on the aforementioned assumption that surface information in the LTM files is specified in object-centered coordinates). It is now straightforward to find the portion of the array that will be the destination of the points depicting the object's parts, since all the array cells have addresses relative to the object's skeleton, and the LTM specification of the proper location of the part is specified relative to the skeleton as well. This eliminates Kosslyn & Shwartz's somewhat cumbersome process of searching over the partially constructed image until attachment points for to-be-generated parts are recognized via their depicted shapes.

5.4. Bottom-up pattern recognition. The position of a receptor in the retina determines the two angular viewer-centered coordinates of a local region of stimulation, and the retinal disparity of corresponding local regions of the stimulus pattern determines its depth (together with information about eye position). Thus the mapping from visual input to the array cells (addressed by their viewer-centered coordinates) is fairly direct. However, an efficient bottom-up pattern recognition system requires a description of the input shape that is insensitive to the orientation, location, projected size, and projected shape of the object, so that the description can be matched against a single or a small number of canonical descriptions of the object's intrinsic shape (Marr & Nishihara, 1978; Pinker, 1984). In the current theory, once the depth of every point has been established, the positions of parts of the objects in world-centered coordinates preserving size and shape constancy are available. If the origin (and possibly axes) of the world-centered coordinate system is then shifted to coincide with the natural axis of the object, each local surface region is specified in object-centered coordinates, so a global object-centered description of the object and its parts for input into the recognition process can be computed with a relatively small number of steps.

5.5. Top-down pattern recognition. Marr and Nishihara (1978) have suggested that when bottom-up procedures are inadequate to delineate the orientation in depth of a part of an object, one might use something like the following procedure: a) select, by bottom-up means, a long-term memory description of the object which specifies the relation between the principal axis (or skeleton) and each part; b) use that description to generate a set of possible two-dimensional projections of the part that are consistent both with the perceived orientation of the main axis of the object and with the spatial relations between the part and the main axis; and c) choose the part orientation from that set that yields the best match between predicted projection and actual input projection. This "image space processor" (and other top-down recognition processes, e.g., Waltz, 1979; Horn & Bachman, 1980; Pinker, 1980a) could be implemented as a template-matching process in the current theory by a) using the LTM shape description to generate a skeletal image; b) using the world/object-centered coordinates to rotate one of the parts in depth; and c) using the viewer-centered coordinates of the resulting pattern, to determine when the rotated part best matches the silhouette of the input pattern.

5.6. Eye movements and attention shifts. Eye movements between objects in 3D space have been found to consist of two separate phases (Graham, 1965): a yoked movement of the eyes bringing the bisector of the angle they form into alignment with the target, and a convergence movement bringing vertex of that angle onto the target. Together with information about the current eye positions, a command for the former motion can be derived directly from the first two viewer-centered coordinates of the target (i.e., the location of the depth string); a command for the convergence motion can be derived simply from the third (i.e., the location of the target cell within the depth string). Similarly, internal attention shifts seem to enhance a region of visual space defined by a range of visual angle and depth (Downing and Pinker, 1985); this would correspond to priming a cluster of adjacent cells in the array defined by the viewer-centered coordinate system.

5.7. Perceptual stability. As mentioned, the world/object-centered coordinates of visual patterns are used to assess the physical layout of scenes. Say people mentally represent their positions in space by linking some portion of the world/object-centered coordinate system to a semantic memory structure for a known world location and direction (e.g., facing north in a familiar room). Now, when they move their eyes, head, or body, they can take a copy of the motor commands and use them to displace the origin of the world-centered coordinate system a corresponding amount and direction within the array. This preserves the perception that the visible world objectively stayed put (since objects are linked to the same world-centered coordinates as before), but also is consistent with the fact that the surfaces in the world that are currently visible, and their relation to the eyes, have changed as a result of the movement (since the array cells are in fact filled with a different pattern than before).

5.8. Perceptual adaptation. It is well-known that with practice, humans can adapt to wearing prisms that distort the visual input in a variety of ways (Dodwell, 1970). In the current model, this could consist of altering the cell-by-cell linkages between world-centered addresses (which are accessed in intersensory and sensorimotor coordination) and the viewer-centered addresses (which are linked to specific field locations), based on discrepancies between the coordinates of objects or limbs in haptic or auditory representational structures and the object/world-centered coordinates in the visual array. Interestingly, Finke (1979) has shown that mismatches between intended and imagined hand locations can cause sensorimotor adaptation, and Kubovy (1981) has conjectured that the class of mathematical functions available for visuomotor adaptation is just the class available for mental image transformations. Both support the current argument that a common array structure underlies both mental images and the visual percepts that tie in to other sensory and motor systems.

6. CONCLUSION

In any field of science, metaphors are a double-edged sword. They can serve a heuristic function, inspiring and organizing experimental research. On the other hand, they can lead one to confuse one's everyday familiarity with the metaphorical object with true explanations of the object under investigation. The metaphor of "a mind's eye looking at a mental picture" has had both roles in the study of imagery. No one denies that the metaphor has inspired fascinating discoveries, such as the study of mental rotation. But some of the most vehement disagreements in philosophy experimental psychology during this century have centered around the purported misuse of the metaphor, such as the absurd notions of homunculi in the skull, pictures painted onto the surface of the brain, and so forth. Happily, the application of computational cognitive science to the study of imagery has taken imagery theory and research out of the realm of metaphor. The array theory and its implementation as a computer simulation have exorcised the sense of paradox that surrounded the notion of images being picture-like entities that are inspected by perception-like processes. I hope to have shown how the paradox of squeezing a stable three-dimensional world into a two-dimensional "mental picture" can also be eliminated by a careful consideration of the ways in which computational processes can access and manipulate information about the geometric properties of objects and space. Such consideration led to a theory that, I hope, preserves the intuitive appeal and the empirical support of the picture metaphor, while being capable of handling the inherent computational problems of representing and reasoning about 3D space. Whether the theory can be convincingly shown to be true is another story, but if we can focus our attention on whether theories are true, rather than on whether they are possible or logically coherent, then the study of imagery has truly made progress.

REFERENCES

Abelson, R.P. Script processing in attitude formation and decision making. In J.S. Carrol & J.W. Payne (Eds.), Cognition and Social Behavior. Hillsdale, New Jersey: Erlbaum, 1976.

Anderson, J.R. Arguments concerning representations for mental imagery. Psychological Review, 1978, 85, 249–277.

Attneave, F. Representation of physical space. In A.W. Melton & E.J. Martin (Eds.), Coding Processes in Human Memory. Washington, D.C.: V.H. Winston, 1972.

Attneave, F. & Block, N. Apparent motion in tridimensional space. Perception & Psychophysics, 1973, 13, 301–307.

Attneave, F. & Pierce, C.R. Accuracy of extrapolating a pointer into perceived and imagined space. American Journal of Psychology, 1978, 91, 371–387.

Bisiach, E. & Luzatti, C. Unilateral neglect of representational space. Cortex, 1978, 14, 129–133.

Block, N. (Ed.) Imagery, Cambridge, MA: MIT Press, 1981.

Boring, E.G. The Gibsonian visual field. Psychological Review, 1952, 59, 246–247.

Brooks, L.R. The suppression of visualization by reading. Quarterly Journal of Experimental Psychology, 1967, 19, 289–299.

Chambers, D., & Reisberg, D. Can mental images be ambiguous? Journal of Experimental Psychology: Human Perception and Performance, 1985, 11, 317–328.

Cooper, L.A. & Shepard, R.N. Chronometric studies of the rotation of mental images. In W. Chase (Ed.), Visual Information Processing. New York: Academic Press, 1973.

Dodwell, P. Perceptual Adaptation. New York: Holt, Rinehart, & Winston, 1970.

Downing, C. & Pinker, S. The spatial structure of visual attention. In M. Posner & O. Marin (Eds.), Attention and Performance XI: Mechanisms of Attention and Visual Search. Hillsdale, NJ: 1985.

Farah, M.J. The neurological basis of mental imagery: A componential analysis. Cognition, 1984, 18, 245–272.

Farah, M.J. Psychophysical evidence for a shared representational medium for visual images and percepts. Journal of Experimental Psychology: General, 1985, 114, 91–103.

Finke, R.A. The functional equivalence of mental images and errors of movement. Cognitive Psychology, 1979, 11, 235-264.

Finke, R.A. Levels of equivalence in imagery and perception. Psychological Review, 1980, 87, 113-132.

Finke, R.A. & Kosslyn, S.M. Mental imagery acuity in the peripheral visual field. Journal of Experimental Psychology: Human Perception and Performance, 1980, 6, 126-139.

Finke, R.A. & Kurtzman, H.S. Mapping the visual field in mental imagery. Journal of Experimental Psychology: General, 1981, 110, 501-517.

Finke, R.A. & Pinker, S. Spontaneous image scanning in mental extrapolation. Journal of Experimental Psychology: Learning, Memory, and Cognition, 1982, 8, 142-147.

Finke, R.A. & Pinker, S. Directional scanning of remembered visual patterns. Journal of Experimental Psychology: Learning, Memory, and Cognition, 1983, 9(3), 398-410.

Finke, R. A., Pinker, S., and Farah, M. J. Reinterpreting visual patterns in mental imagery. Submitted for publication, 1987.

Finke, R.A. & Shepard, R.N. Visual functions of mental imagery. In K. R. Boff, L. Kaufman, & J. Thomas (Eds.), Handbook of Perception and Human Performance, Vol. 2. New York, Wiley-Interscience, 1986.

Fiske, S.T., Taylor, S.E., Etcoff, N.L., and Laufer, J.K. Imaging empathy, and causal attribution. Journal of Experimental Social Psychology, 1979, 15, 356-377.

Fodor, J.A. Psychological Explanation. New York: Random House, 1968.

Fodor, J.A., The Language of Thought. New York: Thomas Y. Crowell Company, 1975.

Freyd, J.J. & Finke, R.A. Facilitation of length discrimination using real and imagined context frames. American Journal of Psychology, 1984, 97, 323-341.

Gardner, H. The Mind's New Science. New York: Basic Books, 1985.

Gibson, J.J. The Perception of the Visual World. Boston: Houghton Mifflin, 1950.

Gibson, J.J. The visual field and the visual world: A reply to Professor Boring. Psychological Review, 1952, 59, 149-151.

Graham, C. Visual space perception. In C. Graham (Ed.), Vision and Visual Perception. New York: Wiley, 1965.

Haugeland, J. (Ed.) Mind Design: Philosophy, Psychology, Artificial Intelligence. Montgomery, VT: Bradford Books, 1981.

Hinton, G.E. Imagery without arrays. The Behavioral and Brain Sciences, 1979, 2, 555-556. (a)

Hinton, G.E. Some demonstrations of the effects of structural descriptions in mental imagery. Cognitive Science, 1979, 3, 231-250. (b)

Hollins, M. Styles of mental imagery in blind adults. Neuropsychologia, 1985, 23, 561-566.

Horn, B.K.P., & Bachman, B.L. Registering real images using synthetic images. In P. H. Winston & R. H. Brown (Eds.), Artificial Intelligence: An MIT Perspective. Cambridge, MA: MIT Press, 1979.

Keenan, J.M. & Moore, R.E. Memory for images of concealed objects: A re-examination of Neisser and Kerr. Journal of Experimental Psychology: Human Learning and Memory, 1979, 5, 374-385.

Kosslyn, S.M. Information representation in visual images. Cognitive Psychology, 1975, 7, 341-370.

Kosslyn, S.M. Measuring the visual angle of the mind's eye. Cognitive Psychology, 1978, 10, 356-389.

Kosslyn, S.M. Image and Mind. Cambridge, MA: Harvard University Press, 1980.

Kosslyn, S.M., Pinker, S., Smith, G.E., & Shwartz, S.P. On the demystification of mental imagery. The Behavioral and Brain Sciences, 1979, 2, 535-581.

Kosslyn, S.M., Pinker, S., Smith, G.E., & Shwartz, S.P. The how, what, and why of mental imagery (Authors' response). The Behavioral and Brain Sciences, 1979, 2, 570-581.

Kosslyn, S.M. & Shwartz, S.P. A simulation of visual imagery. Cognitive Science, 1977, 1, 265-295.

Kubovy, M. Two hypotheses concerning the interrelation of perceptual spaces. In L. D. Harmon (Ed.), Interrelations of the Communicative Senses. 1981.

Marr, D. Vision. San Francisco: Freeman, 1982.

Marr, D. & Nishihara, H.K. Representation and recognition of the spatial organization of three-dimensional shapes. Proceedings of the Royal Society, 1978, 200, 269-294.

Metzler, J. Cognitive analogues of the rotation of three-dimensional objects. Unpublished doctoral dissertation, Stanford University, 1973.

Metzler, J. & Shepard, R.N. Transformational studies of the internal representation of three-dimensional space. In R. Solso (Ed.), Theories in Cognitive Psychology: The Loyola Symposium. Potomac, MD: Lawrence Erlbaum, 1974.

Miller, G.A. & Johnson-Laird, P. Language and Perception. Cambridge, MA: Harvard University Press, 1976.

Neisser, U. Cognition and Reality. San Francisco: W.H. Freeman, 1976.

Neisser, U. Images, models, and human nature. The Behavioral and Brain Sciences, 1979, 2, 561.

Newell, A. & Simon, H. Human Problem Solving. Englewood Cliffs, NJ: Prentice Hall, 1973.

Phillip, W.A., Hobbs, S.B., Pratt, F.R. Intellectual realism in children's drawings of cubes. Cognition, 1978, 6, 15-33.

Pinker, S. Mental imagery and the visual world. Center for Cognitive Science Occasional Paper #4, MIT, 1980. (a)

Pinker, S. Mental imagery and the third dimension. Journal of Experimental Psychology: General, 1980, 109, 354-371. (b)

Pinker, S., Choate, P. & Finke, R.A. Mental extrapolation in patterns reconstructed from memory. Memory and Cognition, 1984, 12(3), 207-218.

Pinker, S. & Finke, R.A. Emergent two-dimensional patterns in images rotated in depth. Journal of Experimental Psychology: Human Perception and Performance, 1980, 6, 244-264.

Pinker, S. & Kosslyn, S.M. The representation and manipulation of three-dimensional space in mental images. Journal of Mental Imagery, 1978, 2, 69-84.

Pinker, S. & Kosslyn, S.M. Theories of mental imagery. In A. Sheikh (Ed.), Imagery: Current Theory, Research and Application. New York: Wiley, 1983, 43-71.

Pinker, S., Nimgade, A., & Wiesenfeld, H. C. Memory for pictures imagined at different sizes, distances, and orientations. Paper presented at the 62nd Annual Meeting of the Western Psychological Association, Sacramento, CA, April 8-11, 1982.

Pinker, S., Stromswold, K., & Beck, L. Visualizing objects at prespecified orientations. Paper presented at the annual meeting of the Psychonomic Society, San Antonio, November, 1984.

Posner, M.I., Snyder, C.R., & Davidson, B.J. Attention and the detection of signals. Journal of Experimental Psychology: General, 1980, 109, 160-174.

Pringle, R. & Uhlarik, J. Chronometric analysis of comparative size judgments with two-dimensional pictorial arrays. Paper presented at the annual meeting of the Psychonomic Society, Phoenix, Arizona, 1979.

32

Pylyshyn, Z. What the mind's eye tells the min's brain: A critique of mental imagery. Psychological Bulletin, 1973, 80, 1–24.
Pylyshyn, Z. The imagery debate: Analogue media versus tacit knowledge. Psychological Review, 1981, 88, 16–45.
Pylyshyn, Z. Computation and Cognition: Toward a Foundation For Cognitive Science. Cambridge, MA: Bradford Books/MIT Press, 1984.
Segal, S.J. & Fusella, V. Influence of imaged pictures and sounds on detection of visual and auditory signals. Journal of Experimental Psychology, 1970, 83, 458–464.
Shepard, R.N. The mental image. American Psychologist, 1978, 33, 125–137.
Shepard, R. N. & Cooper, L. A. Mental Images and Their Transformations. Cambridge, MA: Bradford Books/MIT Press, 1982.
Shepard, R.N. & Judd, 'S.A. Perceptual illusion of rotation of three-dimensional objects. Science, 1976, 191, 952–954.
Shepard, R.N. & Metzler, J. Mental rotation of three-dimensional objects. Science, 1971, 171, 701–703.
Shwartz, S.P. Studies of mental image rotation: Implications of a computer simulation model of mental imagery. Unpublished doctoral dissertation, The Johns Hopkins University, 1979.
Slee, J.A. Individual differences in visual imagery ability and the retrieval of visual appearances. Journal of Mental Imagery, 1980, 4, 93–113.
Spelke, E. S. Where perceiving ends and thinking begins: The apprehension of objects in infancy. In A. Yonas (Ed.), Minnesota Symposia on Child Psychology, in press.
Spoehr, K.T. & Williams, B.E. Retrieving distance and location information from mental maps. Paper presented at the nineteenth annual meeting of the Psychonomic Society, San Antonio, Texas, November 9–11, 1978.
Uhlarik, J., Pringle, R., Jordan, D., & Misceo, G. Size scaling in two-dimensional pictorial arrays. Perception & Psychophysics, 1980, 27, 60–70.
Waltz, D.L. On the function of mental imagery. The Behavioral and Brain Sciences, 1979, 2, 569–570.
Weber, R.J. & Malmstrom, F.V. Measuring the size of mental images. Journal of Experimental Psychology: Human Perception & Performance, 1979, 5, 1–12.

PART 2

IMAGINAL CODING AND THE PROCESSING OF VERBAL INFORMATION

2.1. IMAGERY AND THE REPRESENTATION OF VISUAL INFORMATION

READING MENTAL IMAGES

JON MICHAEL SLACK

OPEN UNIVERSITY, U.K.

ABSTRACT
People often report using mental images to access visuo-spatial information held in long-term memory. A theory of how such information is accessed and the processes involved in reading information off mental images are described. The theory is based on an important distinction in the representation of visual information, that between viewer-centred and object-centred reference frames. Objects are represented in long-term memory in terms of both types of system; mental images correspond to viewer-centred representations and structural descriptions are object-centred. Mental images are often used to access information about spatial relations and visual form because such information is not directly available within structural descriptions. Instead, this information has to be derived from viewer-centred images by means of visual routines.

1. INTRODUCTION

Various experimental studies have shown that mental imagery seems to have a functional role in accessing information in long-term memory relating to visual form and spatial relations (Eddy and Glass, 1981; Glass, Millen, Beck and Eddy, 1985). In answering questions of the form 'What shape is an alsatian's ear?' or 'In which hand does the Statue of Liberty hold the torch?', many people report creating a mental image of an alsatian's head or the Statue of Liberty and then *looking* at the image in order to read off the information necessary to answer the question. The issue which this paper explores is how people are able to translate the visuo-spatial information contained in mental images into information structures that are directly accessible through language. What are the processes involved in reading information off mental images?

This question can only be answered in the context of a theory of mental imagery, and an understanding of the functional relationship between imagery and other facets of cognition, particularly perception and language processing. The following sections outline a theory of mental imagery, an image-processing framework for understanding perception, and the possible relationships between the two. This theoretical background provides the basis for a model of the functional role of imagery in language access to visuo-spatial information.

2. DESCRIBING MENTAL IMAGES

One of the first questions to consider in analysing the processes involved in describing mental images is how they relate to the processes involved in describing visual stimuli.

37

M. Denis et al. (eds.), Cognitive and Neuropsychological Approaches to Mental Imagery, 37–46.
© *1988 by Martinus Nijhoff Publishers.*

This question is derived from a more fundamental one concerning the basic relationship between mental imagery and visual perception. Farah (1985) has explored these questions through a componential analysis based on Kosslyn's theory of visual imagery (1980). Briefly, this theory posits two kinds of structures underlying the functioning of visual imagery; long-term visual memory structures and the *visual buffer*. The former structures store information relating to the form and shape of objects, i.e., their appearances. The second type of structure, represents a medium in which images can be generated and manipulated; it does not store permanent visual information. According to this theory, the conscious experience of a visual image corresponds to a pattern of activity in the visual buffer. Furthermore, there are a number of studies supporting the claim that the visual buffer underlying mental imagery is also involved in visual perception (Farah, 1985; Finke and Schmidt, 1977, 1978; Finke and Kosslyn, 1980). It seems that imagery and perception share a common information processing medium, the visual buffer.

In line with the above claim, Farah (1985) has derived component analyses of the tasks of describing mental images and visual stimuli. These component analyses are shown in figure 1.

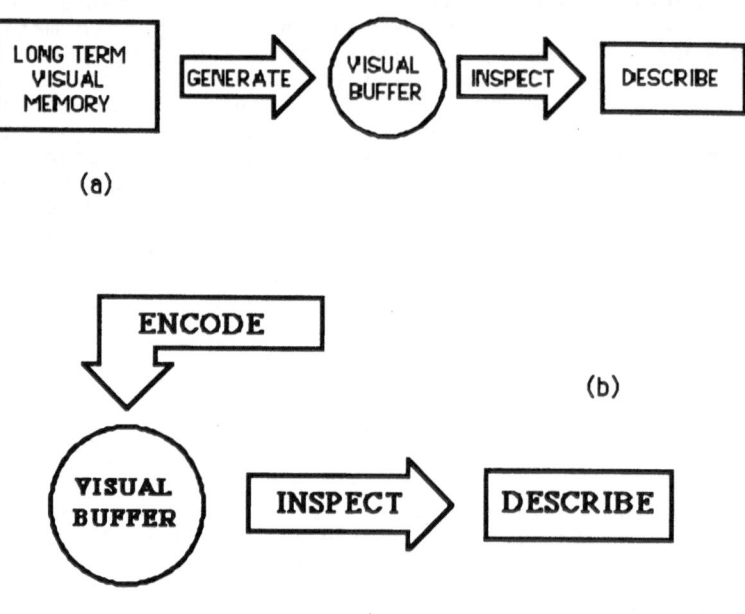

(a)

(b)

FIGURE 1. Task analysis for a) question-answering from memory, and b) description of visual stimuli.

The component processes shown in figure 1a relate to the processes postulated in Kosslyn's theory. The *generate* process creates a mental image in the visual buffer on the basis of the information stored in long-term visual memory. The patterns of activation in the visual buffer can be accessed by the *inspect* process, which converts them into structured perceptual descriptions, identifying the parts of the image and the spatial relations between them. Finally, the *describe* process attaches language to the perceptual description produced by the inspect process.

Farah argues that the component processes necessary for describing visual stimuli overlap with the imagery processes, as shown in figure 1. The only difference between the componential analyses of the two tasks is in terms of the processes involved in activating the visual buffer. In the perceptual task, the contents of the visual buffer are derived through perceptual encoding processes rather than generated from long-term memory structures. According to this analysis, the contents of the buffer are accessed and translated through the inspect and describe processes regardless of the source of the information.

Kosslyn has not elucidated on the precise nature of the inspect and describe procedures, but has suggested that the inspect process makes use of the elementary pattern recognition routines which are required for visual recognition. This paper provides a more explicit description of the two processes by identifying the nature of the underlying perceptual representations and processes. However, before this can be done it is necessary to outline the overall framework of visual analysis within which the explanation is set.

Marr (1982) has proposed an information processing framework within which visual analysis is explained by means of a series of processing stages; the stages being computationally modular and sequential. This framework has recently been augmented by Ullman (1985) through the introduction of the notion of *visual routines*. The early stages of visual processing operate in a bottom-up manner creating low-level representations of the visible world. These representations are called *base representations*. The visual routines operate on these representations to extract properties and spatial relations that are not explicit in the original encodings. The representations resulting from the application of visual routines are called *incremental representations*. The routines are constituted from more elementary processes, and are assembled using a fixed set of basic operations. The perceptual system can create different routines to derive a limitless range of shape properties and spatial relations.

There is a clear overlap between the theoretical constructs proposed by both Kosslyn and Ullman. Kosslyn's inspect process achieves the same ends as one of Ullman's visual routines; it builds explicit representations of visuo-spatial information which is only implicit in the contents of the visual buffer. Viewing the inspect process as a visual routine suggests that the contents of the visual buffer correspond to base representations. However, such representations can be created through either bottom-up encoding processes or top-down image generation processes. This correspondence is explored further in the later sections.

3. THE COGNITIVE REPRESENTATION OF VISUAL INFORMATION

The representation of information relating to visual objects and scenes is not an issue on which researchers have a common understanding. However, certain ideas are gaining general acceptance. One of these is the view that people use hierarchical structural descriptions to represent visual form and spatial relations in long-term memory. In such descriptions there is a node for each object that is linked to lower-level nodes for its parts. These lower-level nodes, in turn, are linked to nodes for their parts, and so on until a level of primitive features like edge segments is reached. One of the central concepts associated with this type of representation is the *object-centred reference frame*. An object is described in terms of a canonical frame of reference imposed on the object. The sizes, positions and orientations of the parts of an object are described relative to this object-based frame. Each node in a structural description has its own associated object-based frame of reference, and the links between two nodes are labelled with the spatial relation holding between their two object-based frames (Marr and Nishihara 1978). One of the major advantages of this form of representation is that an object can be described in terms of a constant set of object-based features and can thus be recognised regardless of its size, orientation and position in the visual field. By imposing a different object-based frame, a different set of object-based features is obtained. This explains why the same visual object can have several phenomenal shapes. For example, a tilted square may also be perceived as an upright diamond. Certain frames seem natural for given objects. For instance, a square, or cube, is most naturally described with respect to an object-based frame aligned with its edges, or sides. However, other object-based frames can be imposed; a square could be described relative to an axis along its diagonal. Experiments have shown that the assignments of such reference systems can be made dynamically (Hinton, 1979a).

Within the theoretical framework presented by Marr, hierarchical, object-based structural descriptions are used to represent 3-D object models. These representations contrast with the type of data provided by the prior, bottom-up stages of visual analysis. The base representations defined by Ullman are *viewer-centred*; the visual features generated within a base representation are retina-based and are dependent on the viewing position. That is, the sizes, positions and orientations of the features are defined relative to the frame of reference derived from a particular view. If the viewpoint changes, the viewer-centred features produced by an object also change, so they do not constitute a consistent shape representation. Moreover, the base representations do not correspond to full 3-D images; they comprise descriptions of the surfaces, their orientations and depths. The final stage of visual analysis involves mapping the viewer-centred base representation onto an object-centred, structural description of the image. In fact, the task of visual recognition can be thought of as building a description of the object consisting of two parts; (1) the structural description of the object with respect to an object-based frame of reference; and (2) the mapping of the object-based frame to the viewer-centred frame (referred to as the *view-mapping* throughout the rest of the text).

4. REPRESENTATION OF MENTAL IMAGES

There is considerable scope for theoretical alignment between Kosslyn's theory of mental imagery and the framework for visual perception outlined above. It has already been suggested that the contents of the visual buffer correspond to base representations. However, the distinction between mental images and other forms of stored visuo-spatial information can be made even more precise. Mental images are viewer-centred representations of visuo-spatial information derived from long-term memory. Thus the visual buffer is best conceptualised as a medium for viewer-centred representations which can be activated either through perceptual encoding, or by top-down image generation. In the former case, the viewer-centred reference frame is derived from the retinotopic coordinate system.

Hinton (1979b) has argued that imagery involves the imposition of a global viewer-centred reference frame on a stored structural description, without the need for a special medium to embody such representations. The elements of the viewer-centred image space can be attached directly to the structural description of an object or scene. In this sense the image space is structured by the associated structural description. However, this is also true of Kosslyn's model. The elements of the visual buffer are activated, in part, according to the structural descriptions stored in long-term memory. The contents of the visual buffer can be accessed through the part-of hierarchy comprising the structural description. When people use imagery to verify a sentence such as *The Statue of Liberty holds her torch in her right hand,* they do not generate an appropriate image and then search image space for the necessary information. Rather, they generate the image and are directed to the required information under the guidance of the structural description from which the image was derived. Hence, within both theories the image space is structured, in terms of its access, by the associated structural description.

The main difference between the two theories of mental imagery is the extent to which the image space is structured, or interpreted. According to Hinton's model, image space is fully interpreted. That is, all the information implicit in the image of an object is also implicit in the underlying stored structural description. However, this implicit information can only be made explicit within the structural description by accessing it through a viewer-centred coordinate system. In Kosslyn's model, on the other hand, the image represented in the visual buffer holds visuo-spatial information which is not implicit in the structural description. This information is derived from the associated image files. The view-mapping which determines the contents of the visual buffer given a particular structural description is information retrieving. This contrasts with Hinton's model where the view-mapping merely determines the particular viewer-centred reference frame imposed on the object; no additional visuo-spatial information is generated.

The major theoretical issue separating the two models is difficult to resolve empirically because it relates to the

nature of the perceptual encoding processes which create structural descriptions. If you accept Ullman's two-stage model for
deriving perceptual descriptions, then Kosslyn's model seems the
more appropriate theoretical position. Once a structural description has been encoded Hinton's model no longer makes
recourse to perceptual encodings with the properties of base
representations. However, the image files within Kosslyn's model
do seem to have the properties of base representations, that is,
they are uninterpreted, visuo-spatial representations. For this
reason, Kosslyn's conception of image space is to be preferred
as the basis for explaining how people read information off
images. Using a theoretical framework which is an amalgam of
Ullman's two-stage model and Kosslyn's theory of imagery, it is
possible to explain language access to visuo-spatial information
in terms of the notion of visual routines. Kosslyn's inspect
process encompasses a set of visual routines which access images
(base representations) to create structural descriptions that
explicitly represent the visuo-spatial information necessary for
language-related tasks. The inspect routine maps visuo-spatial
information implicit in base representations onto explicit
structural descriptions, or incremental representations.

5. LANGUAGE ACCESS TO VISUO-SPATIAL INFORMATION

Given the representation of mental images described above,
it is necessary to explain why people need to use imagery to
access certain forms of visuo-spatial information. It is only
necessary to use imagery when the requisite visuo-spatial
information is not explicitly encoded as a structural
description (this is the only form of visuo-spatial encoding
that is directly accessible through language). There are two
main reasons why such encodings may not be present in long-term
memory. First, the requisite information may be implicit, rather
than explicit, within the structural description representing an
object. This is the case for unusual spatial relations. If you
are asked to decide whether a car's headlamps are closer to the
ground than its door handles, then it is necessary to employ a
viewer-centred reference frame in which both parts of the car
are encoded relative to the ground, that is an image of the car.
This is because the object-centred spatial locations of the two
parts would not be tied to the same reference axis, and it is
not possible to compute relative locations over non-adjacent
levels of the structural description hierarchy. Such
computations are only possible using viewer-centred coordinate
systems.

Another reason why long-term memory encodings may be
inaccessible is that the relevant structural descriptions do not
contain the requisite information in the first place. Attentional processes influence the contents of perceptual encodings, and
structural descriptions are rarely complete representations of
the visual form of an object. Visual features, or properties of
an object which are irrelevant to the cognitive environment at
the time of encoding will not be represented as part of the
object's structural description. However, such features are
encoded in the base representations associated with the object
as these encodings are delivered by mandatory, bottom-up
processes. When it becomes necessary to access these features it

is achieved through activation of the appropriate viewer-centred, base representation. The inspect routine accesses this encoding and generates a suitable structural description (an incremental representation).

5.1. Two access routes to visuo-spatial information

When accessing visuo-spatial information stored in long-term memory it appears that there are two independent routes; the direct route, and the indirect/imagery route. These alternative access routes are shown in figure 2. The direct route, labelled

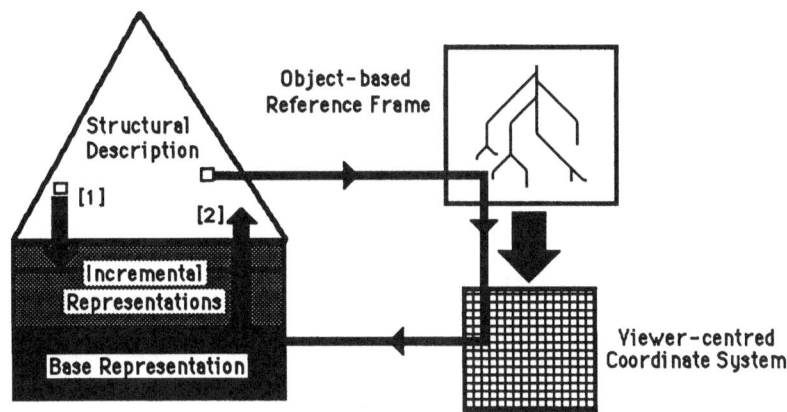

FIGURE 2. Access routes to visuo-spatial information

[1], accesses the information directly as either a perceptually derived, structural description or an incremental representation produced by a previously applied visual routine. This route is used to access information which is organised and encoded in terms of an object-centred reference system.

The second route, labelled [2] in figure 2, is indirect in that the information can only be accessed through the processes of image generation and inspection. As the direct route is not available, it is necessary to construct an appropriate image, structured according to the corresponding object-based reference system, and view-mapping. This creates a viewer-centred encoding which can then be inspected through the application of visual routines. The output of these routines is an incremental representation encoding the requisite visuo-spatial information as an object-centred, structural description (shown by the thicker line in figure 2). This route is used when the direct route fails, and when a viewer-centred encoding is required in order to extract implicit spatial relations.

5.2. Inspect routine

The inspect routine maps visuo-spatial information from viewer-centred, coordinate systems onto object-centred reference frames. Like other visual routines, it comprises a set of more elementary routines which can be combined in different ways to perform different tasks. The main tasks that the inspect routine performs are as follows:

[a] Within the viewer-centred coordinate frame it identifies axes of symmetry, and other principal axes for the component shapes, or parts of an object. These axes form the basis for the object-centred reference systems (Marr and Nishihara, 1978; Leyton, 1986).

[b] It determines the mapping between these principal axes and the axes of the viewer-centred, coordinate systems. In the original perceptual encoding of the object this mapping establishes the core of the view-mapping.

[c] It determines the spatial relations between principal axes when mapped into a viewer-centred coordinate frame. This is achieved through elementary routines which determine the scale, and relative translation and orientation of pairs of axes.

As an example of the functions of the inspect routine, consider the processing necessary to verify the sentence *The Statue of Liberty holds her torch in her right hand*. An image of the Statue would be generated from a particular view-point specified as a default of the view-mapping. The view-mapping would also determine the location in the image space of the principal axes of the torch and the Statue. The elementary translation routine would establish the relative direction of the axis of the torch from the axis of the Statue within the viewer-centred, coordinate space. The identified direction would be expressed as a structural description encoding, which could then be matched against the representation of the sentence.

5.3. Automatic versus effortful access

Glass *et al.* (1985) have recently used a distinction between automatic and effortful access to visuo-spatial information to account for the divergent results from sentence verification tasks using high- and low-imagery sentences. Some high-imagery sentences are verified faster than low-imagery sentences, while other high-imagery sentences are verified slower. The distinction that Glass *et al.* draw on is between verifying sentences by using visuo-spatial descriptions which can be accessed automatically (e.g., The apple is red), or verifying sentences using information relating to relatively unfamiliar objects for which it is necessary to generate and inspect a visuo-spatial image (e.g., The Statue of Liberty holds her torch in her right hand). Both types of sentences would be classed as high-imagery, but they are distinguished in terms of the ease of access of the visuo-spatial information necessary to verify them.

This distinction obviously overlaps with the alternative access routes to visuo-spatial information suggested in section 5.1; automatic access is equivalent to using the direct route where the necessary information is encoded as a structural description, and effortful access is via the indirect route of image generation and inspection. Furthermore, it has been suggested that to describe certain spatial relations it is generally necessary to use the indirect route. It follows from this that sentences requiring access to unfamiliar spatial relations for verification should take longer to process than other forms of high-imagery sentences. This hypothesis is borne out by the results of Glass *et al.* (1985) studies looking at the modality interference effects associated with verifying different types of high-imagery sentences; one type they used involved verifying unfamiliar spatial relations.

6. CONCLUSIONS

The phenomena associated with the experience of mental images seem to be derived from the coordination of two different forms of visuo-spatial representation; viewer-centred and object-centred reference systems. The crucial component of this coordination process is the view-mapping which determines how the elements of one representation system are encoded in the other. The view-mapping is established as a product of perceptual learning, and is by nature many-to-one. That is, many different viewer-centred, encodings of an object map onto a single object-centred representation. Any adequate theory of mental imagery is forced to account for the reverse, one-to-many mapping. What determines the viewing parameters for a particular mental image of an object that a person might generate? The nature of the view-mapping remains one of the crucial problems that imagery researchers have to solve.

However, there are other important issues which the present paper has side-stepped, which also deserve fuller exploration. One of these is the issue of whether image space is fully or only partially interpreted. The present paper is based on the assumption that image space is partially interpreted, as proposed by Kosslyn (1980). Chronometric studies are generally of little use in distinguishing between theories which, while differing in terms of their underlying architecture, make equivalent behavioural predictions.

Finally, the discussion of the inspect routine begs consideration of the nature of the underlying elementary routines. Given the proposed properties of the visual buffer it is not difficult to imagine these routines being built from simple array manipulation processes, or being based on hard-wired connections between neighbouring cells (Trehub, 1977). But again, this issue is dependent on the general form of the architecture of the image processing system. At present, it is only meaningful to specify the functions of the routines in relation to an information processing theory of imagery.

REFERENCES

1. Eddy, J.K., & Glass, A.L. (1981). Reading and listening to high and low imagery sentences. *Journal of Verbal Learning and Verbal Behavior,* **20**, 333-345.
2. Farah, M.J. (1985). The neurological basis of mental imagery: A componential analysis. In S. Pinker (Ed.), *Visual Cognition.* Cambridge, Mass.: MIT Press.
3. Finke, R.A., & Kosslyn, S.M. (1980). Mental imagery acuity in the peripheral visual field. *Journal of Experimental Psychology: Human Perception & Performance,* **6**, 244-264.

4. Finke, R.A., & Schmidt, M.J. (1977). Orientation-specific color aftereffects following imagination. *Journal of Experimental Psychology: Human Perception & Performance*, **3**, 599-606.
5. Finke, R.A., & Schmidt, M.J. (1978). The quantitative measurement of pattern representation in images using orientation-specific color aftereffects. *Perception and Psychophysics*, **23**, 515-520.
6. Glass, A.L., Millen, D.R., Beck, L.G., & Eddy, J.K. (1985). Representation of images in sentence verification. *Journal of Memory and Language*, **24**, 442-465.
7. Hinton, G.E. (1979a). Some demonstrations of the effects of structural descriptions in mental imagery. *Cognitive Science*, **3**, 231-250.
8. Hinton, G.E. (1979b). Imagery without arrays. *Behavioral and Brain Sciences*, **2**, 555-556.
9. Kosslyn, S.M. (1980). *Image and Mind*. Cambridge, Mass.: Harvard University Press.
10. Leyton, M. (1986). A theory of information structure II. A theory of perceptual organization. *Journal of Mathematical Psychology*, **30**, 257-305.
11. Marr, D. (1982). *Vision*. San Francisco: Freeman.
12. Marr, D., & Nishihara, H.K. (1978). Representation and recognition of the spatial organization of three-dimensional shapes. *Proceedings of the Royal Society of London*, **200**, 269-294.
13. Trehub, A. (1977). Neuronal models for cognitive processes: Networks for learning, perception and imagination. *Journal of Theoretical Biology*, **65**, 141-169.
14. Ullman, S. (1984). Visual routines. In S. Pinker (Ed.), *Visual Cognition*. Cambridge, Mass.: MIT Press.

MENTAL IMAGERY AND PERCEPTION:
MODULARITY OR FUNCTIONAL EQUIVALENCE?

MANUEL DE VEGA

UNIVERSITY OF LA LAGUNA, SPAIN

ABSTRACT
   This paper examines the hypothetical sharing of a processing component between apparent motion and mental rotation. The locus of the interface between imagery and perception is placed at the level of "completion" routines of the visual system, particularly those responsible for apparent motion phenomena. A preliminary research was conducted to probe for the existence of a mental rotation mechanism operating in both image rotation and apparent motion. Each trial consisted of an apparent rotation priming (clockwise, counterclockwise, or control) immediately followed by a mental rotation pattern. An interactive effect between kind of priming and angular orientation of the mental rotation pattern was obtained. The results are discussed in terms of Shepard's mental kinematic theory and the modular structure of vision.

1. INTRODUCTION

   An adequate description of the "levels" of equivalence between imagery and perception requires an examination of the functional architecture of the visual system. Recent theoretical models on perception tend to consider it as a very complex functional architecture. The visual system is assumed, by some authors, to be a prototypical modular processor (Marr, 1982; Fodor, 1983). A modular system is composed of a set of "modules", or specialized processing mechanisms which receive a particular kind of input, and generate a particular output, performing specific computations. Following Fodor, I will select some of the functional characteristics of modular systems, which can be applied to visual perception:
   First, modules are "highly specialized computational mechanisms"; that is, they process a very specific kind of stimuli or tasks. Vision is also highly specialized in the processing of patterns of light carrying spatial information from the environment. Secondly, modules are informationally encapsulated. In other words, modules are cognitively non-penetrable to our knowledge, intentions, goals, etc. (Pylyshyn, 1981). Vision is at least partially encapsulated. A large amount of computation occurs in our visual system, mainly in the early stages of processing, without any feedback from central representations. Visual illusions make this point clear, because we continue to perceive the target stimulus

47

M. Denis et al. (eds.), Cognitive and Neuropsychological Approaches to Mental Imagery, 47–56.
© *1988 by Martinus Nijhoff Publishers.*

erroneously in spite of knowing its objective features. Thirdly, modules operate in a mandatory or automatic way. When a module receives an appropriate input the processing necessarily occurs without any possible voluntary control. Most of the early processes in vision are mandatory. We cannot switch off the processing of the objects we are looking at. Even when we shift our attention to a different task (for instance hearing a song or focusing our thinking), the visual system makes computations in a preattentive way.

Doubtless the structure of vision is, at least, partially modular. This modularity seems plausible from an adaptive point of view. Vision is an "on line" processor whose function is to cope with current spatial information under severe time pressure. This is a formidable computation task, which involves segregating three dimensional objects, and figuring out their "objective" shapes, relative position, colors, textures, dynamic patterns, etc., from unstable and ambiguous proximal stimuli. It appears to have an adaptive advantage in performing these operations by means of built-in algorithms or modules, instead of appealing to the - powerful but slow - central processor. Top-down processes which combine proximal data from the receptors and concepts or rules from semantic memory, would be computationally inefficient.

Can we conclude from these arguments that the whole architecture of vision is modular? The answer is critical for the issue of perception-imagery equivalence. If vision is a wholly modular system, then the question of equivalence is devoid of meaning. A strictly data-driven visual system is hardly compatible with the equivalence of mechanisms between both systems. Any visual module involved hypothetically in an imagery task would necessarily be activated from central outputs. But this is a violation of the encapsulation postulate. Therefore, a tentative conclusion is that the mechanisms shared by perception and imagery cannot be modular in the constrained sense used by Fodor.

Whether or not the whole perceptual architecture is modular is mainly an empirical question. A selective search in the current experimental literature shows clear evidence of top-down and inferential processes in the later stages of visual processing. Doubtless, there must be a high order interface between the input processors and the conceptual system. At this level the product of our vision is largely influenced by the activated categories or "constructs" (Yates, 1985). This fact makes some researchers emphasize the thinking-like nature of perception (e.g., Bruner, 1957; Rock, 1983), although this radically "intellectual" notion of seeing cannot be upheld when taking into account the modular architecture of the early visual processor. So where should we look for imagery-perception shared components? I think that neither modules of vision nor a high level interface with the conceptual system are good candidates. Modules are by definition informationally encapsulated, and the high level interface totally lacks interest because almost everything-not only imagery and vision - interfaces at this stage (categorization, integration of visual, auditory and haptic information, etc.). Therefore, we ought to search for the critical interface between imagery and perception at intermediate level components of vision (Finke, 1980). Presumably, at this locus some primitive and highly local top-down phenomena take place. Let's examine this alternative more closely.

There is not a one-to-one correspondence between proximal data and perceptual experience. Sometimes we do not "see" all the patterns projected in our retina. There is a data reduction process from the rich analogical information of distal stimuli to a more "digitalized" or categorical format (e.g., Dretske, 1983; Yates, 1985). But, more interesting in our context, sometimes our perceptual experience goes beyond the proximal stimulus (Grossberg and Mingolla, 1985; Shepard, 1984; Yates, 1985). The physical stimulus tends to be poor and ambiguous (e.g., objects partially conceal one another) and the visual system generates its own noise (e.g., the retina has a blind spot, veins and scotomas). However, our phenomenal experience is continuous and detailed, "cleaning" and "completing" the noisy data. Our visual system probably arrives at this remarkable achievement by means of completion and enhancing routines (de Vega, 1986).

Grossberg and Mingolla (1985), for instance, propose top-down completion mechanisms to explain illusory borders (the segregation of a phenomenal figure in spite of its partially depicted borders). In the same vein Shepard (1984) suggests a trajectory completion mechanism to account for the apparent motion phenomenon, by which people perceive motion when two stationary identical patterns are alternatively presented in different positions. Furthermore, Shepard postulates that the same processor intervenes in the well known mental rotation task. These completion and enhancing routines are intermediate level components of the visual system. I believe that a rich and specific interface between imagery and perception should be expected at this level.

I will focus now on the dynamic transformation component hypothetically underlying both apparent motion and mental rotation. Shepard has proposed a "resonant kinematic" theory, suggesting the same underlying mechanisms for "imagery, perceiving, thinking and dreaming". This "mental" kinematic is used by subjects in at least two situations: firstly, when a poor (or "nonconductive") dynamic pattern is shown. A typical case is apparent motion, in which two identical stimuli are presented alternately. If the temporal and spatial parameters are properly adjusted, then our visual system interpolates a pathway resulting in a phenomenal experience of motion. Secondly, in absence of any physical stimuli subjects perform imagined transformations, apparently applying the same kinematic laws.

Although Shepard defends the imagery-perception equivalence very well, his arguments are mainly theoretical. The only empirical support to the theory is rather indirect. Specifically, he found similar chronometric functions for both mental rotation and apparent motion. Thus, the average reaction time for a mental rotation task increases linearly with the angular disparity between the target stimuli. In the same way, the stimulus onset asynchrony (SOA) required to perceive apparent motion, also increases linearly with the angular separation between the alternative stationary stimuli. Unfortunately, the existence of this functional similarity does not necessarily imply that imagery and perception share components. Instead of a functional equivalence, in principle a functional convergence hypothesis can be defended. Let us suppose the existence of two separate, although similar routines respectively for rotating images, and for figuring out pathways in apparent motion. Both routines would be convergent "solutions" to similar computational problems of transforming mental representations, occurring either at the perceptual level or at the central processor level.

In order to accept Shepard's equivalence hypothesis (and reject the alternative convergence hypothesis) a more straightforward empirical test is required. Consequently, I designed an experiment aiming to probe for an interaction between apparent motion and mental rotation. According to the rationale of interactive experiments, the activation of a common mechanism in a perceptual task would cause an aftereffect in an immediate imagery task, or viceversa (Finke, 1980, 1985; Farah, 1985). Our subjects received several two stage trials: (1) In the priming stage, a set of four alternate identical rectangles were successively shown, resulting in a clear experience of rotational motion. The serial order of the patterns was varied across the different trials, to induce either a clockwise or a counterclockwise apparent rotation. Furthermore, a no motion control condition was added in some trials, in which the four rectangles were simultaneously presented; and (2) Immediately after the apparent motion stage, subjects performed a standard mental rotation task (Cooper and Shepard, 1973). The former task was expected to interact with the latter one, either as a positive priming (facilitation) or as a negative priming (interference). Specifically, the clockwise apparent rotation would facilitate the clockwise mental rotation (letters with orientations of 240 and 300 degrees), while it would interfere with counterclockwise mental rotation (letters with orientations of 60 and 120). Counterclockwise apparent rotation would induce an inverse effect on the letter rotation task. The no motion priming would be neutral in its effect on the imagery task. In summary, the interactive hypothesis predicts two different asymmetry patterns for both clockwise and counterclockwise priming. The former condition would increase latency for orientations less than 180, and/or would decrease latency for orientations greater than 180. By contrast, the latter priming condition would produce an opposite asymmetry.

2. METHOD

2.1.-Subjects. Thirteen undergraduate (six high spatial and seven moderately low spatial) students at the University of La

Laguna at Tenerife participated, satisfying a research requirement for an introductory psychology course. Three of the selected subjects were eliminated (2 low and 1 high spatial), because of their high rate of errors or extreme reaction time patterns in the experimental task.

2.2.-Design. A complete factorial design 2x3x3x2x6 was drawn. The first factor (psychometric scores) was a grouping factor, while the rest were within-subject manipulations. The second factor (temporal block) categorized the whole set of 252 trials into three consecutive blocks, previously balanced. The third factor (perceptual priming) had three levels corresponding to two apparent rotation conditions (clockwise and counterclockwise, respectively) and a control (no motion) condition. The fourth factor was a standard manipulation in the kind of letters (normal versus mirror) in the mental rotation task. Finally, six different letter orientations were generated across trials (0,60,120,180,240 and 300 degrees).

The dependent variable was reaction times for correct responses.

2.3.- Material and procedure. A computer program was developed for the IBM PC, in order to automatically generate the stimuli, collect the chronometric data, and repeat the erroneous trials and reaction time outlyers. The perceptual priming task consisted in the alternate presentation on the computer screen of four identical rectangular shapes. Each pattern occupied approximately 3.5 degrees of visual angle. The serial order of the four stimuli emulated a clockwise rotation (1/3 of the trials), a counterclockwise rotation (1/3 of the trials) or a stationary intermittent cross, in the rest of the trials (figure 1). The SOA and ISI were adjusted in a pilot study in order to induce a realistic experience of apparent rotation. Their approximate values were 80 and 6 milliseconds, respectively. All the experimental subjects reported (in their post-experimental verbatim) a salient experience of rotation.

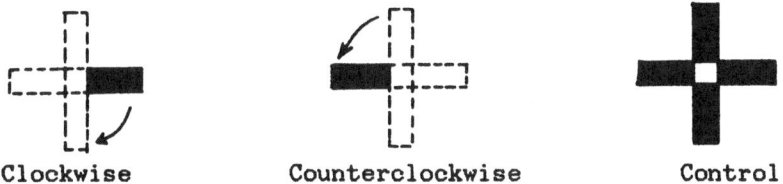

Clockwise   Counterclockwise   Control

Figure 1. Kinds of apparent motion priming

The patterns selected for the mental rotation task were six asymmetric capital letters or digits: J,R,F,4,7,2, and their mirror images. Patterns were presented inside a narrow block (of about 2.5 degrees of visual angle per side) in the middle of the screen.

Each subject was placed in front of the computer screen and supported by a chinrest. He or she performed one session with an approximate duration of 70 minutes, receiving a total of 262 trials, with short resting periods every 24 trials. The first ten trials were for training, and were not recorded for analysis. Every trial began with the perceptual priming task. In order to guarantee the visual fixation and attentional focus on the "moving" pattern, subjects were instructed to mentally count six complete turns in the apparent rotation conditions, or six flashing crosses in the control priming, before pressing a switch. The subject's response stopped the perceptual priming, and was immediately followed by the target letter of the mental rotation task. False alarms (pressing before six cycles) did not stop the priming. The kind of priming was shifted every 28 consecutive trials.

In the second task the subjects were required to categorize "as fast and accurately as possible" the target letter as "normal" or "mirror", by pressing one of two alternate keys. Immediately after the fading of the perceptual priming the frame block was presented and then the target letter. The letter and the frame block remained in sight until the subject pressed one of the two response keys.

3. RESULTS

The initial average rate of errors was 8.8%, although in the second replication the errors were reduced to 1.9%. These second chance errors were excluded from reaction time analysis.

The most significant main effect corresponded to letter orientation and to kind of letter. Reaction time increased with angular orientation, until a maximum was reached at 180 degrees. Higher orientations caused a decreasing trend in reaction time, resulting in a grossly symmetric function $(F(5,45)= 38.69;$ $p<=.00001)$. Moreover, mirror letters produced longer reaction times than normal letters $(F(1,9)= 25.67;$ $p<=.0007)$.

The temporal block showed a small but significant effect $(F(2,18)=4.24;$ Greenh. Geisser $p<=.03)$. The means corresponding to the three blocks were 668, 643 and 592 milliseconds, respectively. No significant effect was obtained for perceptual priming.

A departure from symmetry in the orientation effects when the priming of apparent rotation preceded the letter was predicted. In fact, the interaction priming x orientation was not significant when the three priming conditions were analyzed. In a second ANOVA, the control priming condition was excluded, in order to enhance the eventual differential effect between clockwise and counterclockwise priming. The interaction now almost reached significance $(F(5,45)= 2.16;$ Huynh Feld $p<=.075)$. Visual inspection of figure 2a, suggests some asymmetries, mainly between those orientations closer to 180 degrees (specifically between 120 and 240 degrees). A last ANOVA, confined to 120, 180 and 240 orientations, was carried out. A small but significant effect for the interaction priming x orientation was obtained $(F(2,18)= 3.69;$ $p<=.045)$. The q of Tukey test showed a significant difference between 120 and 240 orientations for the clockwise condition $(q(6,18)=.07;$ $p<=.05)$. This difference supports the interactive hypothesis, because responses for 120 were slower than for 240 degrees. Otherwise, there was a small asymmetry in the expected direction between 120 and 240 orientations of counterclockwise priming, although it did not reach the level of significance.

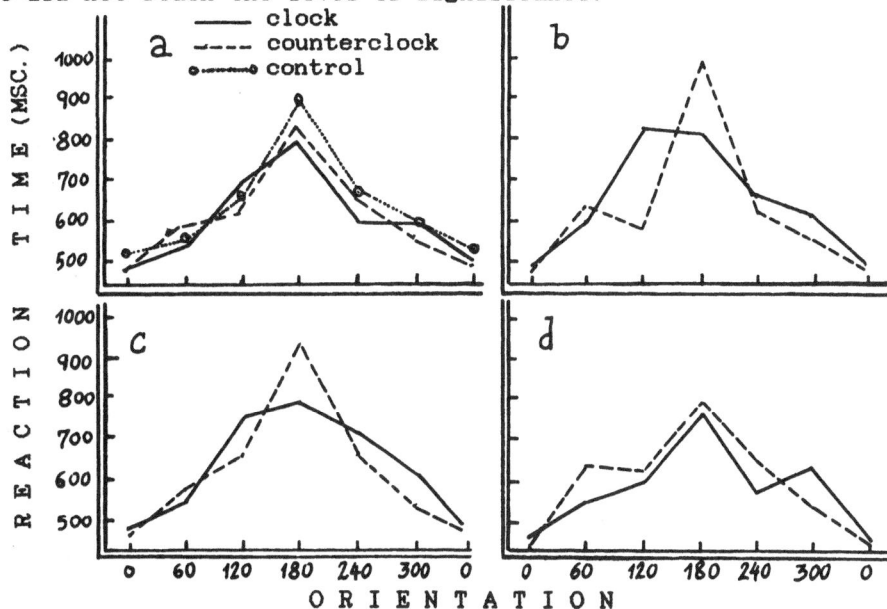

Figure 2. Mean reaction times for each orientation and kind of priming. Total (a), first block (b), second block (c), and third block (d).

Following Hintzman et al. (1981) I calculated a symmetry score, by correlating corresponding points on either side of the axis 0-180 degrees. Three correlations were obtained for each subject, corresponding to the three kinds of priming. Each correlation used twelve pairs of reaction time means (all the pairs 60-300 and 120-240, for the normal and mirror letters, for every temporal block). The lowest symmetry usually corresponds to clockwise priming (average score = .61) while counterclockwise and control priming are associated with high symmetry scores (.75 and .73 respectively). The Wilcoxon test showed a significant difference between clockwise and control symmetry scores (T=1; p<= .01), whereas the contrast between counterclockwise and control did not reach significance.

Other interactive effects involving the kind of priming, were priming x kind of letter ($F(2,18)= 4.59$; Greenh. Geisser p<= .025), and specially priming x orientation x block ($F(20,180)= 3.78$; Greenh. Geisser p<=.0076). The latter three way interaction seems the most interesting. Roughly speaking this interaction shows that the effects of priming on mental rotation is not fixed, but are strongly affected by practice. This explains why the expected interaction between priming and orientation was so weak. Actually, this interaction is modulated by a third factor: the temporal block (figure

2b,c,d).

4. DISCUSSION

The interactive hypothesis proposed here posits a simple and clear-cut effect of perceptual priming on the principal task of reaction time. Specifically, the hypothesis predicted two different asymmetrical patterns for the mental rotation task, depending on the previous clockwise or counterclockwise perceptual priming. By contrast, the no motion priming would not distort the symmetry.

The results clearly support the interactive hypothesis. The perceptual priming induced distortions in the pattern of reaction time shown by the mental rotation task. However the interaction is rather more complex than was expected.

Firstly, asymmetry is rather weak, and confined to large-pathway rotation trials (a priming by orientation interaction). This can be explained easily if we assume that mental rotation is an iterative and discrete set of operations (see for instance, Just and Carpenter, 1985). Consequently, as the angular distance increases more iterative operations are required. Thus, any experimental factor affecting the duration of the discrete rotation stages would appear more clearly in long-pathway rotations due to a simple accumulative effect. Two experiments illustrating the interactive effect of orientation should be mentioned in this context. Pylyshyn (1979, experiment 1), found that complex stimuli are rotated more slowly than simpler ones. However, this effect was larger as the pattern's orientation were closer to 180 degrees (a pattern by orientation interaction). With a very different purpose and design Hintzman et al.(1981, experiment 7), obtained decreasing reaction times for three consecutive sessions of a mental rotation task. These training effects were more striking for orientations closer to 180 degrees.

Secondly, asymmetry is most evident for clockwise priming conditions. This asymmetry involved a selective effect of apparent motion on the imagery task, depending on the direction of mental rotation. Thereafter, our hypothesis is partially supported. However, the counterclockwise priming did not decrease symmetry appreciably. Mental rotation seems more sensitive to clockwise priming than to the reverse. This unexpected result is difficult to interpret from our data. Further research is required to replicate this phenomenon and to explain it.

Thirdly, the effect of priming is unstable and tends to change with subject practice (interaction for priming x orientation x block). Asymmetry, and the hypothetical perception-imagery interaction, is probably stronger in the first moments of the experimental session (figure 2b). Further practice increases the overall similarity of the chronometric functions in all the priming conditions (figure 2c, and d). On a more theoretical level of description, this means that the functional interaction between apparent motion and mental rotation is not a fixed one. What causes this extreme flexibility? Perhaps the subject learns to diminish his or her attention to the priming task as the session progresses, making this task more automatic. Consequently, the experience of apparent motion would be weakened, as would be its effects on the imagery task. However, our subjects reported a persistent experience of motion across the whole set of trials. Furthermore, the experimental procedure was designed to prevent a drop in attention to the priming task.

In summary, the results show specific interactive effects between perception and imagery. In particular, previous exposure to an apparent motion task determines either a facilitation or an interference effect on an imagery rotation task. A similar interaction was obtained by Corballis and McLaren (1982) though their task differed from the present one on two critical features. First, they used as a priming a rotating disk instead of an apparent motion pattern; therefore, their results are not clearly interpretable from Shepard's arguments on mental kinematic. Secondly, Corballis and McLaren's rotating stimulus (a white disk with black letters and numerals) was surprisingly similar to the mental rotation stimuli (the letters F,G, and R); consequently some kind of structural and categorical priming effect should be expected, in addition to the dynamic aftereffect. By contrast, the present interaction supports Shepard's theory of the existence of a functional component, shared by both apparent motion and imagery rotation. This component would be responsible for dynamic processes occurring in both systems, either completing pathways in apparent motion or performing mental transformations in images. The rationale of the experiment is straightforward. If the dynamic process underlying apparent motion and mental rotation are identical, then interactive effects should be expected. Otherwise, there must be a statistical independence between apparent motion priming and any imagery manipulation.

We can now return to the modularity issue. What is the functional status of the common component suggested by our data? Is it a module, or is it a non-modular enhancing mechanism? Shepard does not use the term "module" himself, but he seems close to this notion when he describes the "resonant kinematic" mechanism. The description of this very specialized processor, genetically built-in as a result of phylogenesis, coincides with Fodor's notion of module. However, a critical difference emerges. Whereas Fodor emphasizes the encapsulating nature of modules, Shepard explicitly describes his kinematic mechanism as informationally open. Thus, it can be activated either from current sensory data (as in apparent motion), or from more "cognitive" informational sources (as in imagery). Our experimental data also support the notion of an informationally open processor. In fact, as we have seen, the very notion of a shared component is hardly compatible with some of Fodor's restrictive criteria of modularity. We propose that the dynamic component shared by perception and imagery belongs to an intermediate level of the visual system, where enhancing and completing operations take place. Like modules, the components corresponding to this level are local processors with an evolutionary origin, but, unlike modules, they accept inputs from higher cognitive levels.

This experiment is a preliminary study, that leaves open many questions concerning the sharing of dynamic components between perception and imagery. New research is required to consolidate the results, to exclude possible experimental artifacts, and to extend the hypothesis to other dynamic operations like the interaction between apparent displacement and the scanning of mental images.

REFERENCES

1. Bruner, J.S.(1957). On perceptual readiness. Psychological Review, 64,123-152.
2. Cooper, L.A. & Shepard, R.N.(1973). Chronometric studies of the rotation of mental images. In W.G. Chase (ed.): Visual information processing. New York: Academic Press.
3. Corballis, M.C. & McLaren, R.(1982). Interaction between perceived and imagined rotation. Journal of Experimental Psychology: Human Perception and Performance, 8,215-224.
4. Dretske, F.I.(1981). Knowledge and the flow of information. Oxford: Blackwell.
5. Farah, M.J.(1985). Psychophysical evidence for a shared representational medium for mental images and percepts. Journal of Experimental Psychology: General, 114,91-103.
6. Finke, R.A.(1980). Levels of equivalence in imagery and perception. Psychological Review, 87,113-132.
7. Fodor, J.A.(1983). The modularity of mind. Cambridge, Mass.: The MIT Press.
8. Grossberg, S. & Mingolla, E.(1985). Neural dynamics of form perception: Boundary completion, illusory figures, and neon color spreading. Psychological Review, 92,173-211.
9. Hintzman, D.L., O'Dell, C.S & Arndt, D.R.(1981). Orientation in cognitive maps. Cognitive Psychology, 13,149-206.
10. Just, M.A. & Carpenter, P.A.(1985). Cognitive coordinate systems: Accounts of mental rotation and individual differences in spatial ability. Psychological Review, 92,137-172.
11. Marr, D.(1980). Vision. San Francisco: Freeman and Company.
12. Pylyshyn, Z.W. (1979). The rate of "mental rotation" of images: A test of a holistic analogue hypothesis. Memory and Cognition, 7,19-28.
13. Pylyshyn, Z.W.(1981). The imagery debate: Analogue media versus tacit knowledge. Psychological Review, 88,16-45.
14. Rock, I.(1983). The logic of perception. Cambridge, Mass.: The MIT Press.
15. Shepard, R.N.(1984). Ecological constraints on internal representation: Resonant kinematics of perceiving, imagining, thinking and dreaming. Psychological Review, 91,417-447.
16. Shepard, R.N. & Cooper, L.A.(1982). Mental images and their transformations. Cambridge, Mass.: The MIT Press.
17. de Vega, M.(1986). Percepción visual y conciencia. Paper presented to the Annual Meeting of SEP (Madrid).
18. Yates, J.(1985): The content of awareness is a model of the world. Psychological Review, 92,249-284.

ORNELLA ANDREANI

ISTITUTO DI PSICOLOGIA, UNIVERSITA' DI PAVIA, ITALY

ABSTRACT
    A series of experiments designed to test Paivio's dual-code hypothesis are discussed for their relevance to the controversial issue of pictorial-analogical and propositional models of imagery. The experiments concern the role of different perceptual inputs in short-term and long-term memory, the effects of the level of vigilance, age and education on the use of image or verbal coding; they indicate that information is stored in LTM by a semantic, abstract code with dynamic properties, which can activate either images or propositions. Similar conclusions were obtained in another experiment which compared the representation of a town in description, recall and imagination. The advantages of a unitary system of representation in maintaining and reconstructing information emerge from both lines of research on memory and imagery.

1. INTRODUCTION
    Over the past years our institute has been carrying out research in the field of memory through experimental and longitudinal investigations.
    Some of the empirical findings obtained in a series of experiments designed to test Paivio's (1983) dual-code hypothesis will be briefly presented here with a view to showing the analogies between the controversy on the visual-verbal code in memory research and the debate on pictorial and description-proposition models in imagery research.
    Between 1970 and 1980 we conducted studies on short-term and long-term recall of meaningful material. The analysis of the effects of different conditions of learning (before sleep or in waking state) and different materials (concrete, narrative text vs abstract, scientific text) showed that in the long term, all differences across independent variables disappeared whereas those concerning individual variables maintained their statistical significance. In the first phases we attempted to study the effect of complex personality dimensions, such as introversion/extroversion, interests and values as they related to the type of text (Andreani & Cavagna, 1968, 1969).
    Subsequently, we decided to observe more specific characteristics, namely subjects' coding strategies (Baldi & Pezzini, 1979). Using three types of stimuli (Pictures, Words, Pictures+Words) at two levels of complexity (isolated vs

57

M. Denis et al. (eds.), Cognitive and Neuropsychological Approaches to Mental Imagery, 57–65.

structured items) we found that image coding was superior for
isolated items, while verbal coding was better for organized
material. We   hypothesized that the probability of recall
depends on the availability of both codes (as predicted by
Paivio) in STM, while in LTM different perceptual experiences
and different inputs tend to merge in a single, semantic
system.

The type of material and the first coding are certainly
relevant in the initial phase, but are not the decisive factors
for LTM, which seems to depend on the use of superior, abstract
codes.

2. DIFFERENT PERCEPTUAL INPUTS AND MULTI-COMPONENT CODE

In   these experiments (Amoretti, 1980; Moro, 1980) we
attempted to extend Paivio's theory to other perceptual
modalities: since in real life a large part of behaviour is
activated by voices, sounds, odours, tactile and kinesthetic
experience, why should psychology experiments   be based on
visual or verbal material alone? Surely these different
perceptual inputs are important   cues for discrimination ,
recognition and recall of objects, people and events, and a
model of memory should be tested using various categories of
perceptual modalities.

Hence we constructed series of pictures, sounds, odours and
words, matched for imagery value, frequency and situation.
After a pre-test on another sample, the 4 parallel series of 30
items were presented in rotated order to 4 groups of subjects
matched for memory ability, sex, education. The task required
free association, imagination of a scene and performance on a
recognition test (after 48 hours). This design was constructed
to provide responses to the following issues:

1. Do different stimuli elicit different percentages of
recognition?

2. Do individual differences affect coding more than
perceptual inputs? Do they persist with different inputs? Do
they interact?

3. Do different perceptual inputs activate the production
of specific codes?

Results were as follows:

1. The highest percentage of recognition was elicited by
pictures and words, followed by odours, then sounds. But the
results were not clear-cut, because some stimuli were not
identified (for sounds and odours there are technical
difficulties in eliminating ambiguities). This difficulty,
however, permitted us to look into the strategies and to define
two principal types:

a- exploration at a perceptual level with image coding:
some subjects immediately started with an image, developing a
series of multimodal associations. Ex.: Coffee (odour): "I see
myself at the breakfast table at home... holiday...
pleasant..."

b- exploration at a verbal level with semantic coding:
these subjects were completely unable to evoke associations in
response to odours or sounds until they had identified them
with a verbal label: only after this did they produce verbal
associations with paradigmatic or syntagmatic links. Ex.:

Coffee (odour): ... (latency) ... "Coffee ... milk ... water ... liquid ...drink ... eat".

We defined these strategies as Figural (image) and Semantic (verbal), respectively, and observed that the subjects used them in a very consistent way throughout different sets of stimuli.

2.Individual differences are fairly self-consistent and more significant than differences between perceptual inputs. This calls to mind the distinction between verbalizers and visualizers already formulated by Bartlett (1932), but it might also be a product of development and culture, and vary with situational tasks and instructions.

3.Inputs with different perceptual modalities probably maintain their specifity in STM, and these may be stored in LTM in the same way, particularly if they are related to an emotional experience: in fact we found many flash-bulb memories aroused by odours and sounds in the experiment, and, similarly, in old people's autobiographical memories we found many episodic memories which preserved the form of the original situation (odours, voices, expressive traits of faces and so on).

Our analysis of coding strategies suggests that sense-specific surface information is very often integrated by visual images, since they are related to concrete objects, people, events; but they are stored in LTM by a semantic, abstract code which is in general a linguistic verbal code, but may take the form of many other symbolic languages, such as mathematical symbols, chemical formulae, musical notes, graphs, computer programs.

If specific codes are still present in immediate recall, probably dual-code (Image and Verbal) is typical of intermediate memory when the subject identifies the stimulus; but the principal core of LTM seems to be a semantic code that enables us to remember and reconstruct very complex and difficult material from economical and dynamic schemata for a very long period of time. This does not exclude the retention of some episodic memories located in personal time at the deepest levels of personality, loaded with emotional, affective tones and coded as images of which most, but not all, are visual (the smell of fresh bread, gas, explosion of bombs, the voice of a beloved person, etc.). These vivid memories can be activated either by specific perceptual inputs similar to the original ones, or by verbal and internal stimuli.

This type of memory already described by Tulving (1972) and recently exemplified in many personal reports quoted by Neisser in his "Memory Observed" (1982) is more specific, more static, more prevalent in children, in illiterate subjects, in very old people, and in states of low vigilance (hypnagogic states, rêverie).

3. DIFFERENCES IN VIGILANCE LEVELS AND IMAGERY

Following up our previous results, we carried out experiments to test the hypothesis that a hypnagogic, dream-like state of low vigilance increases the use of imagery (Andreani, Bidone, & Sangiorgi, in press).

Fifty subjects were tested in a state of high vigilance (waking state) and low vigilance (réverie). In the latter condition they were lying in bed in a semi-dark room, with a small light in a corner and soft music in the background, and they were instructed to relax. In both conditions 10 high and low-image value words (rated according to Cornoldi's list, 1974) were presented by a tape-recorded female voice, at a constant rate.

Subjects were instructed "to report anything which came to their minds"; and responses varied from loose free-association to the imagination of structured scenes: order of wake-réverie condition and order of presentation of words were rotated. Responses which varied from loose free associations to the imagination of structural scene, were analyzed for structural complexity, concreteness/abstractness, syntagmatic/paradigmatic aspects, sequences, and intra-individual differences in both conditions. We found significant differences between levels of vigilance, but more significant differences between individuals in their ability to relax, use imagery, produce associations and sequences. Subjects showed consistent cognitive style in a high and low-vigilance state, although in the latter all of them had an increase in imagery.

During réverie nearly all subjects produced a large number of images with many sensorial components, reporting sounds, lights, tactile impressions and intense emotional feelings.

At times, inhibitions were lowered and childhood memories rose to the surface. In the hypnagogic state, abstract words with very low imagery values were transformed into rich, vivid images of concrete scenes with many details. For example, the word "Chance" originated "Dice falling, a witch throwing the dice"; "Aim" produced "An arrow striking target"; "Grace" elicited "Flower ...mummy ... soft hands, fondling touch ..." and so on.

Many images were dynamic, full of movement, which indicated mobility and transformations in imagery, as in a preliminary state of creative processes (cf. movement responses in the Rorschach test). Finally, in the réverie state there were more concrete, syntagmatic associations (which appear to be typical of child language) while in the waking state there were more paradigmatic expressions such as homonyms, antonyms, synonyms, periphrases, and metaphorical passages from concrete to abstract. For instance, "Fire" generated "fireplace, burning fire" in the first case, "energy" or "purification" in the second.

We assume that image code is more primitive; therefore it should be more frequent in children, in illiterate people and dream-like states; but it might also be the preliminary pre-conscious state of a creative process. Certain results from research on age-differences in memory seem to substantiate the first hypothesis.

4. AGE DIFFERENCES

In recent years we have studied a group of 96 elderly people, divided into 5-year groups from 60 to 80, comparing them with a control group of adults (40 years) and for some tests with children (Andreani, 1986).

I will simply summarize the relevant points here:

1. The decline in memory abilities varies across tasks and is negatively correlated with educational level. Old people with a high level of education are slower in learning, but they can remember well if the learning is self-paced and if it is possible to use strategies to reconstruct material.

2. Visual recognition and visual recall show less decline with age than verbal recall (faces are remembered better than names).

3. LTM of recently learned materials shows greater decline than short term and intermediate memory: for instance, in story recall elderly people make substitutions on immediate reproduction which do not modify the meaning of the story, but with an increasing delay they introduce many deformations and substantial changes, probably reconstructing the story on the basis of their previous experience. This result only apparently contradicts the common belief that older people should be better in LTM. They are, indeed, better only for memory of old salient material which has been repeated many times, or which has strong affective values: in a test of memory of historical events (Baldi, 1979) older people perform better or the same as younger adults in recognizing pictures of historical characters or events, but when they give spontaneous recall of historical facts, these are more often connected to personal episodic memories.

We studied autobiographical memories of 96 older people intensively (Spairani, 1980), and again we found a striking difference between educational levels, since highly educated people were able to reconstruct the period of time, the history of their family, the places; in short, they were able to locate the events in a well-defined space-time frame, while less well educated subjects proceeded in a more emotionally toned way, connecting episodes through emotive associations. In short, we might say that these autobiographical memories are always reconstructions, organized around a core of positive evaluation of self-image, with a prevalence of semantic associations in the more educated people, and episodic memory in less educated people.

The results led us to reformulate some conventional points on the growth and decline of memory ability, which are also relevant for the problem of image or semantic code: <u>visual code develops earlier and is preserved longer</u>, since we find that children perform like adults in STM, iconic and echoic memory, incidental learning, spatial memory of positions and routes (Cornoldi, De Beni,& Mazzoni, 1986); but with age there is a sharp increase in encoding strategies connected with conscious goals and social motivations: the use of metamemory increases with formal education and contributes to the development of semantic memory and propositional representation, which is probably the most important factor in explaining adults' better performance.

The controversial issue of levels of processing needs to be reformulated in terms of automatic and conscious processing, which also emerges from neuropsychological research, and depth should be reassessed as richness of elaboration (see Kintsch, 1974; Kintsch & van Dijk, 1978; Baddeley, 1982, for memory of faces). Thus the superiority of image or verbal code appears to be a false issue, since both can ensure LTM if they are embedded in a rich semantic network, but the distinction between the two codes should be retained, since it is supported by hemispheric specialization.

Nevertheless, neither the distinction between automatic/conscious processing, nor the use of visual or verbal code are determined by the task, but rather by the level of expertise and the cognitive style of subjects: some can execute a complex task in an automatic way, while others require greater attention, and use of verbal mediators for memorizing pictures or figural imaging for memorizing words and sentences.

Our experiment with specific perceptual inputs suggests that a specific code could be active at the STM level, the dual code at an intermediate level, but there could be different access paths to a single LTM system, in which perceptual experiences are reorganized in symbolic amodal format, and which could be reactivated from different inputs.

Probably certain experiences (very few) are preserved as episodic memories, with an iconic or acoustic format, and may remain unmodified for years; but, most frequently, they interact with semantic codes and logical reasoning, starting new processes of creative thinking and problem solving .

The prevalence of one coding during retrieval or another depends on the task, the situation, the level of vigilance, the cognitive style, the age and education level of the subject; but usually adult subjects can activate one, or both representational systems (see Marschark & Paivio, 1977; Marschark, Richman, Yuille & Hunt, in press).

5. MEMORY AND IMAGINATION IN THE REPRESENTATIONS OF A TOWN

Recently, we tried to connect our research on LTM memory with data taken from the analogue-propositional debate on imagery, which has been developing in a way similar to the figural-semantic code issue.

We chose the topic of representation of a town at three levels of cognitive processing, perception, memory and imagination, which could be manipulated through the task, assuming that this theme made it possible to explore differences between subjects with various experiential backgrounds as well as the differences in conditions (Vecchio, in press). The sample of 40 subjects consisted of 4 groups of science and humanities students, shop-keepers and housewives, matched for educational level and period of residence in Pavia. The task of representing a town is less artificial than mental rotation or mental manipulation of distances and makes it possible to study mental maps of a macro-space rich in personal and social meaning. The perception of environment has usually been studied for content, but since we were interested in processes, we tried to differentiate three levels through precise task instructions:

1. Description of 4 aerial photos of an unknown town;
2. Memory description of our town, Pavia (free recall);
3. Imagination of a fantasy town.

There was a one-week interval between the three testing sessions.

We conducted two kinds of analysis, thematic categories and descriptive styles, which were compared in the three tasks. The first analysis considered thematic categories in the three conditions: we found that physical aspects always ranked highest for frequency (60%), followed by value judgements and personal references in recall tasks, and historical and economic aspects; in imagination, after physical aspects we found a mixed category others, which included a variety of contents which were difficult to classify.

The high frequency of personal judgements in the description of the photos shows that the description process is not an analogical reproduction of environment, but a reconstruction guided by a schema based on previous experience (knowledge base): if we compare the percentage in each category we find lower percentages of physical aspects in description (25%) than in remembering (39.8 %), while the percentage of judgments is the same (34%). Typical of free recall is the high frequency of these references to social interactions and historical aspects, while in imagination there was an increase in the "other" category (51.8 %) which is difficult to define, but probably contains the distinctive feature of being the expression of "wishful thinking": the fantasy town is often described not in physical, pictorial traits, but as an extension or a projection of an existing model towards a better quality of life. Positive aspects were accentuated or integrated, the negative rejected, so the ideal town has a river, is small, quiet, has ancient and also modern buildings. There is more rational town planning, more greenery, no traffic, more opportunities for meetings and hobbies. True fantasy descriptions with bizarre features were very rare (less than 10%).

In the second analysis, we distinguished spatial descriptions, which underlie the spatial relationship between the elements of the town, non-spatial descriptions, in which elements are listed by categorization (churches, towers, streets, etc.) and intermediate, with some reference to spatial disposition, but rather vague and indefinite.

In the photo description we found the highest frequency of intermediate responses, which often implied a mixed sequence of spatial-non spatial subjective interpretation, with an attempt to identify the town in the picture.

Remembering and imagining are very similar, with 60% of non-spatial descriptions. They can be divided into two modes: categorial (churches, towers, streets) and functional (shopping areas, university).

In the imagination of the town, we found an alternation between vivid snapshots of pictorial details based on a few elements, with successive integrations, but not a global map with analogical features. Some subjects proceeded from the centre to the periphery, or vice versa (from the access roads to the town), but this sort of scanning seems guided by semantic connections of a verbal or affective nature more than by spatial indications; the images seem to develop gradually on the basis of an abstract representation of an ideal town that can activate either an image or a knot along the semantic net. Since the spatial description concerns only limited sectors of the town in all the tasks, we can posit that analogical representation is limited by storage capacity and that memories are organized in a more economical abstract format, which can be reactivated either in propositional or analogical modes.

These data are consistent with our analysis of autobiographical memories in older people, where we found both semantic and episodic memories, and with the results of our previous experiments on multi-component codes and the state of vigilance: on the whole they seem to support the hypothesis of abstract representation in LTM, which may generate verbal description and/or mental imagery according to the diversity of the tasks and the cognitive style of the subjects: the assumption of an abstract format would permit economy of storage and potential plurality of a representation. While not contradicting any of the experimental results, it does seem to offer a unitary frame in which to interpret the data from dual-code research in memory and from the analogical/propositional debate in imagery research.

REFERENCES

1. Amoretti, G. (1980). Processi mnestici attivati da diverse modalità sensoriali: gli stimoli olfattivi. In Atti del XVIII Congresso degli Psicologi Italiani, vol.2, Palermo: Il Vespro.
2. Andreani, O. (1986). The effect of biological and educational factors in the growth and decline of different memory performance with age. Paper presented at the 2nd European Conference on Developmental Psychology, Rome.
3. Andreani, O., Bidone, B., & Sangiorgi, G.(in press). Processi mnestici e immaginativi in stato di veglia e in stato ipnagogico. Archivio di Psicologia, Neurologia e Psichiatria.
4. Andreani, O., & Cavagna, G. (1968). Ricordo dopo condizioni di sonno o veglia. Rivista di Psicologia, 62, 455-498.
5. Andreani, O., & Cavagna, G. (1969).Fattori che influenzano il ricordo a lunga distanza. Annali di Psicologia, 2, 1557.
6. Baddeley, A.D. (1982). Your memory. A user's guide. London: Multimedia Publications Ltd.
7. Baldi, P.L. (1979). Un test di memoria a lungo termine (MLT '77). Costruzione e taratura preliminare su adulti normali. Archivio di Psicologia, Neurologia e Psichiatria, 40, 25-52.
8. Baldi, P.L., & Pezzini, A.R. (1979), Strategie di codifica verbale e iconica. Rivista di psicologia, 72, 43-49.
9. Bartlett, F. (1932). Remembering. Cambridge: Cambridge University Press.
10. Cornoldi, C. (1974). Imagery values for 310 Italian nouns. Italian Journal of Psychology, 1, 211-225.

11. Cornoldi, C., De Beni, R., & Mazzoni, G. (1986). The development of meta-memory strategies and memory. Presented to the 2nd European Conference on Developmental Psychology, Rome.

12. Kintsch, W. (1974). The representation of meaning in memory. Hillsdale,N.J.: Erlbaum.

13. Kintsch, W., & Van Dijk, T.A. (1978). Towards a model of text comprehension and production. Psychological Review, 85, 363-394.

14. Marschark, M., & Paivio, A. (1977). Integrative processing of concrete and abstract sentences. Journal of Verbal Learning and Verbal Behavior, 16, 217-231.

15. Marschark, M., Richman, C., Yuille, J.C., & Hunt, R.(in press). The role of imagery in memory: On shared and distinctive information. Psychological Bulletin .

16. Moro, P. (1980). Processi mnestici attivati da stimoli acustici. In Atti del XVIII Congresso degli Psicologi Italiani, vol.2, Palermo: Il Vespro.

17. Neisser, U. (1982). Memory observed. San Francisco: W.H. Freeman.

18. Paivio, A. (1983). The empirical case for dual coding. In J.C. Yuille (Ed.), Imagery, memory and cognition. Hillsdale,N.J.: Erlbaum.

19. Spairani, M. (1980). Ricordi spontanei e test di memoria di eventi remoti in vecchi dai 60 agli 80 anni.In Atti del XVIII Congresso degli Psicologi Italiani, vol.2., Palermo: Il Vespro.

20. Tulving, E. (1972). Episodic and semantic memory. In E. Tulving & W. Donaldson (Eds.), Organization of memory. New York: Academic Press.

21. Vecchio, L. (in press). Processi percettivi, mnestici e immaginativi nella rappresentazione di una città: Pavia. In E. Bianchi, F. Perussia & M.F. Rossi (Eds.), Immagine soggettiva e ambiente. Milano: Unicopli.

2.2. THE PROCESSING OF LEXICAL INFORMATION

STROOP AND PRIMING EFFECTS IN NAMING AND CATEGORIZING TASKS USING WORDS AND PICTURES

JUAN MAYOR, JAVIER SAINZ AND JAVIER GONZALEZ-MARQUES

COGNITIVE PROCESSES DEPARTMENT, COMPLUTENSE UNIVERSITY, MADRID, SPAIN

ABSTRACT
An experiment was conducted in order to study word and picture processing within the framework of the Stroop and Priming paradigms. Tasks, modalities and semantic relationships were equated for both paradigms. Three experimental conditions were constructed on the basis of the temporal interstimuli interval: previous (Priming), simultaneous (Stroop), previous and simultaneous (Stroop & Priming). Results showed several facilitation and interference reversed effects which are attributed to the interaction between temporal interstimuli sequence, task demands and modality in working memory. Results are discussed in relation to the differential processing of words and pictures and the nature of the representation format.

1. INTRODUCTION
One of the most consistent research lines on mental imagery is the one which attempts to clarify the nature of the representation format (Kosslyn & Pomerantz, 1977). Most paradigms used to evaluate the coding format analyze the processing of information presented in words and pictures (Lupker, 1985). Snodgrass (1984) proposes three criteria in favor of a unitary format of representation: the same processing time for both modalities of stimuli (words and pictures), and similar facilitation and interference effects in both modalities. Experimental results do not completely support these criteria: different processing of words and pictures and different facilitation and interference effects have been found, although not always in the same direction (Smith & Magee, 1980; Glaser & Düngelhoff, 1984). What is the reason for these differences and for these asymmetric trends with reversed effects? It seems obvious that they should be attributed to the type of semantic decisions required in each task which depend, in turn, on the experimental variables manipulated.

Two paradigms (also called tasks, effects, phenomena, or conditions in the literature) are particularly useful in this regard due to their specific manipulation of the relevant variables: Stroop paradigm (Virzi & Egeth, 1985) and Priming paradigm (Lorch, Balota & Stamm, 1986). We will refer to them as paradigms or conditions. Both paradigms allow for the combination of various modalities: word (W) vs. picture (P); tasks: naming (N) vs. categorizing (C) vs. lexical decision; semantic relationships: conceptual congruency (Con) vs. categorical congruency (Cat) vs. incongruency (Inc); and the temporal sequence of the stimuli. Both paradigms use a compound stimulus made up of an irrelevant stimulus and a target stimulus that leads to the response.

It is generally thought that the Stroop (ST) paradigm produces interference effects (e.g., between a color and the name of a color). This initial paradigm has been progressively modified: a picture substituted for the color, naming and categorizing tasks have been combined, the semantic relationship and the stimulus onset asynchrony (SOA) have been varied. The robustness of the effect is maintained even when the color is replaced by a picture (Glaser & Düngelhoff, 1984; Lupker, 1985). Results indicate that the Stroop paradigm can lead to asymmetric effects: words used as

M. Denis et al. (eds.), Cognitive and Neuropsychological Approaches to Mental Imagery, 69–78.

irrelevant stimuli increase the picture naming reaction time (RT), whereas the opposite effect is not found. If the task demands for the categorization of the target, the phenomenon reverses; that is, the presentation of a picture as irrelevant stimulus increases the word categorizing RT, whereas the opposite effect does not occur. According to the response competition hypothesis, the locus of the effect is in the response phase (Posner & Snyder, 1975), whereas according to the semantic decision hypothesis, the locus is in an intermediate processing phase (Glaser & Glaser, 1982).

The Priming (PR) paradigm is usually regarded as leading to facilitation effects. Initially, this paradigm involved the faster reading of a word (e.g., doctor) when it was preceded by a semantically related word (e.g., nurse), compared to when it was preceded by an unrelated word (e.g., butter) (Meyer & Schvaneveldt, 1971). Various aspects of the paradigm have also been modified (see Lupker, 1985): the quality of the stimulus (clear vs. degraded), the task (lexical decision vs. naming vs. categorizing), the semantic relationship (identical vs. related vs. unrelated), the stimulus modality (picture vs. word) and even the stimulus onset asynchrony (SOA) (e. g., Dallas & Merikle, 1976, presented both stimulus simultaneously).

There have been recent attempts to make these two paradigms converge. Glaser and Düngelhoff (1984) used a pre-exposition time of the irrelevant stimulus ranging from 400 to 100 msec.La Heij, Van der Heijden and Schreuder (1985, p. 64) used a word-word modification of the Stroop paradigm that "can be used in a semantic Priming paradigm". The differences between both paradigms can be reduced to the range of responses that they allow for (ST: a few; PR: a lot and unrepeated), to the number of semantic domains (ST: one; PR: various), and to the role of words as targets and distractors (ST: the same words are used as target and distractor; PR: the target word is never used as prime).

The various modifications of these paradigms have led to opposite results: parallel and similar effects on the one hand, and different and reversed effects on the other. The former are usually attributed to the fact that both the basic experimental condition and the required response are the same (two stimuli are presented while subject's response is addressed to one of them). Thus, Stroop and Priming paradigms trigger shared processing mechanisms (automatic processing of the irrelevant stimulus and strategic processing of the target stimulus) (Posner & Snyder, 1975; Den Heyer, Briand & Smith, 1985). The different and reversed effects are attributed to the interaction between the experimental conditions (ST, PR) and the manipulated variables: stimulus modality (W, P), type of task (N, C), semantic relationship (Con, Cat, Inc), and temporal sequence of the stimulus. It is assumed that the experimental conditions and the manipulation of the variables place different demands on the working memory, thus modulating the access to the semantic memory. For example, in the Priming condition, due to the temporal sequence between irrelevant and relevant stimulus, subjects can automatically attend to the target stimulus. In the Stroop condition, subjects have to ignore the irrelevant stimulus, which is present, and make a decision in order to concentrate their attention on the target stimulus (see Figure 1).

We have modified the initial Stroop and Priming paradigms, while keeping the usual variables: task, modality, semantic relationship, and SOA. The novelty of our design comes from two sources: a) identical manipulation of variables in both paradigms (even those that La Heij et al. considered as differentiating between them). The only difference that we maintained was the temporal sequence of irrelevant and target stimuli presentation (in the ST condition, both stimuli are presented simultaneously during 125 msec; in the PR condition, the prime is presented first, followed by an empty interval, and by the presentation of the target); b) the study of the single ST and PR conditions, and their combined effects (ST & PR). While only one irrelevant stimulus is used in the single conditions (simultaneous or previous), two irrelevant stimuli are used in the combined (ST & PR) condition: one previous (Priming-like) and other simultaneous (Stroop-like).

Our first prediction is that the three conditions, ST, PR, and ST & PR will produce the same pattern of facilitation and interference effects. The underlying hypotheses are that both paradigms trigger some common processing mechanisms (automatic for the irrelevant stimulus, and strategic for the target stimulus), and that the effects of the ST & PR combined condition are not additive. We also predict that the manipulation of the variables (modality, task, and semantic relationship) will lead to differential effects in each condition (ST and PR). More specifically, we expect to obtain asymmetries, but of different directions and amplitudes, when we combine: a) the modality (W, P) with the task (N, C); b) the modality with the conditions (ST, PR); c) the semantic relationship (con, cat, inc) with the task (N, C); d) the semantic relationship (con, cat, inc) with conditions (ST, PR); e) the modality (W, P) with the task (N, C), and with the semantic relationship (Con, Cat, Inc). The underlying hypothesis is that these variables do not lead to consistent effects across conditions, but rather depend upon the demands placed on the working memory. These demands varied according to the interaction between the variables and the temporal sequence of the stimuli in each of the three conditions.

Confirmation of our first, but not the second, prediction, will support both Snodgrass' (1984) and La Heij et al's (1985) theses. The former would be supported because we would not find differences depending on the modality (W, P); the latter would receive support because, given the equation of Stroop and Priming criteria, the effects of both conditions would be basically identical. Confirmation of the second, but not the first, hypothesis would provide evidence against both Snodgrass and La Heij et al.'s theses.

Confirmation of both predictions would lead to the partial acceptance of La Heij et al's. thesis and the rejection of the criteria that, according to Snodgrass, would support an unitary format of representation. Nevertheless, confirmation of both predictions would not necessarily lead to the rejection of a unitary format of representation. In fact, it could be argued that the differences predicted between modalities have their basis at a functional level (i.e., different processing of words and pictures), rather than at a semantic level. A unitary format of representation in the semantic memory does not imply equal response latencies that can be attributed to their differential processing in working memory.

2. EXPERIMENT

2.1 Method.

2.1.1. Subjects. Sixteen students from the Psychology Department of the Complutense University of Madrid, aged 20 to 30, were selected to participate in the experiment on the basis of a pre-test performance criterion (i.e., less than 2 errors).

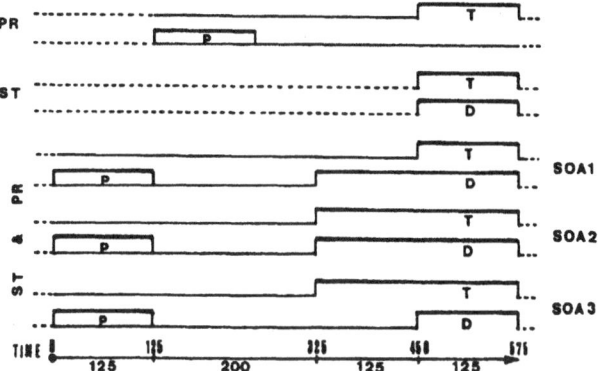

FIGURE 1. Diagram of temporal course of stimuli presentation. (PR = Priming, ST = Stroop, ST & PR = Stroop and Priming combined condition, T = Target, D = Distractor, P = Prime, SOA = Stimulus Onset Asynchrony; time in msec).

2.1.2. <u>Materials and Instruments</u>. Six categories of basic level (table, chair, car, plane, spoon and fork) were used as stimuli. According to the categorical norms of a Spanish sample, the stimuli represented the most typical exemplars of three superordinate categories (furniture, vehicles and silverware). Each stimulus was presented both in word (W) and picture (P) modalities. Eighteen compound stimuli (irrelevant and target) for each of the four series in ST and PR single conditions and other 54 compound stimuli (prime, distractor and target) for each of the twelve series in ST & PR combined condition were used. The stimuli were projected on a screen by using Kodak Carrousel projectors (SAV 2050) with Lafayette shutters controlled by a Hewlett Packard (HP 9825A) computer through a Scanner (HP 3495A). A Campden Instruments Timer (timer counter 565) and a microphone connected to a voice key (Campden Instruments 340) were also used.

2.1.3. <u>Design</u>. Three parallel designs were used, one for each condition. The same 2x2x3 factorial design was used in the Stroop and Priming single conditions. These single conditions were used later as neutral conditions. The three variables were: the task (N, C), the modality of the target (W, P), and the semantic relationship between the relevant and irrelevant stimuli: conceptual congruency (Con) (W and P belong to the same basic category), categorical congruency (Cat) (W and P belong to the same superordinate category), and incongruency (Inc) (W and P belong to different superordinate categories).

A 2x2x3x3x3 factorial design was used in the ST & PR combined condition. Other than the task (N, C) and the modality (W, P), we manipulated two variables of semantic relationship: the Stroop (i.e., the semantic relationship between the target and the distractor), and the Priming (i.e., the semantic relationship between the prime and the target) relationships. The fifth variable manipulated was the SOA, with three levels: in SOA1, the distractor was presented alone during 125 msec, followed by a 125 msec combined presentation of the target and distractor; in SOA2, the target and distractor were simultaneously presented during 250 msec; in SOA3, the target was presented alone during 125 msec, followed by a 125 msec combined presentation of the target and distractor (see Figure 1).

2.1.4. <u>Procedure</u>. The experiment was conducted over three consecutive sessions. Each session was dedicated to one of the three experimental conditions: ST, PR, ST & PR. The order of participation in the conditions was counterbalanced across subjects. In the ST condition, both the relevant and irrelevant stimuli (W-P or P-W) were simultaneously presented during 125 msec. In the PR condition, a prime was presented during 125 msec, followed by a 200 msec interval, and by a 125 msec presentation of the target; in order to equate the latter with the ST condition, only combinations of complementary modalities were used. In the ST & PR combined condition, the global stimulus in each trial was made up with three stimuli: the prime (presented during 125 msec), followed by a 200 msec interstimuli interval, and by another stimulus made up of two stimuli (the distractor and the target); the latter were presented in different SOAs.

In all conditions, subjects' task was either naming (i.e., reading the word or naming the picture of the target stimulus) or categorizing (i.e., classifying the word or the picture of the target) according to the three superordinate categories. For each series of trials, the stimuli were generated at random. The irrelevant and target stimuli were presented in complementary modalities (W-P or P-W). All conditions of semantic relationship were equated (only one of all four posible combinations of incongruency was systematically chosen).

2.2 <u>Results</u>.

Table 1 shows the mean RTs for ST and PR condition depending on the task (N, C), the modality (W, P), and the semantic relationship (con, cat, inc).

Both in ST and PR, naming was faster than categorizing (225 msec, overall mean). A main effect of modality was present only in the PR condition. Main effects of semantic relationship, and the following interactions were all significant in both conditions: Task (T) x Modality (M), Task (T) x Semantic Relationship (SR), and Task (T) x Modality

(M) x Semantic Relationship (SR) (see graphic representation in Figure 2a). Table 2 shows the results of the ANOVA performed on the Stroop and Priming conditions.

TABLE 1. Mean RTs (msec) for task, modality, and semantic relationship in the ST and the PR conditions.

| | STROOP CONDITION | | | | | | PRIMING CONDITION | | | | | |
| | Naming | | | Categorizing | | | Naming | | | Categorizing | | |
	Con	Cat	Inc	Con	Cat	Inc	Con	Cat	Inc	Con	Cat	Inc
WORD	573	575	596	914	916	998	604	601	622	878	884	981
PICTURE	652	703	712	806	799	850	588	621	632	725	691	738

TABLE 2. ANOVA performed on the single Stroop (ST) and Priming (PR) conditions.

| | STROOP | | | PRIMING | | |
	F	df	p<	F	df	p<
TASK	108.65	(1,15)	.001	112.83	(1,15)	.001
MODALITY	0.17	(1,15)	.68	39.58	(1,15)	.001
S.R.	28.93	(2,30)	.001	8.30	(2,30)	.01
TASKxMOD	24.54	(1,15)	.001	88.40	(1,15)	.001
TASKxSR	4.10	(2,30)	.05	3.83	(2,30)	.05
TxMxSR	3.41	(2,30)	.05	3.71	(2,30)	.05

The type of asymmetry usually found in the ST paradigm was present in our data. In the ST condition, the word used as distractor interfered with the picture naming, whereas the picture only weakly interfered with the word reading; in the categorizing task, a reversed Stroop interference trend was observed. No phenomenon of similar characteristics was observed in the PR condition (the difference in RT between W and P is only 4 msec), although a marked effect, similar to the reversed Stroop, was present in the categorization. Overall, there was an interaction between the task and the modality leading to reversed effects for facilitation and interference: in categorization (both for ST and PR), P is always faster than W; in naming, W is faster than P in both conditions (there was a small non-significant difference in PR); see Figure 2b. Mean RTs for ST & PR condition according to all five independent variables are shown in Table 3.

TABLE 3. Mean RTs (msec) in ST & PR condition for task, modality, SOAs, Stroop semantic relationship (on horizontal) and Priming semantic relationship (on vertical).

| | | | SOA1 | | | SOA2 | | | SOA3 | | |
			Con	Cat	Inc	Con	Cat	Inc	Con	Cat	Inc
		Con	514	527	539	625	655	647	603	645	640
	Word	Cat	533	557	567	646	654	666	619	656	686
		Inc	543	543	575	639	669	663	634	670	665
NAMING											
		Con	571	573	582	675	677	711	663	676	679
	Picture	Cat	607	610	615	704	696	731	705	687	740
		Inc	616	608	607	700	707	721	710	719	730
		Con	671	658	771	785	768	897	743	730	866
	Word	Cat	641	662	745	772	782	893	769	738	835
		Inc	744	702	797	814	816	912	787	792	884
CATEG.											
		Con	618	651	735	781	791	849	773	769	863
	Picture	Cat	641	641	705	809	791	880	757	761	842
		Inc	668	681	744	816	850	902	794	778	868

TABLE 4. ANOVA performed on the ST & PR combined condition.

	F	df	p<		F	df	p<
TASK	139.08	(1,15)	.001	TASKxMOD	9.36	(1,15)	.01
MODALITY	0.01	(1,15)	.91	TASKxSR(ST)	18.71	(2,30)	.001
S.R.(ST)	44.96	(2,30)	.001	TASKxSR(PR)	38.15	(2,30)	.001
S.R.(PR)	54.54	(2,30)	.001	TASKxSOAs	4.77	(2,30)	.05
SOAs	36.71	(2,30)	.001	TxMxSR(ST)	4.58	(2,30)	.05
				TxSxSR(ST)	2.63	(4,60)	.05

The most significant data (those in which the semantic relationship between the prime and target and the distractor and the target match) are shown in Figure 3a. Table 4 shows the results of the ANOVA performed on the ST & PR condition.

As found in the previous ST and PR conditions, results from ST & PR condition, where Stroop and Priming effects are combined, indicated that naming was faster than categorizing (132 msec).

As found in the ST condition, the 50 msec difference between W (faster) and P (slower) found in ST & PR was not significant. There was a significant interaction between the task and the modality, although we did not find reversed effects as those found in the ST condition. In the ST & PR condition, both in naming and categorizing, W was faster than P. This result is infrequent in the literature. The Stroop-like asymmetry effect is mainly present in naming; in contrast, the reversed Stroop effect is not present in categorizing (see Figure 3b).

The SOA1 was most facilitating, the SOA2 was most interfering, and the SOA3 was in between the other two. Such an SOA gradient was not present in the naming task, where the SOA1 was the most facilitating, whereas the effects of the SOA2 and the SOA3 were approximately the same.

The semantic relationship replicates the results obtained in the ST and the PR single conditions (compare Figures 2a and 3a): in naming, the gradient goes, from fastest to slowest, as follows: Con > Cat > Inc; in categorizing, the incongruency is also most interfering, but conceptual and categorical congruencies have similar effects. There are significant trends: one for categorical congruency and incongruency to converge in naming (both opposed to conceptual congruency), and other for incongruency and conceptual congruency to converge in categorization (both opposed to categorical congruency).

It should be mentioned that no interactions between the semantic relationship of the distractor and the target (Con, Cat, Inc -- vertical lines in Table 3), or between the semantic relationship of the prime and the target (Con, Cat, Inc -- horizontal lines in Table 3) were found. This result confirms the existence of a parallel semantic processing in these two conditions, even when they were combined in the same condition ST & PR, where their effects were more likely to reverse. In other words, semantic and temporal relationships are independent of each other in Stroop and Priming paradigms.

In order to test wether there were additive effects when Stroop and Priming paradigms were combined, the data from the ST and PR single conditions were used as neutral conditions. Thus, the contributions of Stroop and Priming conditions could be evaluated by subtracting their data from those obtained in the ST & PR combined condition:

(ST effect) = (ST & PR effect) - (PR effect)
(PR effect) = (ST & PR effect) - (ST effect)

Overall, Stroop and Priming had similar or parallel effects, even though Stroop seemed to interfere somewhat more than Priming. These effects are neither additive, nor do they neutralize each other. If the effects had been identical and additive, the combined results would have shown more facilitation or more interference than the results from the neutral conditions. If the effects were opposed and neutralized each

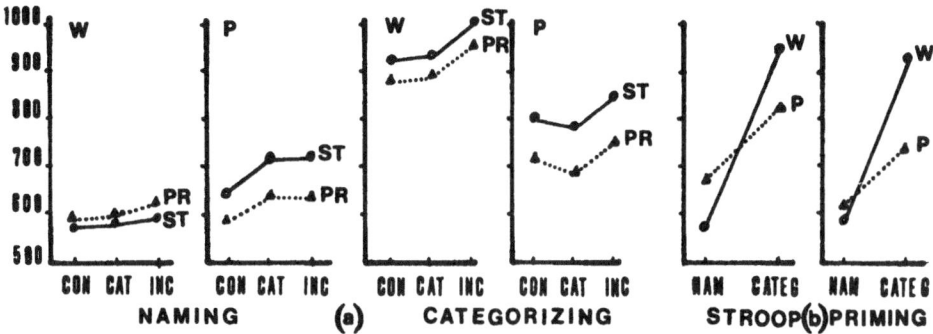

FIGURE 2. (a) Mean RTs (msec) in the ST and the PR conditions for each variable: task, modality and semantic relationship. (b) Interactions between modality and task in the ST and the PR conditions.

other, the combined results would be somewhere between those obtained   in ST and PR neutral conditions.

The effects of the ST & PR combined condition are in the same direction and of the same magnitude as those in the neutral conditions, except for word categorizing. The RTs for the picture modality in the ST & PR combined condition are similar to those found in the ST condition (667-689 msec for N, 796-818 msec for C), whereas the RTs for the word modality are similar to those found in the PR condition (almost identical in N, 614-609; there is a larger difference in C, 749-914 msec) (see Figure 4).

3. DISCUSSION

Our experiment had two main purposes: to clarify the similarities and differences between Stroop and Priming paradigms, and to clarify the nature of the processing mechanisms and the representation format of words and pictures. Regarding the former, and according to La Heij et al. (1985), both paradigms have converged, but results differ as a function of the set of responses, the number of semantic domains, and the role of words as either targets or distractors. Given that we equated both conditions in all the relevant variables, it could be expected that ST and PR conditions would lead to identical results. Actually, we found similarities, but we also obtained significant differences. Among the similarities, we found the same pattern of responses for all semantic relationships (Con, Cat, and Inc) in all conditions (ST, PR, ST & PR) (see Figures 2a and 3a).

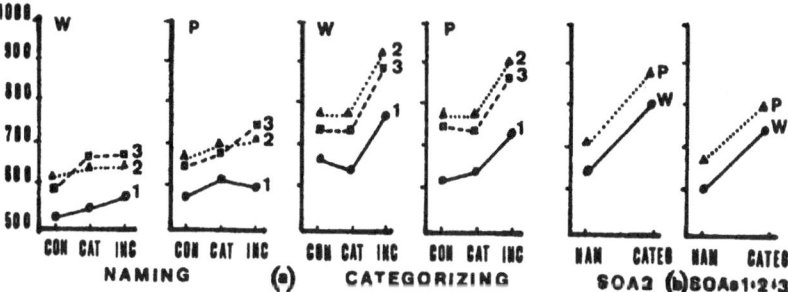

FIGURE 3. (a) Mean RTs (msec) in the ST & PR condition for each variable: task, modality and semantic relationship. (b) Interactions between task and modality in the ST & PR condition for SOA2 and the mean of the three SOAs.

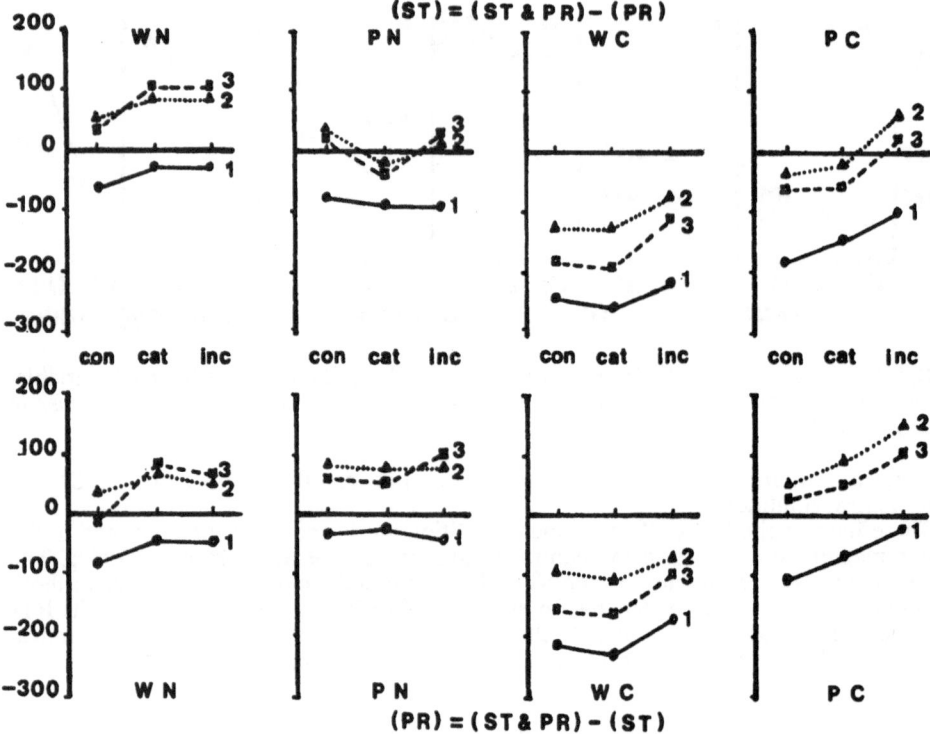

FIGURE 4. Facilitation and interference effects in the different SOAs, tasks and modalities with respect to the neutral PR condition and the neutral ST condition.

We also found that facilitation and interference effects produced by the semantic relationship between the target and the distractor (e. g., Stroop-like effects) in the ST & PR condition, are equivalent to the effects produced by the semantic relationship between the prime and the target (e. g., Priming-like effects). It seems reasonable to attribute these parallelisms to the equation of conditions and variables in both paradigms (even those pointed out by La Heij et al., 1985). Nevertheless, we found differences that cannot be attributed to the criteria established by those authors, but should rather be attributed to the critical difference that we maintained, that is, the temporal difference in the presentation of irrelevant and target stimuli (previous in Priming and simultaneous in Stroop). This temporal sequencing is crucial in the differential processing required by the ST and PR conditions (the first more strategic than the second, which is more automatic). Our hypothesis, an alternative to those exposed by La Heij et al. (1985), receives full support from the following results: 1) word naming is faster in the ST condition than in the PR condition, whereas picture naming is faster in the PR condition than in the ST condition; 2) word categorizing is slower than picture categorizing in the ST and PR single conditions, whereas picture categorizing is slower than word categorizing in the ST & PR combined condition; 3) there are not significant differences in W and P processing time in the ST and ST & PR conditions, although the differences are significant in the PR condition; 4) the ST condition is more interfering than the PR condition in picture naming and in word and picture categorizing (the opposite effect is found in word naming). In summary, ST and PR conditions, that is, the temporal interstimuli differences are independent of the semantic relationship between irrelevant and target stimuli, while interacting with the task demands and the stimuli modalities in working memory.

The second purpose of our experiment was to clarify the nature of the processing of words and pictures, that should help to decide between a unitary or a dual format of representation. Contrary to Snodgrass' (1984) postulates, our results indicated the existence of asymmetries between and within each condition (ST, PR, ST & PR). The most salient asymmetries were the ones referred to as Stroop effect (the P does not interfere with the naming of the W, whereas the W interferes with the naming of the P), and the reversed Stroop effect (the P interferes with word categorizing more than the W interferes with picture categorizing).

Combining the relative speed hypothesis (the presence of the irrelevant stimulus is a necessary and sufficient condition for the Stroop interference) and the hypothesis of a faster access of pictures to their semantic representation in a categorization task, Smith and Magee (1980) predicted that the temporal relationship between irrelevant and target stimuli would prevent the Stroop conflict in the processing of words and pictures. In naming, the pre-exposition to an incongruent stimulus (P) could compensate for its slower processing and would interrupt the reading of the W. In categorization, the pre-exposition to an incongruent stimulus (W) could also compensate for its slower processing and would interrupt the categorization of the P. The manipulation of the temporal interstimuli relationship, while equating the treatment of ST and PR paradigms, sheds some light on these predictions. On the one hand, if the pre-exposition results in the asymmetries of the interference effects (W naming vs. P categorizing), then the asymmetries could be accounted for by the relative speed hypothesis. On the other hand, if no asymmetries are found, then this hypothesis cannot explain the phenomena. Our results indicated the existence of asymmetric effects both in ST and PR conditions that should be attributed to the temporal sequencing of the stimuli. These results are in partial agreement with Smith and Magee's (1980) hypothesis. In contrast to Glaser and Düngelhoff (1984), these results cannot be treated as epiphenomena of the temporal relationship: the trend found in word categorizing is not equivalent to that found in picture naming; similarly, the trend found in picture categorizing is not equivalent to that found in word naming. As opposed to Smith and Magee (1980), the asymmetries are independent from the SOAs. While Smith and Magee (1980) and Glaser and Düngelhoff (1984) assume that the processing of words and pictures is not affected by the manipulation of their temporal sequence of presentation, our results showed a critical interaction between the temporal interstimuli interval (simultaneous presentation in ST and asynchronous in PR) and the tasks and modalities. In addition, the SOA affects the task, but it does not affect the semantic relationship, thus influencing the processing in working memory (Den Heyer, Briand and Smith, 1985). The SOA1 may clearly facilitate the response because the distractor stimulus functions as a prime. The similar behavior of SOA2 and SOA3 supports Glaser & Düngelhoff's hypothesis that the effect resides on the semantic decision phase rather than on the response phase.

The semantic relationship did not result in asymmetries often found in the literature (i.e., the more the semantic similarity, the higher the Stroop-like interference, and the Priming-like facilitation). Our results indicated that in both conditions, the processing is facilitated by the conceptual congruency whereas it is interfered with by the semantic incongruency, in agreement with Dalrymple-Alford's (1972) results. Nevertheless, the categorical congruency leads to asymmetries: in naming, it behaves like incongruency (both in the categorical congruency and incongruency, the two stimuli have different names); in categorization, it behaves like the conceptual congruency (both in categorical and conceptual congruencies, the two stimuli are classified under the same categorical term). These results could be explained according to the notion that semantic similarity facilitates the processing while lack of congruency interferes with it.

These systematic asymmetries that affect words and pictures in different ways are a strong argument against Snodgrass' thesis (1984), whose criteria seem to be either inadequate or insufficient. Nevertheless, the modality (W vs. P) is the only variable where differences do not reach the significance level (neither in the ST nor in the ST & PR conditions). Glaser and Düngelhoff postulate that if there were two independent semantic systems, one for each stimulus modality, the categorization of a word should be interrupted by the picture to the same extent that the picture should interrupt the reading of the word. Since our results did not confirm these postulates, we can argue for the existence of a unitary representation format. If the differences in the processing of words and pictures are only temporary, and the same mechanism underlies both paradigms, then the interference found in Stroop and Priming should be determined by the temporal relationship between the two components (prime-target, distractor-target). Task and modality are the variables that explain the differential treatment received by words and pictures when the temporal sequence of presentation of irrelevant and target stimuli is manipulated. Finally, the obtained differences result from the functional bases of W and P, from the task demands, and from various experimental conditions. Asymmetries and differences are a product of the interaction of all these variables in working memory which, according to our results, is perfectly compatible with the notion of a unitary format of representation in the semantic memory.

REFERENCES

1. Dallas, M., & Merikle, P. (1976). Semantic processing of non-attended visual information. Canadian Journal of Psychology, 30, 15-21.
2. Dalrymple-Alford, E. C. (1972). Associative facilitation and interference in the Stroop color-word task. Perception & Psychophysics, 11, 274-276.
3. Den Heyer, K., Briand, K., & Smith, L. (1985). Automatic and strategic effects in semantic priming: An examination of Becker's verification model. Memory & Cognition, 13, 228-232.
4. Glaser, M., & Glaser, W. (1982). Time course analysis of the Stroop phenomenon. Journal of Experimental Psychology: Human Perception and Performance, 8, 875-894.
5. Glaser, W., & Düngelhoff, J. (1984). The time course of picture-word interference. Journal of Experimental Psychology: Human Perception and Performance, 10, 640-654.
6. Kosslyn, S. M., & Pomerantz, J. R. (1977). Imagery, propositions and the form of internal representations. Cognitive Psychology, 9(1), 52-76.
7. La Heij, W., Van der Heijden, A., & Schreuder, R. (1985). Semantic priming and Stroop-like interference in word-naming tasks. Journal of Experimental Psychology: Human Perception and Performance, 11, 62-80.
8. Lorch, R. F., Balota, D. A., & Stamm, E. G. (1986). Locus of inhibition effects in the priming of lexical decisions: Pre- or post-lexical access? Memory & Cognition, 14, 95-103.
9. Lupker, S. (1985). Relatedness effects in word and picture naming: Parallels, differences and structural implications. In A. Ellis (Ed.), Progress in the psychology of language (pp. 109-142). London: Lawrence Erlbaum Associates.
10. Meyer, D., & Schvaneveldt, R. (1971). Facilitation in recognizing pairs of words: Evidence of a dependence between retrieval operations. Journal of Experimental Psychology, 90, 227-234.
11. Posner, M., & Snyder, C. (1975). Attention and cognitive control. In R. Solso (Ed.). Information processing and cognition: The Loyola Symposium (pp. 55-85). Hillsdale, NJ: Lawrence Erlbaum Associates.
12. Smith, M. C., & Magee, L. E. (1980). Tracing the time course of picture-word processing. Journal of Experimental Psychology: General, 109, 373-392.
13. Snodgrass, J. G. (1984). Concepts and their surface representations. Journal of Verbal Learning and Verbal Behavior, 23, 3-22.
14. Virzi, R. A., & Egeth, H. E. (1985). Toward a translational model of Stroop interference. Memory & Cognition, 13, 304-319.

ALTERNATIVE CODING OF CONCEPTS

F. ALFONSO MEDINA

UNIVERSIDAD COMPLUTENSE, MADRID, SPAIN

ABSTRACT
    Using the technique of priming on a matching paradigm
(Exp. 1), and a sentence verification task (Exp. 2), we
observed facilitation effects of either word primes
(superordinate category noun or prototype noun) or sentence
primes (reflecting perceptual or functional properties of the
categories) on reaction times to pictures and words. Results
showed that the representation activated by the category noun
and by the prototype noun primes yielded similar facilitation
effects. In addition, sentence primes reflecting functional
information lowered reaction times to both pictures and
words. However, sentences containing perceptual information
only facilitated responses to pictures. Discussion of the
results points to the recognition of images and propositions
as two alternative codes for representing concepts, which are
considered "cognitive states" in working memory rather than
fixed entities of the long term store.

1. INTRODUCTION

    The present paper is concerned with experimental
findings that support the hypothesis that at least two
different types of codes are alternatives for the
representation of superordinate semantic categories, that no
one of them is dependent on the other, and that they play
equivalent roles in the comprehension of sentences.
    The traditional conception that the representational
capability of mental images is limited by the concreteness of
the members of the category to which it refers is challenged
here and the rationale is the following :
    Strictly speaking, imagery (Note 1), as a symbol system,
can reach any level of abstraction in its relation with the
represented objects or events. That is, resemblance is a kind
of relation which can be established at infinite levels on
the concrete-abstract continuum. A considerable time ago now,
Arnheim (1969) supported the idea that images can function as
symbols and hence represent things at any level of abstraction. As Kolers and Brison stated : "Abstractness is not an
absolute property of symbols, but, rather, a property of the
way symbols are used..." (Kolers & Brison, 1984, p. 109).
Following this line of thought, we tend to think that the
complexity, rather than abstractness, of the information that
can be contained into a visuospatial format is not dependent
on the structure of the code, but on the way it is used.

79

M. Denis et al. (eds.), Cognitive and Neuropsychological Approaches to Mental Imagery, 79–87.

On the other hand, evidence supporting the propositional view comes exclusively from the linguistic domain and its unavoidable linguistic nature offers grounds to think that propositions can only represent the information coming from the linguistic medium.

One fundamental feature which determines differences between representational codes is the type of relation held between the representing world (symbols) and the represented world (objects, events, beliefs). In the case of imagery, the rules for assigning formats to contents are constructed individually, and thus there is no need for coincidence with other subjects' criteria of resemblance, whereas in the case of propositions these rules are conventions that we assume through language use.

Hence, a priori, both codes are capable of representing the information contained in semantic classes of the highest level of abstraction.

2. EXPERIMENTAL DATA

To test this possibility a few years ago we designed (Medina, 1983) a pair of experiments aimed at comparing the facilitatory effects of the representation activated by the superordinate category name and the prototype name of six natural categories in a semantic priming and matching task with picture and word pairs. The design developed was similar to the one described by E. Rosch (1975, Exp. 3). In our case two independent groups were used to enable comparison between the priming effects of the superordinate category name (CP ; Figure 1a) and the prototype name (PP ; Figure 1b), in relation to a control situation in which a neutral prime was used (NP in both figures ; Note 2). To be more explicit : Neutral prime conditions refer to those trials of the experimental session in which the experimenter pronounces the word "blank" to subjects before presenting the target stimulus, in opposition to prototype and category name primes in which the name of a superordinate semantic category (e.g. "fruit" ; G.I) or the name of a prototype of such category (e.g. "apple" ; G.II) is pronounced by the experimenter. Two seconds after the word has been presented, a pair of words or a pair of pictures is shown. Subjects are asked to indicate by pressing one of two keys whether both pictures or words refer to objects of a same category. For the analysis of the data only yes-responses were considered.

Given that there were no significant statistical difference between both control conditions and that variances were homogeneous across reaction times (RTs) in both groups, a two-way analysis of variance was executed to detect the difference between priming conditions both for word pairs and picture pairs responses. Statistically significant differences were not found in any comparison (CP vs PP for words and for pictures). As can be seen, both figures reflect similar results.

The fact that category name prime and prototype name prime lead to equivalent facilitation effects provides grounds to believe that the mental representation of the category activated has been the same.

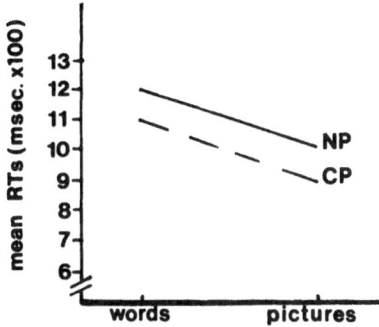
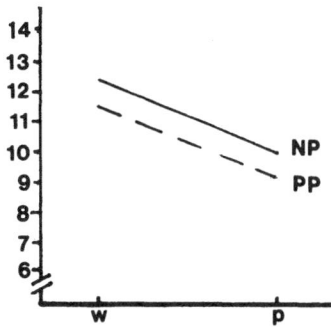

Figure 1a : Mean RTs for yes-
responses to pictures and
words under category prime
and neutral prime conditions.

Figure 1b : Mean RTs for yes-
responses to pictures and
words under prototype name
prime and neutral prime.

But the present data do not allow us to make any statements concerning the nature and the structure of the code,
neither in favor of a propositional nor in favor of an
imagistic format because results showed equivalent facilitation effects for picture and for word decisions. Only the
significantly slower RTs to pictures could be interpreted as
a reflection of the visuospatial nature of the representation. But, from our point of view, they do not provide enough
evidence.

That is why we then directed our attention to recent
studies in concept representation and categorization which
were inspired by previous research in the field of problem
solving. For example, works like those of Barsalou (1983) and
Roth and Shoben (1983) generated broad evidence in favor of
considering the representation of semantic categories as
flexible, variable and context-dependent. It would appear
that the context (verbal and non-verbal) works as a selector
of the properties or the members of the concept that become
relevant for a given moment. In other words, the context
constrains the number of referents that can be applied to a
particular use of a term. From this position, it follows that
concepts should not be considered as fixed mental units of
long-term memory.

In addition, the current state of the art in the study
of goal-driven artificial systems (Newell, 1982 ; Schank,
1982 ; Lenat, 1982) emphasises the active role of the subject
as a director of the conceptualization process, and offers
well founded theoretical reasons to conceive of memory as a
dynamic process capable of building specific schemata for
each context. In the light of the present general framework,
we started thinking about the possibility of testing the
hypothesis that the representational system could select an
adequate code for a concept depending on the nature of the
information provided by a linguistic context.

So we designed an experiment in which the effects of three different types of "abstract" - as described by Glass et al. (1985) - sentences were observed on a semantic decision task on picture and word stimuli.

These sentences are characterized by the use of a noun as the focus of the sentence so that instead of having only one basic level object as referent, it represents a class of possible objects or referents. These nouns are typically considered as belonging to the superordinate level in semantic taxonomies.

In our case, 30 triplets of sentences were constructed to function as verbal priming sentences. Each triplet was formed by a "neutral" priming sentence, that reflects no specific property of the category which is mentioned, a "perceptual" priming and a "functional" priming sentence, that make reference to a state of things in which a visuospatial or a functional property of the same category becomes relevant. Sentences were classified into each type (neutral, functional, perceptual) by ten independent judges. Only one sentence of each triplet was used for a given experimental session. In addition, every sentence was randomly assigned either to a word or a picture verification trial as an item of the corresponding priming condition, so that across the 25 individual sessions every sentence was presented before a picture and before a word an equivalent number of times. However, the same 30 filler items were used for every subject.

Examples :	PRIMING	TARGET (P or W)
Neutral	"SIEMPRE SE OLVIDA EL DINERO" ("He always forgets the money")	"coin"
Functional	"LA PIEDRA VALIA MUCHOS MILLONES" ("The stone was worth many millions")	"diamond"
Perceptual	"ESTA AVE ES MUY FEA" ("This bird is very ugly")	"owl"

In each trial the subjects (N=25) heard one sentence of one of these types through headphones. Immediately after the end of the sentence, they were presented with a slide that had either a written word or a simple drawing referring to a member of a superordinate semantic category (basic level object), and their task was to indicate by pressing one of two keys whether the word or picture fitted or matched the sentence. Note that this type of task requires that subjects not only process the information provided by the context, but that they draw some inferences that enable them to generate an adequate representation allowing them to fulfill the task.

A within subjects design was chosen, such that all subjects received each experimental treatment and the homogeneity of RTs necessary for analysing statistical differences between conditions was ensured. Obviously, effects of item content were not completely avoided. When each subject gets a different set of items, the error term in the analysis of variance reflects both item variability and subject variability (cf. Shoben, 1982 ; p. 306). Furthermore, the facilitation that one sentence can produce for a given stimulus modality should be compensated with the effect produced when the same sentence is presented under the alternative stimulus modality to another subject unless the representation activated by that item sentence is more similar in nature to one of the two stimulus modalities. And that is what we were looking for.

TWO-WAY ANOVA : SIMPLE EFFECTS
(* = significant interactions, $p < .01$)

Stimulus Mode x Neutral   Priming *   Priming x Words   *
Stimulus Mode x Functional Priming   Priming x Pictures
Stimulus Mode x Perceptual Priming *

MULTIPLE COMPARISONS (Wilcoxon test)
(* = significant differences, $p < .05$)

Pairs of
Conditions

NP/W-NP/P	*	
NP/W-FP/W	*	
NP/W-FP/P	*	
NP/W-PP/W		
NP/W-PP/P	*	
NP/P-FP/W	*	
NP/P-FP/P	*	
NP/P-PP/W	*	
NP/P-PP/P		
FP/W-FP/P		W : Words
FP/W-PP/W	*	P : Pictures
FP/W-PP/P	*	
FP/P-PP/W	*	NP : Neutral Prime
FP/P-PP/P		FP : Functional Prime
PP/W-PP/P	*	PP : Perceptual Prime

    As it is shown in the summary table of the ANOVA, significant differential effects of the three types of prime were only found under word responses conditions and the interaction between context and stimulus modality was not significant only when functional information was provided in advance.

    The fact that RTs to pictures did not vary significantly from one linguistic context to another made us think that the subjects, regardless of the information provided, tend to activate a visuospatial representation of the concept mentioned in the prime. This could be taken as proof that the most economical code, even for a superordinate semantic category, is an image of the most representative example(s). However, as is shown in Figure 2a, subjects do not behave in the same way under responses to word conditions. In this case, only functional information works as a facilitatory prime while the representation activated by perceptual and neutral contexts does not seem to help. This difference is highly significant and reflects two distinct conceptual representations : the one activated by the perceptual and neutral primes, which works in a different manner before pictures than before words, and the one activated by the functional context that behaves evenly under both stimulus modalities.

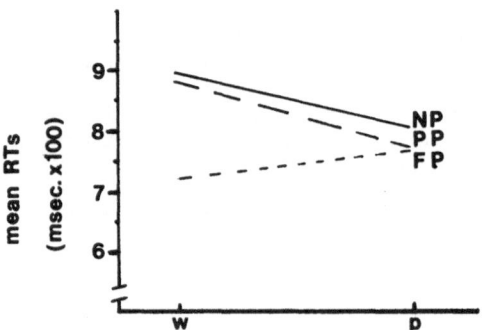

Figure 2a : Mean RTs for yes-responses to pictures and words under the three types of linguistic context (NP, FP, PP).

But, what else can be said about these two codes ?

In the first place, the statistical equivalence between RTs to pictures under neutral and perceptual priming conditions can be interpreted as a reflection of the fact that in both cases the same visuospatial representation is activated. If this is true, that representation cannot be a mental image of a concrete object but rather a summarized (abstract, in other terminologies) image that may preserve some characteristic features of the most typical members of the class. (Remember that the neutral prime provides no information that could be used to infer any particular referent of the sentence, and hence the subject has no means of generating an image of a concrete object.)

In the second place, if we look at the relationship between the nature of the information activated and the code used, functional information seems to be more stable in a concept representation. In other words, it seems to be part of the content in any context (use), as it is shown to be useful for making semantic decisions about words as well as about pictures. For example, Kelter et al. (1984) reported data confirming that functional attributes are used for making picture pair semantic decisions. However, if we were to identify the representation activated by the functional context with a propositional type of code we should be aware that the present data lend support to the analytical but not to the linguistic aspects of such code.

On the other hand, we should recognize the capacity of a visuospatial code to preserve information of different types, versus the relative rigidity of the alternative code to content information of a visuospatial or even highly unspecific (abstract ?) nature, as is shown by the results obtained under neutral priming plus word condition (Figure 2b).

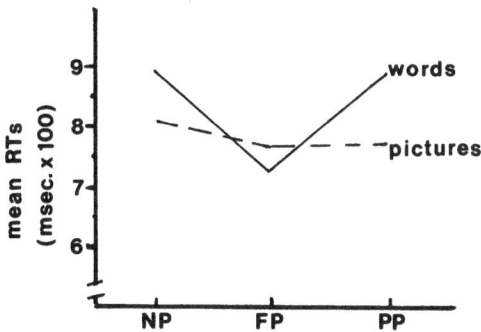

Figure 2b : Comparison of mean RTs to words versus mean RTs to pictures across the different priming conditions.

3. CONCLUSIONS

From our point of view, the present results reflect that concept representation is a driven activity, in the sense that the subjects do not have only one code to represent the meaning of an "abstract" sentence providing information about superordinate semantic classes but, rather, that their cognitive system decides the assignment of one of the alternative formats according to the information which becomes relevant in a certain context, and the goal established by themselves, which in our case is induced by the task.

At the same time, the data obtained led us to think that the two codes could play equivalent roles in the comprehension of sentences. Our data seem to contrast with the position held by Glass et al. (1985) when they state that a visuospatial representation plays an important role in the verification, but not in the comprehension, of sentences. At the same time, we think that it is not convenient to compare the present results with those obtained by Potter, Valian and Faulconer (1977) because there are a few important differences between both procedures. For example, they made no distinction among the sentences used, presentation of the probe was delayed 800 msec, and their subjects, in the experimental condition, received blocks (of 16 trials) of drawings and blocks of words alternated, while in our case no interval was set after presentation of the sentence, and picture and word trials were randomly combined to avoid that subjects anticipate the modality of the probe.

There may be many other theoretical implications of the present results, but, to our knowledge, the most important one is that concepts should not be conceived as fixed - or pre-packaged - entities of long term memory, but rather as cognitive states which are the result of assigning a certain format to the information selected from the input and activated in the data base, for a particular situation. The statement on the selection of an appropriate code to contain the information activated depends, in the first place, on experimental evidence about the existence of at least two functionally different ways of representing it. So far, the psychological study of knowledge representation has not considered this possibility when talking about coding structures that were capable of representing concepts of a high level of abstraction, mainly because mental images were thought of as a type of symbol limited by the existence of a concrete referent to which the image should resemble.

However, this belief, as well as the complementary one that qualifies mental propositions as the unique abstract code "par excellence", is lacking theoretical rigor, and, on the other hand, is refuted by the present results.

At the same time, it seems necessary to specify that our data should not be taken as evidence supporting a dual coding approach (Paivio, 1986) through the identification of the two codes found in our experiment with a verbal code and a non-verbal one, because we have shown that the visuospatial code is able to represent functional information and hence it cannot be considered modality-specific, as Paivio's images are.

Although in our latter experiment functional and perceptual information are isolated and separated from each other, there might be many other situations in which both types of information are required for the conceptual activity. Consequently, the appeal to structures like schemas or scripts, whose main function is to relate different information units, becomes the most adequate position because a) it helps to explain the relation between both codes into the same conceptual representation, and b) it provides a theoretical link with the structure that the information holds in the data base, which - we assume - is amodal (meaning that, within any information processing view, there is no need to posit any kind of format for the stored information when it is not active).

The latter proposal seems necessary if we are to focus our attention in the future on the compatibility of analytical and "analogical" formats within the same representation, and its interaction with long-term memory structures.

NOTES

1. It seems convenient to specify that, in contrast with the framework of most of the papers in this volume, the imagery we talk about has nothing to do with "awareness" or "conscious experience" of mental pictures.
2. Obviously, to qualify a prime as "neutral" is just a declaration of intentions, but in any case, it helps us to understand the role that this type of prime plays in the experimental setting. Similar argument could hold for the functional-perceptual division.

REFERENCES

1. Arnheim, R. (1969). Visual thinking. University of California Press : Berkeley.

2. Barsalou, L.W. (1983). Ad hoc categories. Memory and Cognition, 11, 211-227.
3. Glass, A.L., Millen, D.R., Beck, L.G. & Eddy, J.K. (1985). Representation of images in sentence verification. Journal of Memory and Language, 24, 442-465.
4. Kelter, S., Grötzbach, H., Freiheit, R., Höhle, B., Wutzig, S. & Disch, E. (1984). Object identification : The mental representation of physical and conceptual attributes. Memory and Cognition, 12, 123-133.
5. Kolers, P.A. & Brison, S.J. (1984). Commentary : On pictures, words, and their mental representation. Journal of Verbal Learning and Verbal Behavior, 23, 105-113.
6. Lenat, D.B. (1982). The nature of heuristics. Artificial Intelligence, 19, 189-249.
7. Medina, F.A. (1983). Prototipos y representaciones de categorias semanticas supraordenadas. Informes de Psicologia, 2, 173-194.
8. Newell, A. (1982). The knowledge level. Artificial Intelligence, 18, 87-127.
9. Paivio, A. (1986). Mental representations : A dual coding approach. New York : Oxford University Press.
10. Potter, M.C., Valian, V.V., & Faulconer, B.A. (1977). Representation of a sentence and its pragmatic implications : Verbal, imagistic, or abstract ? Journal of Verbal Learning and Verbal Behavior, 16, 1-12.
11. Rosch, E.H. (1975). Cognitive representations of semantic categories. Journal of Experimental Psychology, 104, 192-233.
12. Roth, E.M. & Shoben, E.J. (1983). The effect of context on the structure of categories. Cognitive Psychology, 15, 346-378.
13. Schank, R.C. (1982). Dynamic memory. Cambridge : Cambridge University Press.
14. Shoben, E.J. (1982). Semantic and lexical decision. In C.R. Puff (Ed.), Handbook of research methods in human memory and cognition. New York : Academic Press.

IMAGES, PREDICATES, AND RETRIEVAL CUES

GREGORY V. JONES

UNIVERSITY OF BRISTOL, ENGLAND

ABSTRACT
Words exhibit systematic differences in the ease with which they evoke mental images, as assessed by subjective judgements. However, they also exhibit very similar differences in the ease with which they evoke predicational information, as assessed either by subjective judgements or by objective performance. These differences are predictive of levels of performance in other domains. One such area is focused on here, that of cued recall. Imagery and predicational explanations of systematic variation among words in retrieval cue power are compared, and it is argued that the predicational explanation is to be preferred.

1. INTRODUCTION

It has been known for many centuries that verbal information is retained in memory remarkably well if mental images are formed of what the words themselves refer to (see Yates, 1966). But one plausible corollary of this rule has been systematically explored only in recent times. This corollary is that the ease with which an individual word evokes a mental image should be a strong determinant of how well that particular word can be remembered. The ease with which an individual word evokes a mental image may be assessed by means of subjective ratings (e.g., Paivio, Yuille, & Madigan, 1968), the word's mean rating often being termed its Imageability (e.g., Richardson, 1980). So is a word's Imageability in practice a strong determinant of memory performance? The evidence from a large body of research (see Paivio, 1971, 1986) shows that, at least at the empirical level, this is indeed the case.

Why is it necessary to insert the qualifying phrase "at least at the empirical level" at the end of the preceding paragraph? The reason has been expressed perhaps most clearly by Anderson and Bower (1973). They pointed out that apparent beneficial effects of mental imagery upon verbal memory may result not directly from the experience of imagery itself, but rather from accompanying improvements in the efficiency with which the words to be remembered access a relatively abstract general-purpose store of knowledge. If this hypothesis is entertained, it can be seen that it leads to the corollary that a powerful determinant of how well an individual word is remembered should be not only the ease with which it evokes a mental image, but also the ease with which it accesses the generalised knowledge base.

At the time at which Anderson and Bower were writing, a problem for their knowledge-based hypothesis was the absence of a satisfactory word variable relating to knowledge access. If their hypothesis were correct, it should be possible to characterise and measure a word variable of this type that should be of comparable effectiveness to Imageability in predicting memory performance. However, an influential subsequent

89

M. Denis et al. (eds.), Cognitive and Neuropsychological Approaches to Mental Imagery, 89–98.

review article (Kieras, 1978) noted that the search for such a "semantic" variable had by then experienced several failures, and therefore in Kieras's view was best abandoned. Following this gloomy prognostication, there has understandably been relatively little further exploration of knowledge-related word variables.

Despite the recent neglect of knowledge-related accounts, it seems to the present writer that there are at least two important areas of cognition where directly image-based accounts of apparent Imageability effects are open to serious question. First, within memory studies it is found that high Imageability words are more powerful retrieval cues than are low Imageability words. Second, within cognitive neuropsychology it is found that patients with deep dyslexia are more likely to correctly read high Imageability words than low Imageability words. These two areas of study are quite disparate, and it is therefore perhaps not surprising that reactions to direct image-based accounts have been rather different in the two areas. In memory studies such an account has had wide currency, and Glass, Holyoak, and Santa (1979, p. 160) are relatively unusual in stating that "Frankly, we do not have a ready explanation for why concreteness actually is more important for the cue word than for the response word". Within cognitive neuropsychology, in contrast, dissatisfaction with any directly image-based account of apparent Imageability effects in deep dyslexia has been expressed widely. In this paper there is space only to consider the retrieval cue area. First however I introduce, as a specific knowledge-based alternative to the notion of Imageability, a word variable that appears to possess relatively wide explanatory powers. This knowledge-based measure may be termed "Ease of Predication" (Jones, 1985) or, for greater conciseness, simply "Predicability".

2. KNOWLEDGE-BASED WORD VARIABLES
2.1. Predicability

The Predicability of a word is intended to be a measure of the ease with which a person can retrieve from memory different pieces of knowledge about whatever it is that the word refers to. The term "knowledge" is meant here to be roughly co-extensive with the cognitive psychology term "semantic memory" (see Chang, 1986). That is, it includes both information commonly allotted to lexical semantics (e.g., that gold is a metal) and that commonly allotted to encyclopaedic entries (e.g., that gold dissolves in aqua regia). Thus when it is stated that Predicability is a measure of the ease of retrieving predicates of that word from memory, it is apparent that "predicate" is used here in an epistemological sense, referring to descriptions or characterizations that comment on the topic which the word itself provides (see Garver, 1967). It should be noted also that the present usage of "predicability" to denote the ease of retrieving predicates from memory is unrelated to the Aristotelian usage of "predicables" to denote the different possible types of logical relation that may hold between predicates and their subjects (e.g., Cohen & Nagel, 1934; for more recent work in this area, see Keil, 1979, and Sommers, 1963).

To obtain empirical estimates of word Predicability, it has been operationalised as the ease with which what the word refers to "can be described by simple factual statements" (Jones, 1985, p. 5). Subjective ratings of this quantity have been collected for 125 words (Jones, 1985) using a procedure modelled as closely as possible upon the procedure used by Paivio et al. (1968) for collecting ratings of Imageability.

Figure 1 relates to the first half-dozen members of an alphabetic listing of the 125 words studied by Jones (1985), and illustrates both Predicability and Imageability values. Although the two variables were measured using similar seven-point scales (lowest = 1, highest = 7), it can be seen that Predicability values are generally lower than Imageability values (over all 125 words, the mean Predicability value, at 4.70, was 0.87 lower than the mean Imageability value, at 5.57). More importantly, however, it is apparent from Figure 1 that variations in the two measures over different words are very closely linked, and this is confirmed by an overall correlation of r(123) = 0.88.

The result described in the preceding paragraph means that the relation between Imageability and Predicability is so close that apparent effects of variation in Imageability are in general equally open to interpretation as effects of variation in Predicability. Contrary to the prediction of Kieras (1978), a semantic alternative to Imageability does exist. How then should one attempt to decide which type of variable is preferable? One immediate advantage of Predicability is that its measurement is not restricted to the realm of subjective judgement. Instead of ratings, assessment can employ objective response measures (see Denis, 1983, for an interesting similar approach). The next section describes such a measure, to be termed Predication Time.

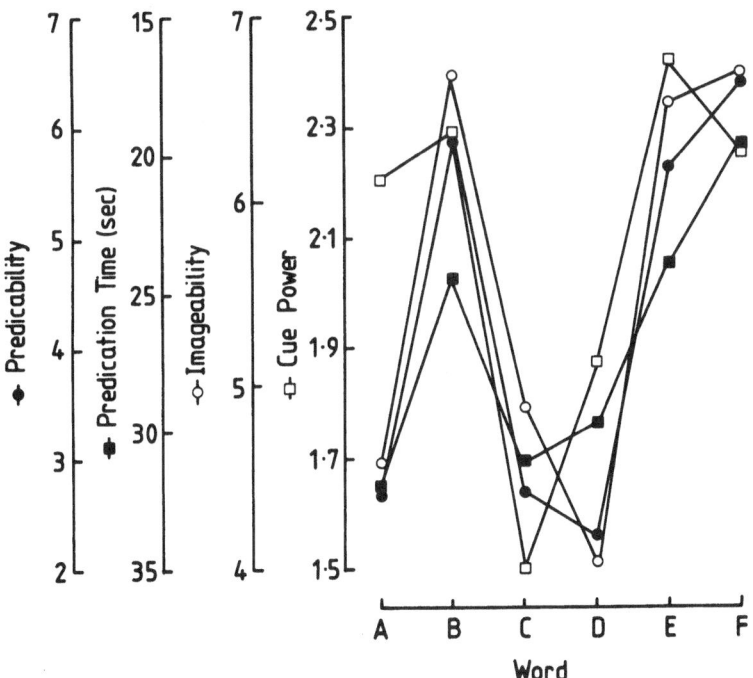

FIGURE 1. Values of Predicability, Predication Time, Imageability, and Cue Power for six words (A = Agility, B = Ambulance, C = Anger, D = Anxiety, E = Army, F = Baby).

2.2. Predication Time

Having previously obtained subjective estimates of the ease with which a word's referent can be described by simple factual statements (Jones, 1985), it was decided to assess this same factor objectively by asking people to actually generate such statements. Generating these statements is sometimes quite a slow process, and therefore counting the number of complete statements generated within a fixed time limit is likely to be a relatively insensitive procedure due to the prevalence of ties. Accordingly the complementary procedure was adopted, of measuring the time taken to generate a fixed number of statements for each word. Predication Time was operationalised as the time (in seconds) taken to generate precisely two statements for each word.

The 125 words assessed for Predicability by Jones (1985) were again used in this study, and are listed in Table 1 (as before, the words "candy" and "kerosene" shown in Table 1 were replaced in the stimulus materials by the British English equivalents of their American English senses, namely "sweets" and "paraffin"). There were three groups of subjects, who gave responses for 39, for 40, and for 46 of the words. Each group consisted of six male and six female undergraduates. The instructions the subjects received were based on those of Jones (1985), and read as follows.

"Words differ in the ease with which what they refer to can be described by simple factual statements. Some words can be put into statements quite easily and quickly, while for others this can be done only with difficulty. The purpose of this experiment is to establish, for a list of nouns, the ease or difficulty with which they can be put into simple factual statements.

As an example, consider the word 'dog'. This could be put into simple factual statements such as the following.

A dog is a type of animal

A dog often lives in a kennel.

The factual statements must refer to the word concerned and not just contain it.

What you have to do is attempt to generate, as quickly as possible, two factual statements, of the above form, for each word shown. In front of you is a pile of cards, each with a noun printed on it. When you are ready to begin the experiment say 'NOW' and turn over the first card and try to generate the two sentences required. When you have written down the two sentences for a word, tap the desk with your writing hand. Then, when you are ready to repeat the procedure for the next word, say 'NOW' and turn over the next card from the pile in front of you and so on until no cards remain.

The trials will be timed, so try to carry out the task as quickly as possible, yet making sure the sentences are as specified".

In only 9 instances out of 1,500 (i.e., 12 x 125) responses did a subject fail to generate the requisite two statements within 90 sec. In each of these instances, the trial was curtailed at that point and a value of 90 sec was entered as the response estimate.

The mean Predication Time is shown for each word in Table 1; I am grateful to Mark Simmons for his help in gathering these data. The mean scores yielded an overall mean and standard deviation of 28.0 sec and 6.9 sec, respectively. The reliability of the mean scores was assessed by randomly dividing each group of subjects into two halves and analysing them separately. The correlations between the two estimates of mean scores took the values $\underline{r}(37) = 0.73$, $\underline{r}(38) = 0.85$, and $\underline{r}(44) = 0.60$.

TABLE 1.   Predication Time (sec) for each of 125 nouns.

Word	Mean	SD	Word	Mean	SD
Agility	32.0	7.6	Ambulance	24.5	7.8
Anger	31.1	11.6	Anxiety	29.6	8.9
Army	23.9	6.4	Baby	19.7	5.9
Beggar	27.4	11.4	Bird	18.3	9.0
Blossom	23.8	6.1	Book	21.3	6.1
Bowl	23.1	6.0	Boy	21.2	5.6
Breast	31.2	15.2	Butter	21.8	4.7
Butterfly	23.0	6.8	Candy	26.3	9.0
Capacity	34.2	12.1	Chair	20.6	8.9
Child	23.0	10.7	Church	23.9	7.2
City	22.6	4.3	Clothing	26.1	7.2
Comedy	31.2	12.8	Comparison	44.9	15.4
Contents	43.7	17.9	Context	49.7	25.5
Corpse	21.4	10.4	Cottage	23.2	9.3
Custom	37.4	12.3	Death	25.4	8.5
Dirt	29.2	7.9	Doctor	24.0	11.2
Door	20.5	4.7	Dream	31.4	8.1
Dress	30.1	12.6	Earth	24.1	8.8
Engine	25.8	8.4	Errand	37.0	14.5
Excuse	44.6	26.3	Fire	19.9	6.7
Flower	25.3	12.3	Friend	34.0	18.5
Frog	19.3	4.9	Fur	21.4	8.6
Girl	21.1	4.5	Glacier	25.1	7.6
Green	19.0	5.5	Grief	29.8	9.9
Hammer	23.1	6.4	Hatred	31.3	14.4
Health	35.7	12.3	Hide	33.4	14.5
History	29.2	9.2	Home	23.9	6.7
Horse	17.5	2.9	Hospital	22.8	5.0
Hostage	34.4	17.3	Humor	32.4	14.9
Industry	38.7	18.6	Ink	21.9	6.8
Jelly	20.7	5.1	Joy	25.4	6.2
Justice	39.9	19.4	Kerosene	21.0	5.7
Kindness	35.2	18.7	King	20.4	5.9
Kiss	32.4	13.5	Lake	26.1	8.9
Love	23.4	10.0	Malice	34.8	11.3
Memory	31.7	3.2	Menace	36.0	20.1
Moment	37.8	15.7	Money	25.1	10.4
Month	25.3	5.8	Mother	35.1	20.6
Mountain	27.4	6.5	Nectar	24.9	8.6
Ocean	26.2	11.6	Opinion	27.5	3.2
Orchestra	26.6	8.8	Paper	18.2	4.2
Party	29.1	7.9	Patent	48.9	21.2
Pencil	22.7	11.1	Person	39.0	25.3
Plant	23.1	11.6	Poetry	30.9	10.2
Power	30.5	9.5	Prairie	33.1	20.4
Pride	36.6	20.2	Priest	27.0	12.9

Word	Mean	SD	Word	Mean	SD
Rattle	26.8	8.6	Revolt	33.9	13.2
River	20.7	6.5	Salad	20.4	6.3
Salute	36.1	11.1	Seat	26.3	12.4
Shadow	28.7	9.4	Ship	19.3	6.1
Sickness	31.5	7.3	Square	22.7	4.4
Star	26.5	8.7	Street	27.3	10.6
Table	21.2	6.5	Theory	40.9	17.0
Thief	24.4	7.5	Time	29.5	17.7
Tobacco	20.9	8.0	Tree	24.9	9.0
Trouble	38.2	16.4	Trumpet	21.8	5.3
Truth	31.3	13.5	Vanity	28.6	7.2
Vehicle	24.6	7.8	Village	25.4	8.0
Violation	39.2	16.3	Virtue	38.8	22.7
Vision	30.3	7.1	Warmth	26.9	11.4
Water	18.9	5.6	Window	25.8	12.2
Wine	20.3	5.9	Woman	28.1	9.2
World	26.0	8.5			

These values suggest that Predication Time is a less reliable measure than Predicability, for which the corresponding correlation was $r(123) = 0.95$ (Jones, 1985). The greater degree of noise in the data for the performance task is probably to be expected, if only because one central aspect of the task - the unique identity of each subject's generated statements - was necessarily an additional source of variation between subjects.

Within the constraints imposed by their reliability, the estimated values of Predication Time agreed closely both with Predicability values (Jones, 1985), $r(123) = -0.72$, and with Imageability values (Paivio et al., 1968), $r(123) = -0.76$ (correlations are negative because a good predicational performance is indicated by a small Predication Time). Values of all three variables for the first half-dozen words of Table 1 are shown in Figure 1 (with the Predication Time axis plotted in descending rather than ascending order).

3. COMPARISON OF WORD VARIABLES

In comparing the imagery variable with the two predication variables, what is the appropriate method of deciding which type of variable is superior? The answer to this question depends upon what is meant by "superior". Two senses that can be distinguished may be termed "empirical superiority" and "explanatory superiority", and it is argued that it is the latter that is the more important. One variable might predict performance on a cognitive task better than another variable does, and thus appear empirically superior. However, careful analysis might reveal that it is in fact the second variable that has greater explanatory potential.

As a hypothetical example, consider two possible predictors of different people's weight gains (or losses) as a result of following a particular diet. The first predictor might consist of an observer's intuitive assessment of each person's likely weight gain. The second variable might consist of the total number of calories consumed by each person. There is widespread agreement that intake of calories is of considerable explanatory importance in accounts of weight gain. It is conceivable, nevertheless, that intuitive assessment might prove superior empirically. This is plausible because such judgements could reflect, albeit imperfectly, differences among individuals not only in calorie intake but also in other potentially relevant factors such as bodyweight and activity level. An analogous situation may in principle occur with word variables. The empirical importance of one variable can appear to be overshadowed by that of another, less fundamental variable because the latter's disadvantage of being only an imperfect measure of the former may be outweighed by its advantage of being also a function of one or more other factors of relevance.

The preceding argument means that in comparing the explanatory importance of the imagery variable with that of the two predication variables, it is insufficient merely to attempt to determine which of them predicts empirical performance the more accurately. This stricture applies not only to correlational but also to orthogonal comparisons. As a specific example one obvious design component for an orthogonal comparison of Imageability and of Predicability would consist of those words whose Imageability values most exceed their Predicability values. But comparison of the norms of Paivio et al. (1968) and of Jones (1985) indicates that the handful of words with the most extreme differences of this kind (viz., anger, joy, kiss, love, and warmth) all relate to a further factor, emotion; each of the five is in fact in the most extreme 10% of words assessed for Emotionality by Brown and Ure (1969). Hence any apparent empirical consequences of belonging to a High Imageability, Low Predicability group might in practice result from membership of a High Emotionality group. It might be objected that the problem can be overcome by controlling levels of Emotionality also. However, even in principle it is not possible to control for other potential confounds whose identities have yet to be recognized. As Cutler (1981, p. 69) remarked when reviewing the number of word variables to which a psycholinguist needs to be sensitive, "If it goes on this way in the eighties, psycholinguists will literally be lost for words."

What, then, is the solution to the problem of empirical indeterminancy among the variables? The answer, it is suggested, may lay in the realm of explanatory adequacy. Note that the logic of the present argument does not dismiss the role of empirical prediction in choosing among word variables, but merely points to its need for supplementation. Prediction (or foresight) is ultimately a step towards explanation (or understanding); see Toulmin (1961). In the next section, imagery and predication explanations are compared in the area of retrieval cue power.

4. RETRIEVAL CUE POWER

It has been known for a considerable time that highly imageable nouns are in general more effective retrieval cues than lowly imageable ones (e.g., Paivio, 1965; Wicker & Thorelli, 1978). Because of the close relation between imagery and predication word variables, it follows that predication also will be associated with cue power. This may be demonstrated using data reported by Rubin (1981) from a paired-associate experiment described by Rubin (1980). In this experiment, each of 76 subjects received one half of the 125 words shown in Table 1 (plus one dummy) as stimulus items and the other half as response items; each of these stimulus-response pairs was tested on three occasions. The subjects were yoked to form 38 super-subjects by interchanging stimuli and responses for successive subjects. The word variable termed "Cue Power" in Figure 1 shows (for each of alphabetically the first six words) the number of times (out of three) that each word was successful when acting as a stimulus, averaged over super-subjects. It can be seen that there is good agreement between Cue Power and each of the other three variables shown in Figure 1. Over all 125 words, the correlation between Cue Power on the one hand and Imageability, Predicability, and Predication Time on the other are $r(123) = 0.67$ (Rubin, 1980), 0.61, and -0.56, respectively.

Parenthetically, one may note that in addition to assessing Cue Power, which he termed a Paired-Associate Stimulus variable, Rubin (1980, 1981) assessed also a complementary Paired-Associate Response variable – the average number of times that each word was successful when in the response role. As expected, correlations with the other word variables were somewhat lower at $r(123) = 0.42$ (Rubin, 1980), 0.31, and -0.32 for Imageability, Predicability, and Predication Time, respectively. In his impressive study, Rubin (1980) in fact investigated the values of 51 variables for each of the 125 words shown in Table 1, values for two-thirds of these variables being newly measured (Rubin, 1981). Rubin (1980) carried out a principal-factor, orthogonal, varimax factor analysis of the intercorrelations among these 51 variables, and found that the second most important factor (after one relating to spelling and sound) was one relating to imagery and meaning. When the factor analysis was repeated with the addition of the Predicability and Predication Time data, it was found that they loaded primarily on this same factor; the correlations between this factor and Imageability, Predicability, and Predication Time were $r(123) = 0.90$, 0.90, and 0.73, respectively (for this analysis, all Predication Times were multiplied by -1 in accordance with the general practice for latency measures of Rubin, 1980, so that better performance is indicated by higher – less negative – numbers). I am grateful to Professor Rubin for kindly making available his data and factor-analysis program in machine-readable form.

Given that both imagery and predication variables strongly influence a cue's power, which type of variable may better be employed in the explanation of cued recall? A long-standing imagery account is that offered by the conceptual-peg hypothesis (e.g., Paivio, 1971 chap. 8). If a person is presented with two words, one of which is to act as a retrieval cue for the other, then it is proposed that the former word functions as a peg to which the latter word must be hooked during encoding and from which it can then be retrieved at recall. To this point, the proposal is essentially a redescription of the basic phenomenon of mental association. To explain why high Imageability makes a cue more powerful, the further proposal is made that this results in the conceptual peg becoming more "solid" (Paivio, 1971, p. 248).

It is argued here that three problems with the conceptual-peg explanation can be discerned. The first is that it is incompletely specified. When it is stated that one peg is more solid than another, the possible interpretation of this metaphor can range widely. A solid peg might for example be one that is well attached to some other structure, or it might be one that is strong, or it might be one that is durable. Each version of the metaphor could suggest a different psychological interpretation. Unless the notion of a "solid peg" is explicated further, it functions merely as a redescriptive synonym for a "good cue".

The second problem with the conceptual-peg hypothesis follows from the first one. Because it is not clear what it means to say that a peg is solid, it is difficult to claim that imagery is expected to make a peg more solid. Why should it not make it less solid? Hence to say that high Imageability makes a peg more solid seems only to redescribe in metaphoric terms the empirical finding that high Imageability makes a cue better, and not to explain it.

The third problem with the conceptual-peg hypothesis is of a different type. Although it has been argued here that the hypothesis is incompletely specified, it is clear that it is based on a node model rather than a link model of memory. In making the peg more solid, Imageability is being hypothesised to influence the representation in memory of the cue itself – Imageability's effect is upon a node, rather than upon a link attached to that node. However, recent work directly comparing node and link models (Jones, 1984) has shown that associative recall is much more accurately represented by link models than by node models. Thus it seems likely that variations in cue power should be explained in terms of variation in the encoding of links, rather than variation in the encoding of nodes. Such an explanation is that provided by the predication approach.

The predicational explanation of variation in cue power is simple. In general, one item can act as a successful retrieval cue for another if a link has been established to this other item's representation in memory. An important type of link from the cue word is a knowledge-based one, forged when one of its predicates turns out to match the other item in some respect. The more readily that predicates of the cue word can be retrieved, the more likely such a link is to be created. Thus highly predicable words should in general act as relatively powerful retrieval cues, as is in fact observed.

5. CONCLUSION

The consequences of knowledge-based differences among words were compared to those of imagery-based differences. The former may be assessed not only by subjective judgement but also by objective performance. In addition, it was argued that the predicational approach provides an improved explanation of variation in retrieval cue power among different words.

REFERENCES

1. Anderson, J. R., & Bower, G. H. (1973). Human associative memory. Washington, DC: Winston.
2. Brown, W. P., & Ure, D. M. J. (1969). Five rated characteristics of 650 word association stimuli. British Journal of Psychology, 60, 233-249.
3. Chang, T. M. (1986). Semantic memory: Facts and models. Psychological Bulletin, 99, 199-220.
4. Cohen, M. R., & Nagel, E. (1934). An introduction to logic and scientific method. London: Routledge & Kegan Paul.
5. Cutler, A. (1981). Making up materials is a confounded nuisance, or: Will we be able to run any psycholinguistic experiments at all in 1990? Cognition, 10, 65-70.
6. Denis, M. (1983). Valeur d'imagerie et composition sémantique: Analyse de deux échantillons de substantifs [Imagery value and

semantic composition: Analysis of two sets of nouns]. Cahiers de Psychologie Cognitive, 3, 175-202.

7. Garver, N. (1967). Subject and predicate. In P. Edwards (Ed.), The encyclopedia of philosophy (Vol. 8, pp. 33-36). New York: Macmillan.

8. Glass, A. L., Holyoak, K. J., & Santa, J. L. (1979). Cognition. Reading, MA: Addison-Wesley.

9. Jones, G. V. (1984). Fragment and schema models for recall. Memory & Cognition, 12, 250-263.

10. Jones, G. V. (1985). Deep dyslexia, imageability, and ease of predication. Brain and Language, 24, 1-19.

11. Keil, F. C. (1979). Semantic and conceptual development: An ontological perspective. Cambridge, MA: Harvard University Press.

12. Kieras, D. (1978). Beyond pictures and words: Alternative information-processing models for imagery effects in verbal memory. Psychological Bulletin, 85, 532-554.

13. Paivio, A. (1965). Abstractness, imagery, and meaningfulness in paired-associate learning. Journal of Verbal Learning and Verbal Behavior, 4, 32-38.

14. Paivio, A. (1971). Imagery and verbal processes. New York: Holt, Rinehart, & Winston.

15. Paivio, A. (1986). Mental representations: A dual coding approach. New York: Oxford University Press.

16. Paivio, A., Yuille, J. C., & Madigan, S. A. (1968). Concreteness, imagery, and meaningfulness values for 925 nouns. Journal of Experimental Psychology Monograph, 76 (1, Pt. 2).

17. Richardson, J. T. E. (1980). Mental imagery and human memory. London: Macmillan.

18. Rubin, D. C. (1980). 51 properties of 125 words: A unit analysis of verbal behavior. Journal of Verbal Learning and Behavior, 19, 736-755.

19. Rubin, D. C. (1981). Norms for 34 properties of 125 words. Journal Supplement Abstract Service Catalog of Selected Documents in Psychology, 11, 19. (Ms. No. 2213).

20. Sommers, F. (1963) Types and ontology. Philosophical Review, 72, 327-363.

21. Toulmin, S. (1961). Foresight and understanding: An enquiry into the aims of science. London: Hutchinson.

22. Wicker, F. W., & Thorelli, I. M. (1978). Stimulus concreteness, response characteristics, and the recognition-recall method in paired-associate learning. Journal of Experimental Psychology: Human Learning and Memory, 4, 136-145.

23. Yates, F. A. (1966). The art of memory. London: Routledge & Kegan Paul.

THE IMPORTANCE OF AGE OF WORD ACQUISITION FOR IMAGEABILITY IN WORD PROCESSING

ANITA VAN LOON-VERVOORN

and MIEP VAN DER HAM-VAN KOPPEN

PSYCHOLOGICAL LABORATORY, UNIVERSITY OF UTRECHT, THE NETHERLANDS

ABSTRACT

In normal and aphasic subjects the retrieval of words in word association appeared to be dependent on imageability (high-imagery words having strong primary responses and few blanks). In normal subjects the relationship between stimulus and response was dependent on the age of acquisition of the stimulus word. In early acquired words (basic lexicon) this relationship referred to commonly experienced episodes (for example, bed-sleep), whereas in later learned words (higher-order lexicon) this relationship was based on verbal definitions (for example, dagger-knife). Aphasic patients were better in retrieving episodic rather than defined relationships, probably because linguistically based knowledge may be more vulnerable to brain damage than the earlier acquired knowledge based on episodic memory.

1. INTRODUCTION

This study is part of a series of investigations into the development and breakdown of lexical representations. The leading theme in these studies is the idea that there are two kinds of lexical knowledge (Marcel & Patterson, 1978; Van Bekkum & De Vries, 1980; Van Loon-Vervoorn, 1985a). The first type of knowledge is based on the sensorimotor interactions with real world entities, the so-called script representations of events (Nelson, 1983), having a strong episodic component (Petrey, 1977). The other type of lexical knowledge is based on verbal definitions in terms of other word meanings and is therefore more linguistically determined. It is assumed that the first word meanings a child acquires are mainly based on the child's sensorimotor interactions with his/her environment (Piaget, 1948; Werner & Kaplan, 1963). These words make up what we have called the basic lexicon, from which a higher-order lexicon is derived during later development (Van Bekkum & De Vries, 1980). The word meanings of this higher-order lexicon are learned by definition, mostly in terms of basic words.

According to this view, imageability as well as age of acquisition are important variables in word processing. The effects of word imagery are well documented in a wide variety of word processing tasks, from which it appears that high-imagery words are processed more easily than low-imagery words. (See Paivio (1971) and Richardson (1980) for reviews of the research in this area). However, the results of studies on age of acquisition are rather conflicting, some studies revealing an age effect, whereas others do not. For example, in picture naming tasks (Carroll & White, 1973) and in category instance naming (Loftus & Suppes, 1972), it has been reported that

M. Denis et al. (eds.), Cognitive and Neuropsychological Approaches to Mental Imagery, 99–107.
© *1988 by Martinus Nijhoff Publishers.*

early acquired words have shorter latencies than late acquired words, whereas in lexical decision, free recall, and word recognition tasks, no effects of age of acquisition were found (Gilhooly & Gilhooly, 1979; Gilhooly & Logie, 1982).

These conflicting results are probably due to an inadequate control of other variables in word processing, such as imageability and frequency, that covary with age of acquisition (Gilhooly & Logie, 1980; Van Loon-Vervoorn, 1985a). To distinguish between the effects of interrelated variables, Gilhooly and his coworkers used a stepwise multiple-regression analysis. However, a crucial problem exists for this analysis when the predictors are interrelated both with each other and with the criterion variable. In this case, the introduction of one predictor in the stepwise analysis includes also the shared variance with the other predictors. The order of introduction of the predictors determines the outcome of the analysis. (See Morris (1981) for some interesting examples and a further discussion of this problem). So, the stepwise multiple-regression analysis does not provide a satisfactory method for determining the relative contributions of interrelated variables to performance. On the other hand, Carroll and White (1973), Morris (1981), and Coltheart and Winograd (1986), resolved the problem of interrelated predictors by using experimental manipulation of the target predictor, in this case age of acquisition, and control of other predictors such as, for example, imageability and frequency. The results of these experiments were conflicting in that Carroll and White found that in picture naming early acquired words elicited shorter latencies than late acquired words, but Morris reported that late acquired words were better recalled than early acquired words, whereas Coltheart and Winograd found no effect of age of acquisition. These latter data are consistent with the results of Gilhooly and Gilhooly (1979) on word recall.

Rather than leaving the effect of age of acquisition an unsettled issue, I want to propose an alternative design to separate this predictor from other predictors in word processing tasks. In this design (first proposed by Stumpel, Van Bekkum, and Van Loon-Vervoorn, 1984), age of acquisition, frequency, and imageability of words, were independently varied in a 2x2x2 design. It was shown that in aphasic patients as well as in normal subjects the age of acquisition of words is a significant predictor in lexical decision and in reading words aloud, in that early acquired words had shorter latencies than late acquired words, whereas imageability only affected reading words aloud. No main effect of word frequency was found. (See also the discussion concerning the facilitating effects of imageability on word production in Marcel and Patterson, 1978).

The experiment reported here may explain the above mentioned contradictory findings concerning the role of age of acquisition in word processing. This experiment involves a word association task, which provides a possibility of discovering how words are related in the mental lexicon. If age of acquisition is a factor in word processing, then we should expect associations to early acquired words to be qualitatively different from associations to late acquired words. Since the meanings of early learned words have a strong sensorimotor component, and the meanings of late acquired words are mainly based on linguistic definition, the associations to early acquired words should be more episodically determined, whereas the associations to late acquired words should be more linguistically based.

2. PROCEDURE
2.1 Design
When age of acquisition (early-late), frequency (frequent-infrequent),

and imageability (concrete-abstract), are orthogonally varied in a 2x2x2 design, the following eight word groups are expected.

```
early acquired, frequent, concrete     (EFC), e.g., tree
early acquired, frequent, abstract     (EFA), e.g., year
early acquired, infrequent, concrete   (EIC), e.g., duck
early acquired, infrequent, abstract   (EIA), ---------
late acquired, frequent, concrete      (LFC), ---------
late acquired, frequent, abstract      (LFA), e.g., power
late acquired, infrequent, concrete    (LIC), e.g., dagger
late acquired, infrequent, abstract    (LIA), e.g., ban
```

The criteria for age of acquisition were based on "De Nieuwe Streeflijst" of Kohnstamm, Schaerlaekens, De Vries, Akkerhuis and Froonincksx (1981). This list contains a set of Dutch words rated by teachers on passive knowledge that six-year old children should have of these words. Early acquired words were sampled from a subset with a teachers' rating of 90% or more (this percentage corresponds to scale value 2.50 on Carroll and White's 1973 rating scale, i.e., words learned before the fifth year). Late acquired words were taken from the subset with a teachers' rating of 40% or less (this percentage corresponds to scale value 4.50 on Carroll and White's rating scale, i.e., words learned after the seventh year). The correlation between the teachers' rating and the age of acquisition of words, rated on an eight-point scale (as used by Carroll and White, 1973), was -.92 for nouns (Van Loon-Vervoorn, 1985b), -.87 for verbs, and -.88 for adjectives (Van Loon-Vervoorn, 1985c). Thus, the teachers' rating can be used as an indication of the age of acquisition of words. In the study by Van Loon-Vervoorn (1985c) it was also shown that "De Nieuwe Streeflijst" is a fairly complete inventory of early acquired words. None of 500 words (nouns, verbs, and adjectives, randomly sampled from a Dutch dictionary) not included in this list, has a mean scale value below 2.50 (i.e., is learned before the fifth year). Words not included in "De Nieuwe Streeflijst" can thus generally be considered as late acquired.

Imageability data were taken from Dutch norms recently established for over 6000 words: 4600 nouns, 1000 verbs, and 500 adjectives (Van Loon-Vervoorn, 1985a). The imageability of these words was rated by students on a seven-point scale, similar to the one used by Paivio, Yuille and Madigan (1968). As concrete words, only words were selected with a scale value of at least 6.00, whereas abstract words have scale values of less than 5.00.

The frequency values of the words were taken from the most recent Dutch frequency count (Uit den Boogaart, 1975). Frequent words were sampled from the subset "over 70 words per 720.000"; infrequent words were taken from the subset "less than 10 per 720.000".

Using these rather stringent criteria, only six out of the eight expected word groups in the 2x2x2 design could be filled. However, more lax criteria would still leave these two cells empty. We may conclude that neither early acquired words, that are both infrequent and abstract, nor late acquired words, that are both frequent and concrete, exist in the lexicon. Put in another way: an early acquired word can only be abstract, when it is also frequently used; whereas a late acquired word can only be concrete, when it is infrequently used. This fact is of some interest in itself.

As a consequence, the effect of the three variables cannot be simultaneously tested in a 2x2x2 design. Therefore, the effect of each variable was separately tested in a two-way analysis of variance with one single factor (the target variable) and a combination of the two other factors as main factors. For age of acquisition, frequency and imageability were combined in such a way that for both the early and the late conditions the combination of frequency and imageability was the same. In this way four groups were compared, namely early and late acquired words, that are either frequent and abstract (EFA and LFA), or infrequent and concrete (EIC and LIC). EFC was left out because its counterpart LFC was missing, and LIA was eliminated because of the absence of EIA. In the same way, frequency was tested against the combined effect of age of acquisition and imageability (EFC and LFA against EIC and LIA), and imageability against the combined effect of age of acquisition and frequency (EFC and LIC against EFA and LIA).

2.2 Materials

In each of the six remaining word groups (EFC, EFA, EIC, LFA, LIC and LIA) the following 10 monosyllabic nouns were selected.

EFC (early acquired, frequent, concrete): bed (bed), blad (leaf), brief (letter), deur (door), hand (hand), kind (child), mond (mouth), raam (window), stad (city), zee (sea).

EFA (early acquired, frequent, abstract): dag (day), ding (thing), jaar (year), keer (time), plaats (place), plan (plan), rust (rest), tijd (time), vraag (question), werk (work).

EIC (early acquired, infrequent, concrete): bijl (axe), dans (dans), fluit (flute), fruit (fruit), gans (goose), hak (heel), heks (witch), kleed (carpet), lach (laugh), noot (nut).

LFA (late acquired, frequent, abstract): dienst (service), eeuw (century), feit (fact), lid (member), macht (power), raad (advice), staat (state), strijd (combat), taak (task), volk (people).

LIC (late acquired, infrequent, concrete): ark (ark), boei (buoy), dolk (dagger), eelt (callus), kaft (cover), kluis (safe), kuip (tub), mok (mug), nar (jester), ruif (rack).

LIA (late acquired, infrequent, abstract): ban (ban), brons (bronze), drang (pressure), durf (daring), faam (fame), hars (resin), list (trick), smart (sorrow), smoes (pretext), toets (test).

2.3 Subjects

Sixty psychology students (30 male and 30 female) and twenty aphasic patients (13 male and 7 female) participated in the experiment. The age of the students ranged from 18 to 25 years, the age of the patients from 30 to 83 years. The aphasic patients differed in extent of aphasia on a Dutch aphasia test (SAN-test: Deelman, Liebrand, Koning-Haanstra, & Van den Burg, 1981). The scores on this test, a combination of a production and a reception score, ranged from the 42nd to the 98th percentile.

2.4 Method

Instructions to the subjects were similar to those used by Sefer and Henrickson (1966): "I'm going to say a word and I want you to say the first word you think of. For instance, when I say 'apple' you may say 'pear' or 'red'. You say the first word you think of whatever it is. Let's take another example: when I say 'vacation', which is the first word which comes into your mind?". After the presentation of three words for training purposes (auto/car, week/week, and zaak/case), the list of words was presented. Order of presentation was randomized and counterbalanced. The experimenter noted the responses.

The normal subjects were encouraged to respond as quickly as possible and not to think up a response deliberately. If no response was immediately available a blank was registered. With aphasics there was no time pressure.

2.5 Scoring
For each stimulus word a response hierarchy was constructed for normal as well as for aphasic subjects. In these hierarchies the strength of the primary response (the response most frequently given), and the number of blanks (no response available), are given. The number of idiosyncratic responses (with a frequency of 1 in the hierarchies), and the overlap of the aphasics' hierarchies with those of normals, were also determined.

3. RESULTS
In free word association the strength of the primary response, the number of blanks, and the number of idiosyncratic responses, are commonly used as dependent variables. The strength of the primary response can be seen as an indication of the availability of a commonal response (as is, of course, the secondary, third, etc. response). When no commonal response comes into the subject's mind, he/she can think up an idiosyncratic response. When this does not occur a blank results.
These three variables are interrelated, so the results for each should be interpreted in relation to the other two.
The analysis of the results will start with the number of blanks, since this number is an indirect indication of the availability of a commonal response and of the ability to think up a more personal response.

3.1 The number of blanks
Table 1 shows the number of blanks per word group for normal subjects (N=60) and aphasic patients (N=20). The three analyses of variance reveal a significant effect of imageability in normal subjects (MS=136.90, $F(1,36)=9.18$, p<.01), as well as in aphasic patients (MS=96.10, $F(1,36)=16.44$, p<.01). These results indicate that concrete words have the smallest number of blanks. Further, an effect of age of acquisition was found in aphasic patients only (MS=48.40, $F(1,36)=7.14$, p<.05), the group showing the lowest number of blanks for early acquired words. No main

TABLE 1. Mean number of blanks, mean frequency of the primary response, and mean number of idiosyncratic responses per word group for normal and aphasic subjects, as well as the overlap between aphasics and normals.

	EFC	EFA	EIC	LFA	LIC	LIA
blanks	1.1	4.7	2.7	6.9	4.9	7.5
primary response	4.2	2.7	3.2	2.5	3.1	2.4
overlap	8.4	4.6	5.3	3.5	6.0	3.9
idio	11.6	12.3	12.2	10.0	9.7	9.4
blanks	0.5	3.3	1.3	4.7	0.6	5.2
primary responses	14.3	18.3	16.8	12.2	25.2	17.3
overlap	8.9	8.1	8.0	6.3	9.9	8.9
idio	14.9	17.6	19.3	21.5	13.3	15.5

effect for word frequency and no interaction effects were found.
It can thus be concluded that in word association the production of a response is facilitated by imagery processes, and that this process is

intact in aphasic patients.

To trace the cause of the age of acquisition effect on word retrieval, three further analyses were carried out on the strength of the primary response, the overlap between aphasic and normal response hierarchies, and the number of idiosyncratic associations. The first two measures may be interpreted as indicators of the availability of a more commonal response to the stimulus word, whereas the third measure may be seen as an indicator of the ability to think up a more personal reaction to the stimulus word, when no commonal response is available.

3.2 The strength of the primary response and the overlap score

The strength of the primary response is the frequency of the most commonal response to the stimulus word. The overlap score is the number of responses shared by the aphasic and the normal group. To compare an arbitrarily chosen group of normal subjects with the control group of this experiment, an overlap score was also established for 20 normal subjects. These normal subjects participated in an experiment on word association with reaction time registration (Van Loon-Vervoorn, Bresser & Nawijn, 1984). In aphasic patients, the overlap score is only affected by word imageability (MS=87.03, $F(1,36)=19.87$, $p<.01$) and not by age of acquisition and frequency. In normal subjects no significant main effects were found. The strength of the primary response in aphasics is also influenced by word imageability (MS=12.10, $F(1,36)=4.31$, $p<.05$). In normals, only a trend for imageability is present (MS=280.90, $F(1,36)=3.54$, $p<.10$). No other main effects were found. In aphasics and to a lesser extent in normals, the availability of a commonal response is determined by imageability.

As can be seen in Table 1, word group LIC has a high mean frequency of the primary response, whereas the LFA group has a fairly low frequency of that response. These differences with the other group means result in a significant interaction between age of acquisition and the combination of frequency and imageability in the analysis of age of acquisition (MS=525.63, $F(1,36)=6.64$, $p<.05$) in normal subjects. This interaction was not significant in aphasic patients. As can be seen in Table 1, the primary response no longer stands out in the LIC group when compared with either of the concrete word groups (EFC or EIC). This is an unexpected result, since Lesser (1973) has suggested that aphasics can respond relatively easily to stimulus words with a clear primary response. In normal subjects the late acquired, infrequent, concrete words have clear primary responses of this type. The fact that aphasic patients cannot take advantage of this, suggests that the lexical knowledge on which these stimulus-response bonds are based is lost in aphasia. In the discussion I will elaborate on this.

3.3 Idiosyncratic responses

Idiosyncratic responses have a frequency of one in the association hierarchies. In aphasics but not in normals, the number of idiosyncratic associations depends on age of acquisition (MS=57.60, $F(1,36)=8.04$, $p<.01$). In the case of an early acquired stimulus, an aphasic patient can think up his/her own private response, when no commonal reaction is available. No effect of frequency and imageability was found in either group. Complementing the data on the strength of the primary response, it appeared that only in normals is the interaction between age of acquisition and the combined effect of frequency and imageability in the analysis of age of acquisition, significant (MS=245.02, $F(1,36)=4.97$, $p<.05$). This interaction is mainly based on the difference between the two late acquired groups (LFA and LIC), as is the interaction effect found for the strength of the primary response (Table 1). When a word is late acquired, in normal subjects, high frequency words, which are automatically abstract, have low bonds with their primary responses, as well as many idiosyncratic associations. However, when a word is late acquired and both infrequent and concrete, the reverse is true.

4. DISCUSSION
   The most important result of this study is the overall facilitating effect of word imageability on word association in normal subjects as well as in aphasic patients, resulting in a decrease of the number of blanks and in an increase of the strength of the primary response in concrete words. In aphasic patients, an effect of age of acquisition was also found, manifesting itself in a decrease of the number of blanks and in an increase of the number of idiosyncratic responses in early acquired words. No effect of word frequency was found in either group.
   At first glance it is tempting to explain the effect of word imageability on word processing in terms of the different word representations involved. Concrete words may have representations that are based on sensorimotor interactions with their referents, whereas abstract word representations are based on verbal definitions, in terms of other word meanings (Johnson-Laird, 1983). However, the results of the present study suggest that this hypothesis may only partly be true. As was shown, late acquired, infrequent, concrete words evoke very strong primary responses only in normal subjects (Table 1), which suggests an interaction between age of acquisition and imageability. Since such an interaction was not found in aphasic patients, we may assume that the imagery effect in word association is not based on a unitary process, but on qualitatively different processing of early and late acquired words.
   A closer look at the relationship between stimulus and response in early and late acquired words in normal subjects is presented in Table 2.

TABLE 2. Primary responses in normal word association to early and late acquired, concrete words (in parentheses the frequency of the primary response).

early acquired	late acquired
bed-sleep(21)	dagger-knife (33)
leaf-tree (31)	safety box-money (30)
see-waves (11)	tub-bath (33)
axe-cut (13)	jester-clown (18)
flute-music (11)	ark-boat (21)
heel-shoe (32)	mug-cup (14)

Early learned words as 'bed' and 'axe' evoke 'sleep' and 'cut' as primary responses, referring to functional aspects of the stimulus word, whereas in the other words the primary response indicates a salient feature of the stimulus (flute-music; sea-water), or refers to a part-whole relationship (leaf-tree; heel-shoe). All these relationships are probably learned through sensorimotor interactions of the child with its environment, i.e., have their roots in episodic memory. The relationship between the stimulus and the primary response in the late acquired words, however, differs clearly from the relationships described above. Most relationships are based on verbal definitions, as in 'bath-tub' and 'mug-cup', or on specification of a superordinate, as in 'ark-boat' and 'dagger-knife'. Only in the case of 'safe-money' a kind of functional relationship is specified. However, it is questionable whether this particular relationship would always be based on personal experience.

So, in word association there seems to be a change in the relationship between stimulus and response, dependent on the age of acquisition of the stimulus word. In early acquired words these relationships usually refer to commonly experienced episodes, especially in concrete words, whereas in later acquired words this relationship is usually based on verbal definitions, even if the stimulus words are concrete (Petrey,1977; Van Loon-Vervoorn, in preparation).

Aphasic patients have less difficulty in responding to early acquired words (less blanks, more idiosyncratic associations), than to late acquired words. So they are better in retrieving episodic relationships than defined ones. That this concerns the retrieval of relationships between words, rather than word retrieval alone, can be deduced from the fact that aphasic patients can easily respond with 'knife' to 'scissors', whereas they fail to respond with 'knife' to 'dagger' (Van Loon-Vervoorn, in preparation). This may be explained by a loss of knowledge based on linguistic definition (higher-order lexicon), and a relatively intact knowledge based on episodic memory (basic lexicon).

REFERENCES
1. Bekkum, I.J. van, & Vries, L.A. de (1980). Een functiepsychologische benadering van de afasiebehandeling. In: A. Jennekens-Schinkel, J.J. Diamant, H.F.A. Diesfeldt, & R. Haaksma (red.), Neuropsychologie in Nederland (pp. 377-402). Deventer: Van Loghum Slaterus.
2. Carroll, J.B., & White, M.N. (1973). Word frequency and age of acquisition as determiners of picture naming latency. Quarterly Journal of Experimental Psychology, 25,85-95.
3. Coltheart, V., & Winograd, E. (1986). Word imagery but not age of acquisition affects episodic memory. Memory and Cognition, 14, 174-180.
4. Deelman, B.G., Liebrand, W.B.G., Koning-Haanstra, M., & Burg, W. van den (1981). SAN test, een afasietest voor auditief taalbegrip en mondeling taalgebruik. Lisse: Swets & Zeitlinger.
5. Gilhooly, K.J., & Gilhooly, M. (1979). Age of acquisition effects in lexical and episodic memory tasks. Memory and Cognition, 7, 214-223.
6. Gilhooly, K.J., & Logie, R.H. (1980). Age of acquisition, imagery, concreteness, familiarity, and ambiguity measures for 1944 words. Behavioral Research Methods and Instrumentation, 12, 395-427.
7. Gilhooly, K.J., & Logie, R.H. (1982). Word age of acquisition and lexical decision making. Acta Psychologica, 50, 21-34.
8. Johnson-Laird, P.N. (1983). Mental models. Cambridge: University Press.
9. Kohnstamm, G.A., Schaerlaekens, A.M., Vries, A.K. de, Akkerhuis, G.W., & Froonincksx, M. (1981). Nieuwe Streeflijst Woordenschat voor 6-jarigen. Lisse: Swets & Zeitlinger.
10. Lesser, R. (1973). Word association and availability of response in an aphasic subject. Journal of Psycholinguistic Research, 2, 355-367.
11. Loftus, E.F., & Suppes, P. (1972). Structural variables that determine the speed of retrieving words from long term memory. Journal of Verbal Learning and Verbal Behavior, 13, 770-777.
12. Loon-Vervoorn, W.A. van (1985a). Voorstelbaarheidswaarden van Nederlandse woorden. Lisse: Swets & Zeitlinger.
13. Loon-Vervoorn, W.A. van (1985b). De Nieuwe Streeflijst als maat voor de verwervingsleeftijd van woorden. Nederlands Tijdschrift voor de Psycho-

logie, 40, 44-47.

14. Loon-Vervoorn, W.A. van (1985c). De Nieuwe Streeflijst als maat voor de verwervingsleeftijd van woorden II. Nederlands Tijdschrift voor de Psychologie, 40, 503-506.

15. Loon-Vervoorn, W.A. van (in preparation). Age of acquisition as a determiner of stimulus-response relationships in word association.

16. Loon-Vervoorn, W.A. van, Bresser, A., & Nawijn, B. (1984). Verwervingsleeftijd, frequentie en voorstelbaarheid als determinanten van woordassociatie-latenties. Intern Rapport Psychologisch Laboratorium Rijksuniversiteit Utrecht.

17. Marcel, A.J., & Patterson, K.E. (1978). Word recognition and production: reciprocity in clinical and normal studies. In: J. Requin (ed.), Attention and Performance VII (pp. 209-226). Hillsdale New Jersey: L. Erlbaum Ass.

18. Morris, P.E. (1981). Age of acquisition, imagery, recall, and the limitations of the multiple-regression analysis. Memory and Cognition, 9, 277-282.

19. Nelson, K. (1983). The conceptual basis for language. In: Th. B. Seiler & W. Wannenmacher (eds.), Concept development and the development of word meaning. Berlin: Springer Verlag.

20. Paivio, A. (1971). Imagery and verbal processes. New York: Holt, Rinehart & Winston.

21. Paivio, A., Yuille, J.C., & Madigan, S.A. (1968). Concreteness, imagery, and meaningfulness values for 925 nouns. Journal of Experimental Psychology, Monograph Supplement, 76, 1, part 2.

22. Petrey, S. (1977). Word association and the development of lexical memory. Cognition, 5, 57-71.

23. Piaget, J. (1948). Language and thought of the child. London: Routledge and Kegan Paul.

24. Richardson, J.T.E. (1980). Mental imagery and human memory. Old Woking Surrey: Unwin Brothers Ltd.

25. Stumpel, H.J., Bekkum, I.J. van, & Loon-Vervoorn, W.A. van (1984). Woordherkenning bij afasie. Verslag ZWO-project, nr. 13-33-008.

26. Uit den Boogaart, P. (1975). Woordfrequenties. Utrecht: Oosthoek, Scheltema & Holkema.

27. Werner, H., & Kaplan, B. (1963). Symbol formation: an organismic-developmental approach to language and the expression of thought. New York: Wiley.

FREQUENCY, IMAGERY VALUE, AND TYPES OF FEATURES IN NATURAL CATEGORIES

HERMINIA PERAITA

UNIVERSIDAD NACIONAL DE EDUCACION A DISTANCIA, MADRID, SPAIN

and PILAR FERRANDIZ

UNIVERSIDAD COMPLUTENSE, MADRID, SPAIN

ABSTRACT

The data presented here are part of a wider research program which focused on the general model of features (Medin and Smith, 1981, 1984). In this study the objective was to try to relate the theoretical field of image formation with that of conceptual representations (Denis, 1982). Several semantic categories were analyzed to obtain lists of the cognitive units or features from different samples of subjects. An analysis was conducted on the nature of these features, and we thus attempted to verify whether the attributes that represented a concept with the greatest strength are identical to those that have the greatest image value, as measured on a five-point scale. No systematic correlations between the image value of the features and frequency were found. Nonetheless certain trends should be pointed out. The taxonomical features in the superordinate categories have a low image value, whereas in the basic level features the value is higher.

1. INTRODUCTION

This paper is a part of a research program on conceptual representation, specifically on the representation of natural categories, persons and social categories in the theoretical framework of a general model of features, not in its classical definitional version but in the present day probabilistic one. Nor will we deal here with the theoretical bases on which both models are centered since their treatment and evolution are reviewed in Smith and Medin (1981), Medin and Smith (1984), Barsalou and Medin (1986), or with the results we have obtained in this line of research (Peraita, 1985a, 1985b; Ferrándiz & Peraita, 1984).

Our aims are the following: first, to connect or relate the topic of image generation and activation as a possible support for conceptual representations, and secondly, to provide additional support for the major working hypothesis as suggested by Denis (1982a, 1982b, 1983) in the framework of figurative/non-figurative semantic feature theory. At the same time our aim is to analyze from a critical point of view, the role, value and function of one of the most common techniques to measure mental imagery: the image value of linguistic input.

M. Denis et al. (eds.), Cognitive and Neuropsychological Approaches to Mental Imagery, 109–118.
© 1988 by Martinus Nijhoff Publishers.

As has often been stated, models of semantic memory and conceptual representation, as well as the different modalities of scheme theory, have generally neglected the subject of representational codes or formats, and have not taken into account the function of mental images. Just the opposite has happened in research in linguistic processing and problem solving in which attempts at an empirical approach are frequent. Recall for example the sentence verification paradigms for obtaining different reaction times depending on whether or not the sentence content elicits visual images.

Another area of this verification paradigm is one in which what is submitted for verification (truth or falsehood) is a sentence that implies a comparative relationship. Lastly the classic designs comparing drawings and sentences, in which a drawing is compared to the semantic content of a descriptive sentence of a given situation, should be mentioned. Here the emphasis has begun to shift not so much to the "dichotomous" propositional interpretations versus those based on images, but to the different strategies subjects employ.

As started by Denis (1982a) and more recently by Glass, Millen, Beck and Eddy (1985) the results achieved through the verification paradigm either in its classical modality or in the selective interference one, have often been contradictory. Some authors have found that when the linguistic inputs have high image values, they are more rapidly processed than when the opposite is the case. From this fact they infer facilitation in linguistic processing on the part of the analogical code underlying the input. Others have found just the opposite: the higher the image value, the longer the processing time (Glass, Eddy & Schwanenflugel, 1980; Eddy & Glass, 1981).

From our point of view, the image value is the central theoretical construct on which such research is based. The empirical status of image value seems to be well established since most research on linguistic processing, memorization, reading times, etc., tries to obtain correlations between image value and certain behavioral indicators. Our starting point is the hypothesis of the existence of a psychological activity in the subject that allows him/her to evaluate or estimate the intensity of certain types of linguistic inputs for generating mental images, visual or other. However this process takes place without the nature of such psychological activity being clearly known, nor the reason why some words have higher image value than others.

In spite of this, there is at present some research which challenges the notion that image value refers to only one meaning and draws attention to the difficulty of knowing whether or not the subject has access to what the experimenter is asking him/her when the former evaluates image values of different kinds of inputs on a scale (Goldberg, 1986).

Other authors, in view of these contradictory results, suggest studying in depth the concrete vs. abstract dichotomy, generally considered as parallel and equivalent to high vs. low image value, since they consider that not all concrete words have the same access and processing characteristics. At the same time, they posit that the abstract words can depend on the context, and their degree of abstraction is not static or immutable (Glass et al., 1985).

In view of such disparity of criteria and results, we have taken as a focus those perspectives of research which, such as the one by Denis (1982a), obtain coherent results in the framework of the relationship between images and semantic and/or conceptual representations. His proposals are based upon the existence of a subset of features, out of the set of features representing a concept, to which image processes can be applied. These would be the figurative features that supposedly maintain a structural analogy with perceptual experience. Since the image value of words and sentences seems to be an important factor in the processing of the linguistic material, it could perhaps depend on the actualization of the features or figurative components of the underlying concepts. This should provide a means of predicting the image value of a word by the richness of the corresponding concepts in figurative-perceptual features (Denis, 1982b). This is probably related at the same time to the dimension of generality-specificity or hierarchical level. As we descend the hierarchy, the figurative features will be more numerous. Considering all the above, Denis's proposal is to give credibility and operativity to the concept of word image value, which could be predicted from the analysis of the figurative features that form the underlying concepts.

Taking as a starting point of view Denis's basic proposals and other similar arguments, we have investigated certain natural categories already used in research of this kind (Rosch et al., 1976; Dubois, 1983, 1986; Tversky & Hemenway, 1984; Peraita, 1984; Ferrándiz & Peraita, 1984).

We have categorized the set of attributes with which the subjects more frequently defined natural categories, in order to test whether there is an immediate correspondence between perceptual or figurative attributes and image value. At the same time we tried to analyze if the other types of features with which we characterize concepts (functional, taxonomic and evaluative), obtain significantly different image values from those obtained by the figurative ones, or if on the contrary, to these other sets of features image processes can be applied. We have also analysed the different global image values of the categories as regards their membership in biological classes and their generality level.

The goals of this research were the following:
1. To test wether the attributes that represent certain natural categories with greater strength are the ones that have a higher image value (relationship between frequency and image value).
2. To test on the one hand, if the features that have a higher image value are figurative or if, on the other hand , they are also functional, classifying, etc. (relationship between image value and type of features).
3. To test whether biological categories are more salient, from the imagery point of view, than artefactual categories, and whether basic level categories are more salient than superordinates.

2. METHOD

Subjects. A total of 47 subjects (University students) were selected, 18 men and 29 women, whose ages ranged from 20 to 28 years. The group had an average age of 22.

Materials. The items were 18 names of categories (see table 1), 8 biological and 10 non-biological, and their corresponding lists of features. These categories were used by us in a previous work and selected according to suggestions made by Rosch et al. (1976). The features were obtained in our previous work by means of a task of free listing attributes with temporal restriction. They were selected and classified according to the class they belonged to. These are: "is a" group for taxonomic features; "has" or "is" for figurative perceptual properties, and "can" for other kinds of properties (mainly, utility, purpose, action).

We adopted a 5 point scale (0, none; 1, little; 2, average; 3, quite a lot; 4, a lot) to evaluate the capacity of sentences to elicit visual images in subjects' minds.

Procedure. One hundred and sixty-two written items were presented by means of cards, in the form of a sentence asserting a relationship between a concept and a given property (e.g. "a bird has feathers"). Previously the 18 categories were rated by the same subjects but in different sessions. They had to circle the image value they gave to each of these items. The order was randomized both for the names of categories and for the features.

3. RESULTS

As is shown in table 1, the Spearman correlations (calculated over items) between global imagery value and composite imagery value (that is, mean imagery value of corresponding features) for biological and non-biological categories were in both cases $r_s = 0.40$, non-significant at $P<.05$. The image value given by the subjects to the names of the categories did not correlate with the mean value of the features or attributes corresponding to each of the categories. However the global image value is, in all cases, higher than the composite image value, and furthermore the composite values are higher for the levels A_2 and B_2 than for the superordinate ones (A_1 and B_1), and higher too for the biological categories (A_1 and A_2) than for the non-biological ones (B_1 and B_2) (table 1).

In table 2 we present two biological categories with the frequencies for each feature and their image values together with the correlations between both. The superordinate level will be discussed first (A_1). We only observed higher positive correlation than the critical value for the concept "bird", $r_s = 0.76$, $P<.01$. At the subordinate level (A_2), of the four correlations, only one was significant, for the concept "apple", $r_s = 0.72$, $P.<.01$.

In table 3 we present the non-biological categories (B_1 and B_2) with the frequencies for each feature and their image values together with the correlations between both. In relation to the superordinate level (B_1) we find only two significant correlations in the concept "musical instrument", $r_s = 0.77$, $P<.05$, and "vehicle", $r_s = 0.64$, $P<.05$, and with respect to the subordinate level (B_2) we obtain positive correlations for "guitar" and "trousers", $r_s = 0.77$ and $r_s = 0.75$, both $P<.05$.

In table 4 we present the average image value of the features that indicate inclusion in a class ("is a"), perceptual properties ("has"), and likewise for the functional ones. The differences were not statistically

TABLE 1: GLOBAL IMAGERY VALUES AND COMPOSITE ONES FOR EACH
GROUP OF CATEGORIES. SPEARMAN CORRELATIONS BETWEEN BOTH.

CATEGORY		NUMBER OF FEATURES	GLOBAL IMAGERY VALUE	COMPOSITE IMAGERY VALUE	CORRELATION BETWEEN GLOBAL AND COMPOSITE IMAGERY VALUES
A_1	TREE	7	3.02	2.42	
	FISH	9	2.75	2.51	
	BIRD	11	3.28	2.57	
	FRUIT	6	3.20	2.49	
					$r_s = .40$ N.S.
A_2	PINE	11	3.27	2.59	
	TROUT	9	2.85	2.39	
	EAGLE	14	3.15	2.89	
	APPLE	13	3.22	2.42	
B_1	MUSICAL INSTRUMENT	7	3.02	2.38	
	TOOL	6	2.41	2.29	
	CLOTHES	5	2.78	2.57	
	FURNITURE	6	2.85	2.41	
	VEHICLE	8	2.98	2.40	
					$r_s = .40$ N.S.
B_2	GUITAR	7	3.32	2.67	
	HAMMER	7	2.52	2.38	
	TROUSERS	8	3.22	2.54	
	TABLE	8	2.85	2.33	
	CAR	9	3.12	2.29	

significant. We found the same non-significance for the group "can" or "can
be used for", and the two other groups, "has" and "is a".

4. DISCUSSION

As has been stated in the results, we did not find the anticipated
relationship between the image value of the features and their frequency
for most of the categories, natural or artefactual, contrary to what has
been obtained by other authors (Denis, 1983).

The most frequent features are often classifying ones ("is a"
relation), and there are no significant differences between their
image values and those of the figurative ones. In the non-biological
categories the most frequent are functional. On the other hand and contrary
to what we anticipated, these two kinds of features also have image values
whose distribution is very similar to that of the perceptual ones.
Regardless of this, there clearly exist certain tendencies that must be
pointed out:
1. The classifying attributes in the superordinate categories have average

TABLE 2: SOME EXAMPLES OF BIOLOGICAL CATEGORIES

FEATURES	FREQUENCY* IN %	MEAN IMAGERY VALUE	CORRELATION
BIRD (SUPERORDINATE CATEGORY)			
IS A FLYER	77.05	3.13	
HAS A BEAK	45.56	3.09	
HAS FEATHERS	44.32	2.96	
HAS WINGS	41.23	3.13	
IS AN ANIMAL	30.92	2.04	r_s= .76
HAS TWO LEGS	28.89	2.00	
CAN SING	19.58	2.81	P<.01
IS A BIRD (AVE) **	15.46	2.77	
CAN FEED ON INSECTS	15.46	1.57	
CAN LIVE IN NESTS	10.30	2.77	
CAN LAY EGGS	9.27	1.98	
APPLE (SUBORDINATE CATEGORY)			
IS A FRUIT	73.19	2.83	
COMES FROM THE APPLE TREE	47.42	2.49	
IS EDIBLE	46.39	2.96	
CAN BE RED	34.02	2.77	
IS TASTY	25.77	2.89	
CAN BE JUICY	24.74	2.85	
CAN BE FLESHY	24.74	2.62	r_s= .72
CAN BE GREEN	22.68	2.15	
CAN BE YELLOW	22.52	2.45	P<.01
HAS STEM	23.71	1.62	
HAS PIPS	17.57	1.83	
HAS A PEEL	13.40	2.17	
CAN HAVE WORMS	11.34	1.85	
FISH (SUPERORDINATE CATEGORY)			
IS AQUATIC	52	2.96	
IS AN ANIMAL	38.14	2.02	
HAS FINS	38.14	2.53	
HAS SCALES	32.27	2.47	r_s= -.25
IS EDIBLE	30.92	2.17	
HAS GILLS	22.68	1.91	N.S.
CAN LIVE IN RIVERS	19.58	2.68	
CAN LIVE IN THE SEA	19.58	2.91	
IS A SWIMMER	16.49	2.98	
EAGLE (SUBORDINATE CATEGORY)			
IS A BIRD (AVE)	48.45	2.83	

TABLE 2 (cont.)

IS PREDATORY	41.24	2.49	
IS CARNIVOROUS	38.14	2.57	
IS A GOOD FLYER	34.02	3.26	
IS BIG	30.93	2.98	
HAS A STRONG BEAK	27.84	2.72	$r_s = .29$
HAS BIG WINGS	26.80	3.15	
HAS CLAWS	22.68	2.96	N.S.
IS A BIRD	21.65	2.55	
HAS FEATHERS	18.59	3.02	
HUNTS ANIMALS	16.49	2.89	
LIVES ON THE HIGH PEAKS	16.49	3.09	
IS FAST	15.46	3.28	
HAS SHARP VISION	12.37	2.66	

*Percentage of subjects that produce each feature.
**In Spanish there are two terms for bird: "pajaro"/"ave".

TABLE 3: SOME EXAMPLES OF NON-BIOLOGICAL CATEGORIES

FEATURES	FREQUENCY IN %	MEAN IMAGERY VALUE	CORRELATION
MUSICAL INSTRUMENT (SUPERORDINATE CATEGORY)			
CAN BE USED TO COMPOSE MUSIC	41.23	2.91	
CAN BE STRING	41.23	2.43	
CAN BE WIND	36.84	2.23	
CAN BE PERCUSSION	31.95	2.30	$r_s = .77$
CAN BE USED TO PRODUCE SOUND	30.93	2.91	
CAN BE METAL	10.30	2.17	P < .05
CAN BE WOODEN	10.30	2.33	
VEHICLE (SUPERORDINATE CATEGORY)			
IS A MEANS OF TRANSPORTATION	72.16	2.87	
IS A MEANS OF LOCOMOTION	35.05	2.68	
HAS WHEELS	32.99	2.68	
CAN BE MADE OF METAL	22.08	2.17	$r_s = .64$
HAS AN ENGINE	20.62	2.85	
CAN GO ON THE ROAD	10.31	2.70	P < .05
CAN USE OIL	9.28	1.66	
CAN USE GAS	9.28	1.62	
CAR (SUBORDINATE CATEGORY)			
HAS FOUR WHEELS	58.76	2.67	
IS A VEHICLE	43.30	2.22	
IS A MEANS OF TRANSPORTATION	42.27	2.30	

TABLE 3 (cont.)

HAS AN ENGINE	41.24	2.10	
NEEDS GAS	22.68	2.17	r_s= .37
HAS A STEERING WHEEL	19.59	2.07	
IS FAST	15.46	2.52	N. S.
HAS SEATS	10.31	2.42	
HAS A TRUNK	9.28	2.07	

TABLE (SUBORDINATE CATEGORY)			
IS MADE OF WOOD	59.79	2.51	
HAS SEVERAL LEGS	46.39	1.83	
CAN BE USED TO EAT ON	45.36	2.40	
CAN HAVE FOUR LEGS	43.29	2.45	r_s= .08
IS A PIECE OF FURNITURE	31.96	2.60	
CAN BE USED TO LEAN ON	26.80	2.13	N. S.
CAN BE USED TO PUT THINGS ON	10.31	2.40	
HAS A HORIZONTAL BOARD	14.43	--	

TABLE 4: MEAN IMAGERY VALUES FOR EACH TYPE OF FEATURE AND CATEGORY

	CLASSIFYING	PERCEPTUAL	FUNCTIONAL	TOTAL
A_1	2.30	2.51	2.48	2.43
A_2	2.79	2.57	2.49	2.61
B_1	2.52	2.22	2.30	2.34
B_2	2.54	2.28	2.50	2.44
TOTAL	2.53	2.39	2.44	2.45

or low image values (table 4), but when they refer to subordinate categories the image value is much higher ("a fish is an animal" vs. "a trout is a fish").

2. In general, the parts (or qualities) of a natural object that are not directly visible from the outside, because they are inside the object, also present lower image values: "an apple has pips", "it can have worms", "fruit has vitamins", "a fish has gills" (tables 2 and 3).

3. As we have previously indicated in the results, although we have not obtained significant differences between the global image values and composite ones, these latter values tend in general to be higher in the subordinate levels than in the superordinate ones, and higher also in the biological categories than in the non-biological ones.

We believe that in the framework of figurative vs. non-figurative features as support to imagery processes, and for the authors who have adopted a componential point of view (structural and static), some issues remain unresolved: does the decomposition of meaning into discrete elements, components of features, capture the full meaning of words? Because concepts are not isolated entities, but are parts of semantic fields and other relational systems, is it possible to activate and evaluate, from the point of view of imagery, only one isolated concept of a feature without interference? Why do the taxonomic or classifying features that are conceptual and not perceptual in nature (not directly observable) have such high imagery values? And what about the problem of generalization of the results, in the light of the special sets of concepts used? Do all concepts/categories have features to which can be applied imagery processes?

We are afraid that we are faced with the same problems in this research framework as in theories of semantic features and that we must adopt alternative frames for feature decomposition such as inferential links, meaning postulates or prototype and schema theory.

5. CONCLUSIONS AND FURTHER QUESTIONS

The basic hypothesis (subset of figurative features) or basic schema from our point of view is disconfirmed, at least in part, because of:

1. Very weak variations in the global imagery values of terms used. Perhaps a bias in the selection of these terms?

2. Similar terms, belonging to the same group and taxonomic level, like "bird" and "fish" (A_1) or "pine" and "apple" (A_2), "guitar" and "table" (B_2), obtain very different correlations between the frequency of their attributes (supposedly figurative to a great degree) and their imagery value. How is this possible?

3. The classifying features ("is a" relations) have imagery values similar to figurative and functional ones. The present data reveal a lack of systematicity.

4. The features that are not "direct" (like "useful", "dangerous") are apparently assigned imagery values which do not differ greatly from the perceptual, supposedly "direct" ones.

5. The same occurs when the generic name of the category is presented to the subjects and not just the isolated features. The high imagery values obtained in these cases show that global schematic representation is possible.

6. Perhaps it would be necessary to make a more detailed analysis of some imagery values of some categories and subsets of features.

7. And finally, could not it be that the subject (when making an estimation of the imagery value of a word) is really applying linguistic knowledge (grammatical, semantic and pragmatic) of the word, and that it is the knowledge about its concreteness-abstractness, familiarity, meaningfulness, or associativity, that influences the estimation? (Holyoak, 1974; Goldberg, 1986).

REFERENCES

1. Barsalou, L.W., & Medin, D.L. (1986). Concepts: Static definitions or context dependent representations? Cahiers de Psychologie Cognitive, 6, 187-202.

2. Denis, M. (1982a). Images and semantic representations. In J.F. Le Ny

& W. Kintsch (Eds.), Language and comprehension. Amsterdam: North-Holland.

3. Denis, M. (1982b). On figurative components of mental representations. In F. Klix, J. Hoffmann & E. Van Der Meer (Eds.), Cognitive research in psychology. Berlin: VEB Deutscher Verlag der Wissenschaften.

4. Denis, M. (1983). Valeur d'imagerie et composition sémantique: Analyse de deux échantillons de substantifs. Cahiers de Psychologie Cognitive, 3, 175-202.

5. Dubois, D.(1983). Analyse de 22 catégories sémantiques du français: Organisation catégorielle, lexique et représentation. L'Année Psychologique, 83, 465-489.

6. Dubois, D.(1986). La compréhension de phrases: Représentations sémantiques et processus. Thèse de doctorat non publiée.

7. Eddy, J.K., & Glass, A.L. (1981). Reading and listening to high and low imagery sentences. Journal of Verbal Learning and Verbal Behavior, 20, 333-345.

8. Ferrándiz, P., & Peraita, H. (1984). Frecuencia, valor de imagen y tipos de rasgos, en categorias biológicas y no biológicas. Revista de Psicología General y Aplicada, 2, 1257-1278.

9. Glass, A.L., Eddy, J.K., & Schwanenflugel, P.J. (1980). The verification of high and low imagery sentences. Journal of Experimental Psychology: Human Learning and Memory, 6, 692-704.

10. Glass, A. L., Millen, D. R., Beck, L. G., & Eddy, J. K. (1985). Representation of images in sentence verification. Journal of Memory and Language, 24, 442-465.

11. Goldberg, L. R. (1986). The validity of rating procedures to index the hierchical level of categories. Journal of Memory and Language, 25, 323-347.

12. Holyoak, K. J. (1974). The role of imagery in the evaluation of sentences: Imagery or semantic factors? Journal of Verbal Learning and Behavior, 13, 162-166.

13. Medin, D.L., & Smith, E.E. (1984). Concepts and concept formation. Annual Review of Psychology, 35, 113-118.

14. Peraita, H. (1984). El nivell basic de categorització: Un estudi comparatiu basat en l'analisi dels atributs de nou taxonomies. In Siguán M. et al. (Eds.), Estudi experimental del bilingüisme. Barcelona: Fundació Caixa de Pensions.

15. Peraita, H. (1985a). Representación de categorias sociales, roles o profesiones, en una muestra de sujetos adultos de un medio rural. Informes de Psicología, 73-84.

16. Peraita, H. (1985b). Representación de conceptos: Rasgos y esquemas. Infancia y Aprendizaje, 31-32, 187-202.

17. Rosch, E., Mervis, C.B., Gray, W., Johnson, D., & Boyes-Braem, P. (1976). Basic objects in natural categories. Cognitive Psychology, 8, 382-439.

18. Smith, E.E., & Medin, D.L. (1981). Categories and concepts. Cambridge, MA: Harvard University Press.

19. Tversky, B., & Hemenway, K. (1984). Objects, parts, and categories. Journal of Experimental Psychology: General, 113, 169-193.

2.3. SENTENCE AND TEXT PROCESSING

IMAGERY AND PROSE PROCESSING

MICHEL DENIS

CENTRE D'ETUDES DE PSYCHOLOGIE COGNITIVE
UNIVERSITE DE PARIS-SUD, ORSAY, FRANCE

ABSTRACT
    This paper presents an overview of major theoretical and methodological issues associated with the study of the relationships between imagery and prose processing. It reviews and discusses findings from a research program on visual imagery and text processing, which demonstrate the positive effects of imaginal strategies on memory for narratives and texts describing characters. Recent experiments involving texts describing geographical configurations illustrate the relevance of order of description in processing and memory for text. Future orientations in the field of imagery and text processing are outlined.

1. INTRODUCTION

    This paper focuses on the relationships of imagery to the processing of prose, mainly texts, an issue which has only begun to be explored actively in recent years. First, I will point out a number of general issues associated with the study of imagery and text processing. Secondly, I will report and discuss the findings from a research program devoted to the role of imagery in reading and memorizing prose materials. Lastly, I will indicate future lines of research which may prove fruitful to the study of text processing.

2. THEORETICAL AND METHODOLOGICAL ISSUES

    When researchers are confronted with the question of imagery and the processing of texts, they are simultaneously faced with a number of issues, and must make a number of theoretical and methodological decisions in consequence. Two of these general issues will be discussed first, then I will turn to three specific ones.
    (1) The first issue may be qualified as general inasmuch as it is the type of issue that researchers inevitably encounter when investigating the interactions of imagery with the processing of any sort of meaningful verbal material. It concerns the assumptions one makes as regards the theoretical role of imagery in the construction of text meaning. Is visual imagery elicited by sentences in a text completely identifiable with the meaning of these sentences ? Or, on the contrary, are other, non-imaginal processes involved in the elaboration of meaning ? If such is the case, will imagery be viewed as a psychological event without any functional

M. Denis et al. (eds.), Cognitive and Neuropsychological Approaches to Mental Imagery, 121–132.
© *1988 by Martinus Nijhoff Publishers.*

significance ? Or is imagery indispensable to those processes upon which meaning is constructed ? Or again, does it have some sort of additional role, distinct from the role of these processes ?

In short, there is no way the researcher can avoid taking a theoretical position as concerns text processing, especially with regard to the non-imaginal processes implied in text processing itself. Furthermore, more specific assumptions as to the nature of these processes must be made. They may be seen in terms of "verbal" processes, which would be the case if the dual-coding approach is applied to the question of text processing. In this view, the construction of the meaning of concrete texts is dependent on the joint functioning of a verbal system and an imagery system (Paivio, 1971, 1986). Alternatively, non-imaginal processes may be considered to be responsible for the construction of "proposition-like" representations. This is the case if the aim is to insert imagery into current propositional models of text processing. In these models, meaning as a whole is represented in the propositional textbase ; imaginal processes do not contribute to meaning proper, but rather supplement meaning with a pictorial-spatial "model" of the situations described (e.g., van Dijk & Kintsch, 1983 ; Perrig & Kintsch, 1985).

(2) The second general issue concerns the way researchers operationalize imagery processes when introducing them as independent variables in the study of text processing. If the classical distinction first proposed by Allan Paivio (1971) is adopted, three major variants in paradigms are available.

The first operation consists in comparing different sorts of texts or different versions of the same text having differential degrees of likelihood to elicit visual images. For instance, in one version, the adjectives associated with nouns will refer to properties easily expressed through visual imagery, whereas in the other version, each of these adjectives will be replaced by one referring to an abstract property, not easily convertible into a visual image. The major question is whether this operation will affect the memory of adjectives, the memory of the nouns they accompany, the memory of the sentences in which they are inserted, and so on. The difficulty inherent to this sort of operationalization is almost immediately apparent. From one version to the other, not only the image-evoking value of certain words varies, but their meaning varies as well. Thus, differences in recall may result from either the differential involvement of imagery or differential semantic content or both.

The second paradigm, which has long been the most widespread, consists of varying reading instructions. In one condition, subjects are instructed to read the text while generating detailed visual images of its content (the characters, their actions, etc.). In the other condition, control subjects are instructed to read without being given any imagery instructions. Note that this paradigm does not imply that control subjects do not also make use of some imagery. Simply, imagery instructions are taken as a means of maximizing the probability that subjects will use imagery-based strategies while reading. However, very careful wording of the imagery instructions is needed, since these may inadvertently create expectancy effects that may affect processing and recall.

The third paradigm relies on the use of individual imagery differences. All the subjects are exposed to exactly the same text, and are given identical reading instructions which do not refer to imagery in any way. This procedure minimizes the difficulties associated with potential expectancy effects. On the other hand, this method of investigation poses the problems of the measurement of individual imagery characteristics. Which tests or questionnaires will be best suited to this purpose ? Which components of imagery abilities are relevant in the reading of prose ? In addition to subjects' imagery abilities per se, should subjects' proficiency to make use of these abilities, as well as subjects' metacognitive beliefs as concerns the usefulness of imagery in reading tasks, be taken into account ?

(3) In addition to these two general problems, which arise in practically all investigations of imagery in cognitive processing, some problems are more specifically linked with the study of text processing.

The first is concerned with the variety of the types of text one may use in experiments. Narratives have been widely employed. Most narratives strongly elicit visual imagery for characters, scenery, and interactions among characters and with objects. Since narratives were the "typical" sort of text investigated in text processing studies, it is not surprising that they were also the first type of text used by imagery researchers.

Other sorts of texts have been investigated more recently, such as those termed "descriptive" texts. Description is mainly involved when a list of properties connected to a given object is presented. For instance, texts may describe characters, real or fictional, both as concerns their physical characteristics, as well as their psychological or moral features. Another typical sort of description involves spatial configurations, such as geographical materials. Clearly these types of "descriptive" texts possess structural characteristics which are different from those of narratives. While narratives necessarily have a chronological structure, the description of an object is apparently not subjected to such sequential constraints. Put in another way, descriptions portray scenes or objects which are static, and each new piece of information incorporated into the representation simply enriches it ; in the case of narratives, each new piece of information supplied by the text and incorporated in the representation transforms it. If imagery is involved in reading, undergoing enrichment or transformations would not be equivalent.

Lastly, imagery may well be implicated in the processing of texts which "prescribe" actions to the readers. Obviously, many problems one encounters when studying imagery in relationship with text processing will have to be qualified by the type of text used, which also has consequences on the types of processes assumed to be involved.

(4) When considering the hypothetical effects of imagery on prose comprehension and memorization, another important question is to determine the exact level at which such effects are likely to intervene. More specifically, imagery may be reasonably expected to facilitate memory for rather low-level elements, such as sentences, or even episodes. But is imagery of any use in the construction of higher-level structures, such as text macrostructure ? Recent evidence has been presented by Marc Marschark (1985) and Walter Perrig (1986), suggesting that in the processing of concrete prose, the locus of imagery effects is essentially the organization and recall of lower-level elements, whereas imagery is apparently not involved in the thematic organization of texts. Looking for imagery effects thus requires that researchers make theoretical assumptions as concerns the level at which they expect such effects to be found.

(5) Another question concerns the aspects of the processing researchers predict or wish to evidence. In the vast majority of studies, what authors "track" are rather long-term effects of imagery, mainly effects on retention. That is, their analysis bears on a set of data collected at a phase of the experimental procedure when the processes under study are no longer active. It may also be of interest to capture manifestations of imagery processes not after they have developed, but while they are developing, that is, during the processing of the text. Tracking imagery while it is on line, and collecting objective, though indirect, measures of it, is a stimulating challenge, and I will suggest that reading times, when appropriately analyzed, provide a valuable indication of certain aspects of on-line imagery activity.

3. IMAGERY AND THE PROCESSING OF TEXT : EXPERIMENTAL EVIDENCE
Narratives

The second part of this paper presents a selection of experimental results from a research program conducted in our laboratory over the last several years (Denis, 1982, 1984, 1986, 1987). As was the case for most researchers, my first studies bore on the role of imagery in the processing of narrative materials. The texts I used were stories about an automobile trip, a farmer's ride to a village, and the like. Characters and events were described with numerous concrete details. Subjects were instructed to read texts carefully, at their own pace, without rereading. They were told that they would have to answer questions at the end of the experiment. In fact, subjects had to complete a retention test on characters and events presented in the text. Each item referred to a fact that had been explicitly stated in the text.

In these studies, imagery was manipulated essentially at the individual level, with the aim of investigating whether subjects who are spontaneously inclined to elaborate visual images while reading a concrete text would exhibit specific behavioral features in this situation. Would they exhibit superior retention of the text than poor imagers ? Would they show differential reading patterns at the encoding phase ? The basic theoretical assumption underlying my research was that if visual imagery is used during reading, it operates as a cognitive instrument which furthers additional encoding of semantic information, complementing the propositional textbase constructed from the text by the readers. High imagers would then "capitalize" more on this additional encoding than low imagers.

In these studies, Marks' (1973) Vividness of Visual Imagery Questionnaire (VVIQ) was used to discriminate among subjects in terms of their likelihood to elaborate images from verbal descriptions. It was assumed that high VVIQ scorers would have a greater tendency to elaborate visual images of prose content, while low scorers could be considered as being less prone to such elaboration.

Results showed that overall high imagers had higher retention scores than low imagers. This finding was consistent with a number of data in the imagery literature showing that imaginal encoding enhances the retention of verbal materials. At this point, results were consistent with the assumption that imaginal processing increases the likelihood that semantic information is encoded in memory.

However, in this series of studies, the aspect which essentially attracted my attention was the consequence of imagery on reading times. It is a longstanding finding in imagery research that imaging is a process which requires time. My reasoning, then, was that if imagery takes time, the total reading time of a text likely to elicit visual imagery should comprise the time specifically devoted to the elaboration and inspection of images. This led me to hypothesize that texts containing concrete descriptions and episodes would evoke larger "amounts" of imagery activity, and hence would require more time to read than texts devoid of any concrete descriptions and episodes, assuming an equivalent level of text difficulty.

Now, is it reasonable to expect that operations capable of assessing the absolute amount of time devoted to imagery by a reader can successfully be carried out ? Given the possibility that imagery processes at least partly develop in parallel with semantic processing, my assumption is that such an aim is unrealistic. What however remains possible, and logically sound, is to make some sort of differential (rather than absolute) measure of this sort. If we examine people who share the fact of being good readers and who in addition have comparable world knowledge and cultural backgrounds, but who differ in terms of their likelihood to transform verbal information into visual images, it then is reasonable to expect that if imagery actually weighs upon reading times, high imagers will tend to devote a relatively greater amount of time to the elaboration and inspection of their images. If we assume that the other abilities involved in reading are equally distributed across both high and low imagers, then the longer time devoted to imagery activity should be reflected in longer total reading times for high imagers than for people who have low tendencies to convert verbal information into visual images.

The hypothesis that high imagers take more time to read concrete prose than low imagers was confirmed in several successive studies using different sorts of narratives. This finding lends weight to the argument that high imagers' higher retention of text content is dependent on the greater amount of imagery activity they develop during reading. The extra time devoted to reading by high imagers at least partly reflects the extra imagery processing they are engaged in when reading imageable material.

The results of a control condition designed to evaluate the alternate interpretation that high imagers have longer reading times simply because they are slow readers, or slow information processors in general, showed that high and low imagers did not differ in their reading times when they were asked to read a highly abstract, non-imageable text. It thus seems reasonable to conclude that the differences in reading times for narratives do indeed reflect differences in time devoted to imagery. Furthermore, there was no difference between high and low imagers on a retention test for the abstract text. Thus, individual imagery characteristics apparently affect processing of text only insofar as this text is likely to elicit visual imagery.

Additional experiments were conducted in which we attempted to influence imaginal processing during text reading through instructions. Subjects were presented with a narrative and were instructed to read it as fast as possible. The assumption was that such instructions should incite high imagers to decrease their amount of imagery activity. Results showed that high imagers had significantly shorter reading times than previously, whereas low imagers' reading times were not modified. The slight decrease in retention scores was not significant. In another experiment, subjects were asked to construct visual images of characters and events for every sentence while they read the narrative. These instructions increased moderately high imagers' reading times, but considerably increased low imagers' reading times, the end result being no significant difference in overall reading times between high and low imagers. Furthermore, imagery instructions substantially improved retention scores, yielding equivalent high performance for high and low imagers.

Texts describing characters

This type of research, using the individual differences paradigm, was then applied to a fairly different type of text. I turned towards "descriptive" texts, more specifically, ones portraying characters. These texts do not have the same sequential nature as the narratives previously used. Although their structure is sequential, in that different features of the portrait are presented one by one, constraints on the order in which the features are introduced are not as strong. In addition, the texts contained passages with different degrees of concreteness. Highly concrete passages provided a physical description of the characters ; they were thus expected to elicit visual imagery in a steady fashion. Other, less concrete passages described psychological and moral features of the characters ; these statements were assumed to be less easily convertible into visual images.

Examination of the reading times in self-paced reading conditions clearly confirmed the results obtained with narratives : high imagers' reading times were consistently longer than those of low imagers. After fast reading instructions, both high and low imagers reduced their reading times to comparable values, whereas imagery instructions led both groups of subjects to increase their reading times to maximal, similar values.

In the imagery condition, however, low imagers lengthened their reading times much more for concrete than for less concrete passages. This finding probably reflects the fact that people not spontaneously inclined to imaging nevertheless are capable of engaging themselves in imaginal processing when required to do so, but this apparently is easier for them with materials more likely to elicit images. On the other hand, high imagers lengthened their reading times in similar proportions for both kinds of passages. Another interesting finding is that when looking at retention scores, high imagers benefitted from imagery instructions as concerns both concrete and less concrete passages, while low imagers benefitted from this extra processing only as concerns concrete passages. This finding suggests that low imagers, when asked to engage in imaginal processing, are only able to do this efficiently to the extent that the material lends itself to this kind of processing.

In these experiments with descriptive texts, the overall pattern of results was highly similar to that obtained in the experiments dealing with narratives. Apparently, what is critical here is that the texts elicit visual representations, whatever the sequential constraints associated with the processing of the texts.

Texts describing geographical configurations

More recently, I extended this research to other types of descriptive texts, that is, texts describing geographical configurations. These are texts where during reading it is highly likely that imaginal processing has some role to play. However, imagery was not the only variable of interest in this new series of studies, conducted with Guy Denhière. A critical variable was the one mentioned previously, that is, the order in which features appear in the description.

At the beginning of the experiment, the subjects were briefly shown a blank map of a fictitious island (Figure 1). Subjects were then asked to read a short text which described all the features on each location. A sentence by sentence self-presentation of the text was used. Sentences were displayed on a monitor, and subjects' reading times for each

128

sentence were recorded. After reading the text, subjects were again given the blank map and were requested to write the name of each feature at the correct location.

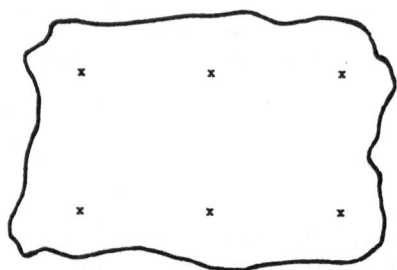

Figure 1.- Blank map of island

Note that at this point of the research program, individual imagery characteristics were not considered as a factor in the study. Our initial purpose was to delineate general patterns in the processing of such a text. As a consequence, reading times did not lend themselves to an analysis in terms of the hypothetical components resulting from imagery activity, but were simply taken as reflecting the overall amount of processing for each sentence. Variations in reading times were related to the main factor, namely, the serial position of the sentences in the description.

We devised two versions of the description, corresponding to two different orders, which themselves may be considered as two among the 6! possible orders of description of the six features (Figure 2). Text 1 was what may be termed a "linear" description. It corresponded to a horizontal scanning of the upper row, followed by similar scanning of the lower row. This order of description may be considered as rather "systematic", and it was assumed to fit the expectations of most readers. In Text 2, by contrast, the order of description was considered as "weakly systematic", in that it completely deviated from linearity. One anchor point was the feature at the extreme west end of the upper row ; the other anchor point was the feature at the extreme east end of the lower row. Note that in both Texts 1 and 2, each feature is precisely located, and both texts provide the same information on the configuration.

Reading times for Text 1 were rather homogeneous, about 10 s per sentence. There was a somewhat longer reading time for sentence 4, which corresponds to the introduction of a new anchor point. The reading times for Text 2 were quite different. While reading times for sentences 1 and 2 did not substantially differ from those of the same sentences in Text 1, there was a significant increase in reading times of subsequent sentences. Overall reading times for sentences 4-6 were almost twice as long as those in Text 1. These chronometric data certainly reflect the greater cognitive load resulting from processing conditions requiring that the

Text 1

1. In the extreme north-west part, there is a mountain.

2. To the east of the mountain, there is a forest.

3. To the east of the forest, there is a lake.

4. In the extreme south-west part, there is a meadow.

5. To the east of the meadow, there is a cave.

6. To the east of the cave, there is a desert.

Text 2

1. In the extreme north-west part, there is a mountain.

2. To the east of the mountain, there is a forest.

3. To the south of the mountain, there is a meadow.

4. In the extreme south-east part, there is a desert.

5. To the west of the desert, there is a cave.

6. To the north of the desert, there is a lake.

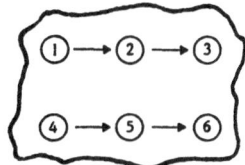
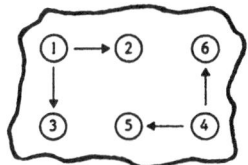

Figure 2.- Two orders of description

readers adapt themselves to a non-systematic description, with reference to a second anchor point, which is not the one expected by the readers, and with alternative use of horizontal and vertical scannings. In short, Text 1 probably fits most readers' descriptive schemes (which was our assumption), while Text 2 does not correspond to any likely descriptive strategy. In addition, the construction of a mental map, or image, of the island is probably made more difficult, and less efficient, from Text 2 than from Text 1.

As concerns recall following the processing of Text 1, retention is at its maximum for the first features mentioned, and then decreases steadily to the last feature. There is no indication of any recency effect. This suggests that encoding of the text implies successive incorporations of the new features to the mental representation (presumably, the visual image) that readers construct for the configuration. Features incorporated first are apparently more efficiently integrated in the representation than are the features encountered later, when the representation is more "loaded" in information. Recall frequencies for Text 2 are overall lower than those for Text 1, which is true even for those features mentioned at the very beginning of the text (for which reading times were quite comparable in both versions). This suggests the existence of interfering effects, impairing the retention of features which nevertheless have been processed in a way similar to Text 1.

In this research program, we integrated a number of variations on the processing conditions, both at the encoding phase and at the recall phase. Here, I will only report a condition where we specifically explored the contribution of visual imagery to the construction of the "mental map" of the island. Our assumption, in this respect, was that visual imagery is the most likely candidate in the construction of the spatial models that subjects elaborate for such configurations.

The first experiment was replicated by simply providing subjects with imagery instructions. Subjects were required, during the reading of each sentence, to form a visual image of the island and "put" each feature at its appropriate location in the image. Again, we recorded reading times as well as recall.

The first interesting result was that overall reading times were very similar to those recorded in the previous experiment. Not only were reading time patterns for a given text similar in both experiments, but more importantly the absolute values of mean reading times were quite similar to those of subjects who were not explicitly instructed to image while reading. While it is generally difficult to interpret the absence of a difference, a tempting assumption is that this result reflects that imaginal processing required from the readers in the new experiment was in fact developed spontaneously in the first experiment. It should be recalled that people possess some sort of knowledge about the efficiency of visual imagery as an encoding strategy (cf. Denis & Carfantan, 1985). Thus it is likely that readers in fact use those strategies that they know or believe to be the most efficient in some context. Overall, recall frequencies tended to be higher in the condition with imagery instructions than in the previous condition. This difference, however, was not statistically significant.

In a further experiment, conducted with Jean-Noël Laurent, the original condition (i.e., reading without imagery instructions) was replicated, but variations in the amount of visual imagery during the processing of texts were manipulated in terms of individual differences in imagery abilities. We compared subjects who obtained high scores on visuo-spatial tests (such as the Minnesota Paper Form Board) to subjects with low scores. Not only did high scorers on these tests have significantly shorter sentence processing times for Text 1, but, more interestingly, the relative increase in their processing times for Text 2 was far smaller than was the case for low scorers, which clearly suggests that their spontaneous inclination to elaborate visuo-spatial representations placed them in better cognitive conditions when they had to deal with poorly structured verbal material. People with low visuo-spatial abilities are hampered relatively more than others in a situation where visual imagery is likely to be an appropriate strategy.

The role of images as "functional sites" encoding spatial information is certainly essential to people's representations of familiar as well as unfamiliar environments. It is relevant here to recall that in memory for geographical information, maps and schemas have been shown to function as efficient "advance organizers" of spatial information transmitted by instructional texts (e.g., Dean & Enemoh, 1983).

4. EXTENSIONS

In the final section, I will mention three new orientations which seem to hold the most promise for research on imagery and text processing.

(1) We are currently engaged in a program designed to analyze how people not only <u>recall</u> geographical information transmitted by prose, but also perform inferential computations on visual images of spatial configurations they have been informed about from prose alone (comparing distances, determining relative positions of features, and so on), in comparison with similar computations performed on representations constructed from actual perception of the configurations. More specifically, the investigation bears on the "mental scanning" of distances between different points in geographical configurations. Previous research has demonstrated that the duration of mental scanning between two points of a previously perceived configuration is proportional to the distance which separates these points on the configuration (cf. Finke & Pinker, 1982 ; Kosslyn, Ball, & Reiser, 1978). Will such chronometric regularities appear in the case of a mental representation derived from a verbal description ? Will the structural isomorphism of the representation to the actual configuration be demonstrated in the same way as when the subject was initially engaged in perceptual exploration of the configuration ?

(2) There is another way of looking at the question of the relationships between imagery and the description of spatial configurations, which consists in studying these factors in text <u>production</u> tasks. Verbal descriptions of configurations occur frequently in daily life, for instance when someone has to describe a route or a territory to another person who does not know anything about it. How will describers use their own internal representation of a configuration in order to elaborate their discourse ? How will they convert their "mental map" (which is hypothetically spatial in nature) into a discourse (whose structure is essentially linear) with the purpose of helping another person to construct in turn an internal representation as similar as possible to their own representation ? These are questions we are now beginning to tackle, with the hope they will extend our knowledge of the relationships between our internal models of the outside world and the way we externalize these models in order to communicate them to others.

(3) The third and final direction deals with the control that readers or listeners exercise over their own imagery during the processing of descriptive texts. As mentioned previously, it is likely that mental imagery developed by subjects during the processing of descriptive texts relies on some sort of metacognitive knowledge or belief about imagery processes and their potential use. Undoubtedly, this is another important aspect of individual differences as concerns processing of texts likely to elicit visual images. That is why approaches to people's knowledge of imagery processes should be more closely related to research on

situations where people have to select processing strategies suited to the constraints they identify in the situation.

REFERENCES
1. Dean, R.S., & Enemoh, P.A.C. (1983). Pictorial organization in prose learning. Contemporary Educational Psychology, 8, 20-27.
2. Denis, M. (1982). Imaging while reading text : A study on individual differences. Memory and Cognition, 10, 540-545.
3. Denis, M. (1984). Imagery and prose : A critical review of research on adults and children. Text, 4, 381-401.
4. Denis, M. (1986). Visual imagery : Effects or role in prose processing ? In F. Klix & H. Hagendorf (Eds.), Human memory and cognitive capabilities : Mechanisms and performances (pp. 237-244). Amsterdam : North-Holland.
5. Denis, M. (1987). Individual imagery differences and prose processing. In M. A. McDaniel & M. Pressley (Eds.), Imagery and related mnemonic processes : Theories, individual differences, and applications (pp. 204-217). New York : Springer-Verlag.
6. Denis, M., & Carfantan, M. (1985). People's knowledge about images. Cognition, 20, 49-60.
7. van Dijk, T.A., & Kintsch, W. (1983). Strategies of discourse comprehension. New York : Academic Press.
8. Finke, R.A., & Pinker, S. (1982). Spontaneous imagery scanning in mental extrapolation. Journal of Experimental Psychology : Learning, Memory, and Cognition, 8, 142-147.
9. Kosslyn, S.M., Ball, T.M., & Reiser, B.J. (1978). Visual images preserve metric spatial information : Evidence from studies of image scanning. Journal of Experimental Psychology : Human Perception and Performance, 4, 47-60.
10. Marks, D.F. (1973). Visual imagery differences in the recall of pictures. British Journal of Psychology, 64, 17-24.
11. Marschark, M. (1985). Imagery and organization in the recall of prose. Journal of Memory and Language, 24, 734-745.
12. Paivio, A. (1971). Imagery and verbal processes. New York : Holt, Rinehart & Winston.
13. Paivio, A. (1986). Mental representations : A dual coding approach. New York : Oxford University Press.
14. Perrig, W.J. (1986). Imagery and the thematic storage of prose. In D. G. Russell, D. F. Marks, & J.T.E. Richardson (Eds.), Imagery 2, (pp. 77-82). Dunedin, New Zealand : Human Performance Associates.
15. Perrig, W., & Kintsch, W. (1985). Propositional and situational representations of text. Journal of Memory and Language, 24, 503-518.

IMAGERY AND INTEGRATIVE PROCESSING

WERNER WIPPICH

FACHBEREICH PSYCHOLOGIE, UNIVERSITÄT TRIER, F.R.G.

ABSTRACT
The vast majority of research on the comprehension and memory of text has neglected the topic of imagery or has denied it any functional role. We report the results of three experiments that challenge this conclusion. The so-called semantic integration of propositions is seen to be heavily influenced by the concreteness of sentences. Contrary to the context availability hypothesis, this conclusion holds when texts are preceded by meaningful descriptions. Imagery may have a functional role at various levels of text processing, including an item-specific surface level as well as an integrative higher-order situation model level.

1. INTRODUCTION

Our own works in the imagery field have been heavily influenced by Paivio's dual coding model and have their roots in the memory domain. We have tried to elaborate the model, combining it with the levels of processing approach, organizational concepts, and featural/propositional accounts of semantic memory (Wippich, 1980, 1981). For episodic memory, we have preferred processing-oriented views and have thereby distinguished between verbal and imaginal coding processes (Paivio, 1971). Compared to purely verbal encoding (mostly with abstract information), imaginal encoding processes contribute specificity and distinctiveness to the episodic memory trace, which in itself is hardly a controversial assumption.

However, episodic memories cannot be fully described by levels of processing or simple imaginal attribute codings. Besides item-specific imaginal effects (see also Einstein & Hunt, 1980), we considered it necessary to postulate relational imaginal effects, accounting for concreteness effects in subjective organization or sentence memory, amongst others. This is an organizational conception that should be added to levels of processing views. In our research, we have tried to distinguish between verbal relational and imaginal relational forms of organization. Within various transfer situations, we have consistently found positive transfer with concrete information and imaginal organization instructions, and negative transfer with abstract information and verbal organization instructions. These and other results have been interpreted as evidence for a second-stage imaginal process: Imaginal attributes (first-stage encodings) may be related by organizational processes (second-stage) into memory units that can be

133

M. Denis et al. (eds.), Cognitive and Neuropsychological Approaches to Mental Imagery, 133–142.
© 1988 by Martinus Nijhoff Publishers.

used efficiently and flexibly in new situations and for other purposes. Verbal attributes may be related by verbal processes, resulting in more rigidly structured and less transferable higher-order memory units.

2. IMAGERY AND INTEGRATIVE PROSE PROCESSING

Whereas the relational encoding function of imagery seems to be well-established within word-list experimentation, a more neglected research-topic is the relational use of imagery in prose processing. Up to now, imagery has not been well-accepted within mainstream prose processing research. There are various reasons for this. First, many people find it implausible that prose messages can be encoded as a continuously changing stream of mental images. Secondly, the most influential models of text processing had relied almost exclusively on abstract-propositional representation assumptions (e.g., Kintsch & van Dijk, 1978). Thirdly, it has been argued that mental imagery is well-suited to making rather meaningless or isolated information more meaningful. With more meaningful materials, such as prose passages, this function of imagery is seen as being irrelevant (see, for example, Marschark, 1985). Finally, and this was our empirical starting point, there have been demonstrations of apparently similar processing results with abstract and concrete prose.

Take, for example, the well-known demonstrations of so-called semantic integration by Bransford and his co-workers. Bransford & Franks (1971) asked their subjects to listen to a set of sentences that together defined so-called complex ideas. In their initial experiments, a complex concrete idea such as "The blue-eyed girl looked out the window that was facing the large garden" contained four simple elements or propositions ("The girl was blue-eyed", for example). Acquisition sentences contained one, two, three, or four of such elements from any one of four different complex ideas. At incidental recognition testing, subjects received sentences, containing one, two, three, or four elements of each idea, some of them previously heard ("old"), some of them new. Their confidence that a sentence had been presented at acquisition was reported to vary directly with the number of elements of a particular complex idea that it contained (a so-called linearity effect). Furthermore, there was little discrimination in evaluating "old" and "new" test sentences containing an equal number of elements. Finally, so-called noncases, containing elements that mixed various idea units together, were considered to be new information by the subjects, and rejected.

As a plausible interpretation, Bransford & Franks (1971) proposed that the subjects had lost information on the specific acquisition sentences (no old-new discrimination). Instead, subjects had abstracted or integrated the propositional content to construct holistic semantic ideas. The correlation between the confidence ratings and the number of elements of test sentences was taken to imply that recognition judgments had been based upon the degree of overlap between a test sentence and the semantic relations that had been constructed into holistic idea complexes. The rejection of noncases was seen as evidence that information not consistently overlapping with these constructed ideas is easily identified as new.

As these initial experiments dealt exclusively with concrete information, one may regard the findings as entirely consistent with an imaginal organization position. Franks & Bransford (1972), however, reported similar results with abstract information (such as "The arrogant attitude expressed in the speech led to immediate criticism"). Thus, the authors concluded that the synthesis of information into holistic representations occurs in the case of both concrete and abstract information and does not depend upon any form of mental imagery. Thus, the concept of imaginal relational processes was called into question for prose memories (see also Richardson, 1985).

3. EXPERIMENT 1: AN EXTENDED REPLICATION

As Bransford & Franks had done two separate experiments, we decided to plan a further study, comparing concrete and abstract ideas directly within the same experiment (Wippich & Bredenkamp, 1979). We used the same materials and procedures as Bransford. Additionally, the instructions at recognition testing were varied. Since this manipulation did not change our results and conclusions, I will only report those results that are directly comparable to the work of Bransford. As can be seen from Table 1, the results of the Bransford group have been essentially replicated.

TABLE 1. Mean "recognition confidence" as measured by a 10-point scale ranging from +5 (very confident that the item was seen before) to -5 (very confident that the item was not seen before). Data from Wippich & Bredenkamp (1979).

		Four	Three	Two	One	Noncases
Con-crete	old	4.94	2.53	2.05	-0.03	-4.65
	new	3.38	2.93	1.62	-1.21	
Ab-stract	old	2.45	2.53	1.36	-0.16	-0.63
	new	3.53	2.60	0.98	-0.83	

Since we found similar linearity effects for concrete and abstract test sentences, containing from four to one propositions, and rather poor discriminations among "old" and "new" information, the results seem to corroborate the position of Bransford and his co-workers. But there was one important exception. As may be seen from Table 1, our subjects performed rather poorly on abstract noncases (51 % of false alarms), whereas false positives were rare with concrete noncases (4 %). Since other researchers have reported similar concreteness effects for noncases (Moeser, 1975; Kamil, Schultz & Bernbach,

1980), we had serious doubts about the so-called semantic integration of abstract sentences. If subjects accept abstract noncases that are clearly incompatible with presumably constructed ideas, the whole process of construction seems to be at stake. As others have expressed even more general concerns about the utility of the Bransford/Franks-type paradigm (e. g., James & Hillinger, 1977; Moeser, 1982), we decided to take a new look on the concreteness dimension with regard to integrative prose processing.

4. EXPERIMENT 2: INSTRUCTIONS TO INTEGRATE SENTENCES

This time, we were more directly concerned with integrative processing. Subjects heard either concrete or abstract sentences that had been taken from the Bransford-Franks pool. We presented them four of the so-called "ones", that is, sentences containing one proposition of the complex idea (such as "The girl was blue-eyed" or "The attitude was arrogant"). According to Hupet & LeBouedec (1977), integration should be facilitated if sentences are given in the order in which they constitute an idea unit. Therefore, sentences from three units were either presented in a meaningful order or in a randomly mixed order. Thus, the 2x2 between-subjects design consisted of two factors: Concreteness of sentences and Presentation order.

Subjects had been informed of potential relations among the simple sentences and were asked to integrate information "belonging together". Having heard the sentences two times, subjects were asked to recall all the information that "went together" in one sentence or at least on one line. Finally, they received three main concepts from each unit (such as "girl" or "attitude") plus three "new" related distractors for recognition. Subjects had to mark "old" concepts and to mark those concepts that belonged to the same idea complex with the same sign.

The main results can be seen in Table 2. Consider first the

TABLE 2. Mean recognition, recall, and "integrative" performance for concrete and abstract sentences.

	Concrete	Abstract
Hit rate	0.95	0.85
False alarm rate	0.19	0.58
Recall	0.82	0.51
Integration (given hits)	0.92	0.62
Integration (given recall)	1.00	0.84

simple recognition and recall findings (e.g., the first three lines of Table 2). As can be seen, there were strong and significant concreteness effects on these measures (and no effects of presentation order), thus corroborating our expectations for item-specific encoding advantages of concrete information. To examine integrative processing, we derived several measures that took into account the strong concreteness effects in simple memory testing. All of these measures indicated significant concreteness effects. For example, given recognition of "old" concepts (hits), subjects were perfectly successful in grouping together recognized concepts if they belonged to the same concrete idea unit. Even if we disregard the high false alarm rate for abstract information and consider only those abstract concepts that had been recognized as "old" (hits), subjects had some difficulties to mark those recognized concepts that belonged to the same abstract idea unit. Furthermore, for recall we found an interaction: Whereas integrative processing of concrete information was independent of presentation order, abstract information processing was facilitated by a meaningful presentation order. But even in the latter case, the integration of recalled abstract information did not raise to the level of concrete information integration. This result was predicted, as well. With word-lists, strong dependence on presentation order was only observed for the recall of abstract information, giving rise to our hypothesis that imaginal processing may be more flexible and less dependent on external cues.

Do these findings indicate a functional role for imagery in integrative prose processing? Our results had been deduced from a certain theoretical perspective, and thus it is legitimate to argue that they are not at variance with these theoretical stances. It can be argued that there are confoundings of the concreteness variable with other, potentially relevant predictors of recall and integration (such as the comprehensibility, for example). But this line of reasoning is also behind theories predicting no differences in integrative processing with abstract and concrete information (and having used the same materials).

5. EXPERIMENT 3: CONTEXT AVAILABILITY AND INTEGRATION

To test the validity of our hypotheses more strictly against other alternatives, a further investigation was conducted. First, one of the currently most influential alternative interpretations for our data is the so-called context-availability position (Kieras, 1978; Schwanenflugel & Shoben, 1983). According to this largely nonimaginal view, concrete information has simply much more overlap with semantic memory information than abstract information. It is easier to comprehend since there is less structure to be built in episodic memory. And it is easier to retrieve since there will be abundant retrieval paths from semantic memory to the new, episodic information. Concreteness effects should be at a minimum, if the processing of abstract information is made more meaningful by embedding abstract information within relevant contextual information.

Second, fashions of theorizing about prose processing are rapidly changing. Former, predominantly "propositional" formulations by Kintsch & van Dijk (1978) have been criticized as "too elementaristic". A new generation of theories attempts to describe the construction of mental representations basically with the help of more holistic structures such as mental models or situation models (Garnham, 1981; Johnson-Laird, 1984). Van Dijk & Kintsch (1983) themselves actually describe the results of text processing at essentially three levels, called the surface level, the propositional representation or text-base, and the situation model. By using different dependent variables, we aimed at a more precise investigation of what level or levels concreteness effects are to be expected, as there is no clear evidence on this problem (Perrig & Kintsch, 1985).

In our last experiment, concreteness was varied as before, but this time as a within-subjects variable. That is, subjects read simple concrete and abstract sentences, belonging to five concrete and five abstract idea units. Sentences of one unit were always presented in a meaningful order. As an example for concrete information, the subjects read the following four sentences: "The girl was blue-eyed", "The girl looked out the window", "The window was facing the garden", "The garden was large". A corresponding example for abstract information is given by the following four sentences: "The attitude was arrogant", "The attitude was expressed in the speech", "The speech led to criticism", "The criticism was strong". In order to manipulate the variable of context availability, some subjects received a brief introduction before reading the four sentences. Concerning the "attitude episode", for example, the following context preceded the information: "The coalition reacted to the reproaches of the opposition leader, after having registered agitation in the public". The following introduction was written for the "girl episode": "Fritz, having inspected the surroundings of the vacation house, informed his parents, still out of breath". According to the context availability position, one should expect at least diminished concreteness effects in text processing, if context embeddings are made explicit.

Besides context, we varied two further factors: Sentences were presented either "separately" (that is, only one sentence was visibly available at one time) or "simultaneously" (previously presented sentences of one unit remained in view with a new sentence presentation). Furthermore, subjects were given either simple understanding instructions for each sentence or instructions to connect all given information in each unit. We will only briefly comment on the effects of these independent variables. Subjects were warned that they would be questioned afterwards (form not specified). The presentation of each sentence was self-paced. Encoding times were recorded but will not be reported here.

In order to measure retention of surface level information (and, according to our view, consequences of item-specific processing), we used a recognition scenario. The subjects had to make judgments on all 50 old abstract and concrete main concepts and on an equal number of similar distractors. The results can be seen on the first two lines of Table 3. As expected, we found clear and strong concreteness effects with this measure (without any interactions). In addition, there was also a positive effect of a simultaneous presentation procedure, especially if this form of presentation was used in combination with context information. The latter results are of lesser importance. Nevertheless, they show that at least some of our manipulations besides concreteness had been successful (in the sense of being influential). Despite this efficiency of our design and investigation, it is noteworthy that there was only a main effect of the concreteness variable, as has been mentioned previously.

To measure integrative processing at a presumably text-base level, we used a reconstruction task. The subjects received all 50 old concepts from the sentences in order to attribute them to lines, representing the 10 idea units. With different calculations, we always found strong concreteness effects without any interactions (see Table 3). The given value in

TABLE 3. Mean recognition, "integrative", and inference performance for concrete and abstract materials.

	Concrete	Abstract
Hit rate	0.84	0.67
False alarm rate	0.13	0.22
Integration index from reconstruction test	0.74	0.37
Accept correct inference	0.79	0.72
Accept false inference	0.13	0.26
Accept correct plus reject false inference	0.68	0.56
Forced choice inference	0.93	0.84

Table 3 reflects the mean performance on all concrete or abstract idea units. That is, a subject could only receive a score of 1.00, if she or he had written all main concepts of each idea unit on one line. But even the selection of the best performances on an abstract and concrete idea unit did not affect our conclusions. Contextual information did not reduce this integration effect. In addition to these results, instructions to connect the sentences as well as simultaneous presentation conditions were helpful to integrative processing, especially if given in combination. Furthermore, instructions to connect semantic information were more successfully applied in combination with contextual information. The latter results again show the sensitivity of our design and of the integration index.

Finally, to assess integrative processing at a presumably situation model-level of representation, we measured the ability of the subjects to draw inferences from the texts. Subjects had to judge from each unit one plausible (such as "The attitude caused the criticism") and one false inference (the converse of the plausible inference, e.g., "The criticism caused the attitude"). Inferencing was tested in a single-item judgment procedure, where the order of plausible and false

inferences to the same unit had been randomized, and then was
tested in a forced-choice procedure. In the latter case, the
subjects had to choose between one plausible and false inference for each unit. At single-item testing, there was again a
concreteness effect without any interactions (see Table 3).
This effect was stronger when only those items had been evaluated as correct, where the subjects had accepted the plausible inference, and additionally rejected the corresponding
false inference (see Table 3). Furthermore, instructions to
connect semantic information from related sentences were helpful again. The latter effect was more pronounced in combination with given contextual information.

At forced-choice testing, we again found a significant concreteness effect (see Table 3). But this and only this time,
there was also a triple interaction involving the concreteness
variable. Abstract information inferencing reached the level
of correct inferences from concrete texts, if and only if
sentence presentations had been made simultaneously and in
combination with instructions to connect related information
from the sentences.

The main results may be summarized briefly. We found strong
concreteness effects at various levels of text processing. At
a surface level of representation, concepts from concrete
texts were recognized much better than concepts from abstract
texts. Corresponding to a text-base level, the reconstruction
of idea units was seen to be more complete and more precise if
the subjects had to work with concrete (versus abstract)
concepts from the texts. And the ability to make inferences
from text (presumably a performance that depends on a situation model) was clearly superior with concrete materials. It
remains to be seen if these results can be generalized to
other sorts of texts and to other testing conditions. For
example, with longer and perhaps more natural texts, Marschark
(1985) was not able to find any differences in the remembering
of concrete versus abstract texts. In our data, there were
some hints that concreteness effects may be missing at a
macro-level of text processing under certain testing conditions (a forced-choice procedure in inference testing) and
processing conditions (simultaneous sentence presentations
plus instructions to connect related information). On the
other hand, the context availability hypothesis must be rejected as a major alternative to an imaginal interpretation of
our data. Providing our subjects with short introductions to
the texts did not reduce any effects of the concreteness
variable.

6. CONCLUSIONS AND PERSPECTIVES

The results that have been reported are positive as concerns
the functional role of imagery within the domain of text
processing. If imagery research is to stay with us, it is
important to demonstrate the usefulness of imagery for practical purposes aside from word-list experimentation. At a minimum, we were able to show that largely nonimaginal views in
the area of semantic integration research are clearly deficient.

It remains to be seen if the reported concreteness effects are really based on images, especially on relational-imaginal processing. Subjects' reports seem to be consistent with this view. I still find it plausible that images are involved in text-processing, at a surface level as well as at integration levels. But I do not think that subjects really store images to a large extent as a consequence of concrete text processing (see Kieras, 1978). Images may be useful in extracting and combining main ideas, for example, but only some information may be stored in the format of mental images.

We are currently trying to specify the basis of the reported concreteness effects. The third experiment that has been described will be replicated. In addition to the "normal" procedure, we will make use of a secondary visuo-spatial suppression task. This distraction task should involve the hypothetical imaginal system. It will be used at the encoding stage or at retrieval. Our expectations are clear-cut: If our results do not depend on the storage of mental images, one should expect equally strong concreteness effects with or without a visuo-spatial distraction task at retrieval. On the other hand, if integrative processing of concrete information at encoding is based on the activation of mental images, such distraction tasks should selectively hamper the processing of concrete information at encoding. Furthermore, a selective impairment of concrete information-processing at encoding should be more pronounced with higher levels of processing (such as a text-base or a situation model).

REFERENCES

1. Bransford, J.D. & Franks, J.J. (1971). The abstraction of linguistic ideas. Cognitive Psychology, 2, 331-350.
2. Einstein, G.O. & Hunt, R.R. (1980). Levels of processing and organization: Additive effects of individual item and relational processing. Journal of Experimental Psychology: Human Learning and Memory, 6, 588-598.
3. Franks, J.J. & Bransford, J.D. (1972). The acquisition of abstract ideas. Journal of Verbal Learning and Verbal Behavior, 11, 311-315.
4. Garnham, A. (1981). Mental models as representations of text. Memory & Cognition, 9, 560-565.
5. Hupet, M. & LeBouedec, B. (1977). The given-new contract and the constructive aspect of memory for ideas. Journal of Verbal Learning and Verbal Behavior, 16, 711-721.
6. James, C.T. & Hillinger, M.L. (1977). The role of confusion in the semantic integration paradigm. Journal of Verbal Learning and Verbal Behavior, 16, 711-721.
7. Johnson-Laird, P.N. (1984). Mental models. Cambridge: Cambridge University Press.
8. Kamil, M.L., Schultz, E.E. & Bernbach, H.A. (1980). Linguistic integration during recognition testing. Bulletin of the Psychonomic Society, 16, 353-355.
9. Kieras, D. (1978). Beyond pictures and words: Alternative information-processing models for imagery effects in verbal memory. Psychological Bulletin, 85, 532-554.

10. Kintsch, W. & van Dijk, T.A. (1978). Toward a model of text comprehension and production. Psychological Review, 85, 363-394.
11. Marschark, M. (1985). Imagery and organization in the recall of prose. Journal of Memory and Language, 24, 734-745.
12. Moeser, S.D. (1975). The integration of verbal ideas. Canadian Journal of Psychology, 29, 106-123.
13. Moeser, S.D. (1982). Memory integration and memory interference. Canadian Journal of Psychology, 36, 165-188.
14. Paivio, A. (1971). Imagery and verbal processes. New York: Holt, Rinehart, and Winston.
15. Perrig, W. & Kintsch, W. (1985). Propositional and situational representations of text. Journal of Memory and Language, 24, 503-518.
16. Richardson, J.T.E. (1985). Integration versus decomposition in the retention of complex ideas. Memory & Cognition, 13, 112-127.
17. Schwanenflugel, P.J. & Shoben, E.J. (1983). Differential context effects in the comprehension of abstract and concrete verbal materials. Journal of Experimental Psychology: Learning, Memory, and Cognition, 9, 82-102.
18. Van Dijk, T.A. & Kintsch, W. (1983). Strategies of discourse comprehension. New York: Academic Press.
19. Wippich, W. (1980). Bildhaftigkeit und Organisation. Darmstadt: Steinkopff.
20. Wippich, W. (1981). Die duale Kode-Theorie und die Konzeption der Analysestufen. Zeitschrift für Semiotik, 3, 295-310.
21. Wippich, W. & Bredenkamp, J. (1979). Bildhaftigkeit und Lernen. Darmstadt: Steinkopff.

METAMEMORY-MEMORY CONNECTIONS AND THEIR DEVELOPMENT
UNDER IMAGINAL ENCODING CONDITIONS

SILVIA MECKLENBRÄUKER

FACHBEREICH I - PSYCHOLOGIE, UNIVERSITÄT TRIER, F.R.G.

ABSTRACT
   The main purpose of the present study was to investigate the relationship between children's knowledge about effects of imagery on memory, and their memory performance. Developmental trends in this relationship were also examined under different encoding conditions and in two different learning tasks: associative and prose learning. No substantial connections between metamnemonic knowledge and recall performance were observed. The assumption that children with better knowledge about imagery will be better able to benefit from an imaginal encoding mode was not supported.

1. INTRODUCTION
   To date imagery research dealing with the influence of imagery on children's memory has primarily been concerned with the effects of imagery instructions and/or the consequences of varying learning materials (cf., e. g., Levin, 1981, 1983; Pressley, 1977). There is a lack of studies, however, which investigate children's - and also adults' - knowledge about imagery phenomena. Denis & Carfantan (in press) conducted a study on young adults' knowledge about imagery. Their results indicate that young adults have an excellent knowledge about the effects of imagery on learning and memory, but very few have an accurate understanding of the inner mechanisms of image processing, such as those revealed by mental rotation and mental scanning. The main purpose of the present study was to investigate age-related changes in children's knowledge of the effects of imagery on memory, and to examine developmental trends in the relationship between such knowledge and memory performance in two different memory tasks: in a simple associative and in a more complex prose memory task.
   In general, results demonstrate positive effects of imagery on children's associative and prose learning. Providing pictorial elaborations in a paired-associate learning task, i. e., presenting the pair-mates in the form of interactive pictures, improves memory compared to an unelaborated presentation mode throughout childhood (cf. Pressley, 1977). There is also little doubt that illustrations which overlap text facilitate children's recall of the content of this text (cf. Levin, 1981; Levin & Lesgold, 1978). Although preschoolers can take advantage of an imagery strategy if provided with pictures, the ability to benefit from instructions to generate images shows a developmental trend, with younger children profiting

143

M. Denis et al. (eds.), Cognitive and Neuropsychological Approaches to Mental Imagery, 143–152.

less than older ones (cf. Pressley, 1977). Available evidence
indicates that imagery instruction effects in children's prose
learning appear to lag a few years behind similar effects in
associative learning (cf. Pressley, 1977). By 5 to 6 years of
age, children can benefit from simple instructions to generate
interactive images when they learn picture or object pairings.
By 7 to 8, they can apply the strategy to purely verbal material. In prose memory, however, instructions to generate images of a story's content fail to facilitate recall of children younger than 8 or 9 years of age. Even 9-year-olds still
need training to benefit from imagery instructions.

Several factors may account for the efficiency of imagery in
learning and memory tasks (cf. Marschark, Richman, Yuille, &
Hunt, in press). First, information can be processed by two
systems, a verbal and an imaginal system (a dual coding approach, see Paivio, 1971). Furthermore, compared to purely
verbal encodings, imaginal encoding processes contribute specificity and distinctiveness to the memory trace. A third
class of interpretations of imagery effects has been based on
the apparent unitary organization of imaginal information.
Imagery is seen as a process particularly suited to interre-
lating units of information into higher-organized structures.
Separate pieces of information, e. g., stimulus and response
items in paired-associate learning, can be combined in a
complex image and can be represented as an integrated unit in
memory. In prose learning an imagery strategy may help to
organize the content by forcing integration of information
that otherwise would only have been encoded in fragments (cf.
Levin, 1981). The concept of imaginal relational processes,
however, has been called into question for prose memories
(cf., e. g., Richardson, 1985).

In educational practice, the use of illustrations and imagery-based learning strategies (e. g., Levin, 1983) are considered to be valuable methods designed to improve prose processing in children. Research results, however, are not as clear-
cut as is often depicted in the literature. With simple narrative prose, imagery instructions often did not improve recall
and, when they did, effects were often minimal (cf. Levin,
1981). Furthermore, effects of imagery are dependent on many
factors (cf. Levin, 1983; Levin & Lesgold, 1978), for example:
class of prose material, organization of text (imagery effects
are assumed to be less pronounced when texts are well organized), type of pictures, and, most important, learner characteristics. In order for pictures to "work", they must activate
certain information processing skills within the learner (cf.
Levin, 1981). An imaginal encoding mode seems to be an optional processing mode, not an obligatory one. One of the main
aims of our study was to test the assumption that children's
ability to profit from imagery may partly be influenced by
their knowledge about imagery.

Children's knowledge about imagery is part of their metamemory, i. e., their knowledge about memory states and processes
(Flavell, 1978). Although a stable and high correlation between metamemory and memory behavior is not always to be
expected (cf. Flavell, 1978), it was one of the most frequent

arguments in favor of studying metamemory that, in general, there should be a close relationship between metamemory and performance in various memory tasks.

Empirical results are mixed. Many studies yielded only moderate or low correlations between metamemory and memory (for a review, see Cavanaugh & Perlmutter, 1982). However, in a meta-analysis of existing correlational findings, Schneider (1985) comes to a different conclusion. His comprehensive analysis of the metamemory-memory behavior relationship yields a complex but generally more positive pattern than recently was assumed in the literature. A substantial metamemory-memory link, however, is not likely to be obtained under all conditions. Available evidence suggests that the relationship between metamemory and memory may be stronger for older children, and that subtests involving task-specific metamnemonic knowledge may be among the best predictors of memory behavior (see Schneider, 1985). Therefore it seems reasonable to assume that children who have better knowledge about imagery will also be more capable of benefitting from an imaginal encoding mode. This relationship should be stronger for older children, or it may even be substantial for older children alone.

Our study consists of two experiments, a paired-associate and a prose learning experiment. In both experiments, imagery was manipulated by varying both learning material and instructions. Memory was tested immediately and one week later. In addition to task-specific metamnemonic knowledge, i. e., knowledge about imagery, we also assessed our subjects' general metamnemonic knowledge. Furthermore, measures of verbal and nonverbal intelligence and of reflection-impulsivity of cognitive style were included in order to test whether task-specific knowledge would be a better predictor of memory performance than these other variables. Reflection-impulsivity of cognitive style was also assessed as an indicator of general information processing strategies. We assumed that the metamemory-memory connection should be stronger for reflective children because their metamnemonic knowledge is more likely to evoke certain metacognitive strategies.

2. THE PAIRED-ASSOCIATE EXPERIMENT (EXPERIMENT 1)

60 kindergartners, 60 second graders, and 60 fourth graders participated in Experiment 1. They were tested individually in three sessions. Different groups of subjects received standard learning instructions, instructions to generate separate images of the pair-mates, or instructions to generate interactive images involving pair-mates. The two imagery instruction groups were given an example on which they could practise, but received no training. The type of learning material (pictures vs. words) and the mode of presentation (elaborated vs. unelaborated) were varied in a within-subject design such that each child had to learn four different types of items: separate (i. e., unelaborated) words, separate pictures, verbal claborations (i. e., sentences involving pair-mates, e. g., "the fish plays guitar") and pictorial elaborations (i. e., interactive pictures of pair-mates, e. g., a colored drawing which shows a fish playing guitar). Older children received

more study items than younger ones. The dependent measure was the number of correctly recalled response items after one presentation of the pair-mates.

Recall results largely confirm previous findings. As was expected (cf. Pressley, 1977), kindergartners only benefitted from an interactive imagery instruction when they learned pictorial material, but not verbal material. Contrary to previous findings, an interactive imagery instruction did not significantly improve recall performance in second graders. There was, however, a tendency in the expected direction. Fourth graders only benefitted from an interactive imagery strategy on immediate recall of unelaborated items. As in previous research, children of all age groups clearly benefitted from pictorial elaborations provided by the experimenter. In immediate recall, pictorial elaborations were recalled best, followed by verbal elaborations, and separate pictures. Separate words were recalled worst (significant main effects of Elaboration and Picture, no interaction). This pattern of results holds for all age groups. The advantage of pictures compared to words - both for elaborated and unelaborated presentation modes - was greatest for kindergartners. This result is not consistent with views taken by Reese (1970) and some findings which support them (cf. Pressley, 1977). Reese (1970) suggested that the ability to benefit from pictorial elaborations increases with age. In delayed recall, children of all age groups profited from pictorial elaborations, but only fourth graders benefitted from verbal elaborations. Kindergartners and second graders remembered pictorial elaborations better than the three other types of material, which did not differ.

Children's general metamnemonic knowledge was tapped by a metamemory battery consisting of eight items, most of which were originally developed by Kreutzer, Leonard, & Flavell (1975). Each item was given a score of 1 (correct answer with relevant argument) or 0. Children's knowledge about imagery was assessed by asking them to rank the four versions of an item used in this study in terms of the easiest to the most difficult to learn, that is, the four versions of an item (separate words, separate pictures, pictorial elaboration, and verbal elaboration) were presented and had to be ranked. In order to test the consistency of judgments, several items had to be judged. Furthermore, task-specific knowledge was assessed both before and after the learning task in order to gain information about possible changes in knowledge as a consequence of experience with the task and in order to test the assumption that stronger metamemory-memory links are obtained with post-learning metamnemonic knowledge. Only knowledge of characteristics of the learning material was assessed since pre-tests had indicated that questions about the effects of various instructions and about possible interactions between instructions and type of material were too complex for the kindergartners.

Our results clearly show that even preschoolers have metacognitive awareness of the importance of pictorial elaborations. As can be seen from Table 1, both preschoolers and school children knew that pictorial elaborations are easiest and separate words are most difficult to remember. An age-related improvement in task-specific knowledge from kindergarten to second grade was observed. Although even the school children underestimated the memorability of verbal elaborations, they were more aware of the importance of them (see Table 1), and were more consistent in their judgments than the

Table 1. Mean rankings of the four presentation modes of an item (only children with relatively consistent judgments). PE = pictorial elaboration, VE = verbal elaboration, P = unelaborated picture, W = unelaborated word; 1 = easiest to remember, 4 = most difficult to remember.

Grade	First assessment				Second assessment			
	PE	VE	P	W	PE	VE	P	W
KG	1.52	3.17	2.08	3.25	1.51	2.95	2.32	3.22
2nd	1.54	2.87	2.37	3.22	1.56	2.69	2.46	3.29
4th	1.68	2.48	2.54	3.28	1.73	2.41	2.53	3.33

preschoolers. Furthermore, more second and fourth graders than kindergartners gave the "correct" ranking (i. e., pictorial elaboration > verbal elaboration > unelaborated picture > unelaborated word). Thirty-five percent of the fourth graders (of those with relatively consistent judgments), 33 % of the second graders, but only 9 % of the kindergartners were perfect.

A measure of a child's task-specific knowledge was obtained as follows: Since even the preschoolers' rankings were relatively consistent (as concordance coefficients showed), we calculated the rank order correlation (Kendall's tau) between a child's mean ranking and the "correct" ranking. A combination of the concordance and the tau coefficients was used as an indicator of a child's task-specific knowledge. Contrary to our expectations, results consistently show no relationship

Table 2. Table of frequencies relating pre-learning task-specific knowledge (good vs. poor) to immediate memory performance (good vs. poor).

		Kindergarten		Second grade		Fourth grade	
		Knowledge		Knowledge		Knowledge	
		Good	Poor	Good	Poor	Good	Poor
Mem-	Good	13	18	14	17	13	18
ory	Poor	10	19	21	8	14	15

between children's task-specific metamnemonic knowledge and
their recall performance. Contingency analyses indicate no
systematic differences or even negative associations (see
Table 2). This finding holds for all age groups, pre-learning
and post-learning knowledge, all instructional conditions, and
for recall of pictorial and verbal material. Furthermore,
substantial correlations between general metamnemonic knowledge and memory performance were not obtained. A positive
metamemory-memory link was not even observed for reflective
children.

3. THE PROSE LEARNING EXPERIMENT (EXPERIMENT 2)

As in Experiment 1, 60 kindergartners, 60 second graders,
and 60 fourth graders participated in three sessions. We used
a 3 (instructions) x 2 (picture vs. no picture) design with
repeated measures on the second factor. Subjects received
standard learning instructions, simple imagery instructions
(i. e., instructions to generate separate images according to
the content of each sentence), or complex imagery instructions
(i. e., instructions to image the content of a story as in a
film). A complex imagery instruction is assumed to be comparable to an interactive imagery instruction in a paired-associate learning task and should promote integrative text processing. Children in the imagery groups were told that the
proposed strategy would help them remember the stories, and
they were given an example to practise this strategy. They
received no strategy training. Subjects heard four short stories under intentional learning conditions, whereby different
stories were used in the different age groups. Kindergartners
heard stories consisting of 18 idea units (i. e., simple
clauses). The stories told to the second and fourth graders
contained 21 and 24 idea units, respectively. The stories were
constructed according to the formal story grammar used by
Stein & Glenn (1979). Half of the stories each child heard
were illustrated. Colored drawings depicted the content of six
idea units, one out of each category (setting, initiating
event, internal reaction, attempt, consequence, and reaction)
of the story grammar. Children had to recall the stories and
subsequently were asked 'explicit' and 'implicit' questions.
The 'explicit' questions asked for information explicitly
stated in the text, whereas in order to answer the 'implicit'
questions children had to draw inferences and/or to integrate
information from different parts of the story.

The recall protocols were scored for the number of idea
units recalled. As expected, kindergartners recalled more idea
units from illustrated than from nonillustrated stories, both
in the immediate (25 % vs. 21 %) and in the delayed test (23 %
vs. 21 %). The effect was rather small in magnitude, but it
must be taken into account that the pictures depicted only
part of the stories' content. Pictures had no effect on the
number of correctly answered 'explicit' questions (83 % and 79
%), but led to more correct answers to 'implicit' questions
(69 % vs. 62 %). This result may be due to the organizational
function of imagery, since children had to integrate information in order to answer 'implicit' questions. Surprisingly,

neither second graders nor fourth graders could remember more idea units from illustrated stories than from nonillustrated ones (41 % and 40 % in immediate recall and 38 % and 39 % in delayed recall for second graders; 53 % and 53 % in immediate recall and 43 % and 42 % in delayed recall for fourth graders). Our data show that pictures weakly facilitated second and fourth graders' recall performance for some of the stories, whereas illustrations had a slightly detrimental effect for other stories. Therefore it is reasonable to assume that at least some of the illustrations used were not optimal.

The result that neither kindergartners nor second graders could benefit from complex imagery instructions is in line with previous findings (cf. Pressley, 1977). The finding that the fourth graders could not profit from this strategy either is not surprising, since available evidence indicates that 9- to 10-year-olds need training to benefit from it. Furthermore, complex imagery instructions did not improve recall of illustrated stories where the pictures may have served as continued concrete reminders to visualize the stories' content (cf. Dunham & Levin, 1979, for a similar finding). Separate imagery instructions impaired immediate recall performance in kindergartners and delayed recall performance in second graders. Presumably, an instruction to generate many tiny images hinders an integrative processing of the text.

In assessing children's knowledge about imagery we were not primarily interested in whether they are aware of the positive effects of pictures on prose recall. Rather, we wanted to know whether they base their judgments on quantitative aspects (e. g., three pictures are better than one, or any irrelevant picture is better than no picture) or whether they mainly take into account qualitative aspects of pictures (e. g., three pictures depicting important ideas are more useful than three pictures illustrating less important ideas). Children had to rank the following six types of illustrations in terms of their usefulness for prose memory: 3 pictures depicting important and 3 depicting less important ideas, 3 similar pictures of the protagonist, 1 picture of the protagonist, no picture, and 1 irrelevant picture. Since this task turned out to be too difficult for the kindergartners, pair-wise comparisons were also required. Again, task-specific knowledge was assessed twice, after the immediate and after the delayed recall test, respectively. Each time, two stories had to be judged.

There were two measures of task-specific knowledge. First, one point was given for each correct answer in making the paired comparisons. Second, rank order correlations were calculated between a child's ranking and the "correct" ranking. This measure, however, was only taken into account for the school-age children (see above). Our results show only small improvements in knowledge from kindergarten to second grade, but a notable change from second to fourth grade. For example, only one second grader was perfect in the ranking task (first assessment) as opposed to 19 fourth graders. Accordingly, nearly all kindergartners (91.5 %) and second graders (85 %) based their judgments on quantitative or irrelevant aspects (e. g., this picture is so beautiful), whereas about 60 % of the fourth graders emphasized qualitative aspects.

What about the relationship between task-specific metamnemonic knowledge and memory perfomance in prose learning? Contingency analyses indicate no connections for kindergartners
and fourth graders, and moderate but significant positive
connections (ϕ = .30 and ϕ = .27 for immediate and delayed
recall) for second graders (see Table 3). This finding holds
for all instructional conditions.

Table 3. Table of frequencies relating task-specific knowledge (first assessment) to immediate recall performance (number of correctly recalled idea units).

		Kindergarten		Second grade		Fourth grade	
		Knowledge		Knowledge		Knowledge	
		Good	Poor	Good	Poor	Good	Poor
Re-	Good	16	14	19	11	15	16
call	Poor	16	14	10	20	15	14

For kindergartners and fourth graders, substantial correlations between general metamnemonic knowledge and memory performance were not obtained, either. For second graders, however, not only task-specific knowledge but also general metamnemonic knowledge and cognitive style were positively related
to memory performance.

4. SUMMARY AND PERSPECTIVES
In general, our results do not support the assumption that
children with better knowledge about imagery will be more
capable of benefitting from an imaginal encoding mode. A
moderately positive relationship between task-specific metamemory and memory performance was obtained only for second
graders' prose learning. This finding is surprising, since a
positive metamemory-memory link was assumed to be more likely
in older children and/or in a simpler memory task. Further
research should focus on whether this connection in second
graders remains significant after the impact of other potentially relevant predictors of memory performance, such as
general metamnemonic knowledge or cognitive style, has been
partialled out. The present results are only preliminary. A
latent variable causal modeling approach will be applied to
study the relationship between metamemory and memory more adequately. Furthermore, we will examine the question of whether
imagery improves recall of important ideas and/or of less
important ideas of stories. This question is an interesting
one as regards the distinction between prose-learning strategies that seem to be well suited to the processing of the main
ideas of a text (macrostructure strategies), and strategies
that seemingly are intended for the processing of details
(microstructure strategies) (cf. Levin, 1982).

A good deal of research remains to be accomplished on the relationship between children's knowledge about imagery and memory performance in different tasks and on the development of this relationship. Particularly studies with upper elementary school children appear to be promising for future research in this field since in several tasks substantial meta-memory-memory links have been obtained for seventh or eighth graders alone (see Schneider, 1985).

A very interesting question concerns the relationship between children's knowledge about imagery and their imagery abilities. Denis & Carfantan (in press) showed that young adults had an excellent knowledge about the usefulness of imagery in learning and memory. This was true for subjects with high and low imagery abilities. According to the authors, this result lends support to the idea that subjects' statements about the usefulness of imagery should not be taken as reliable indicators of the likelihood that they will make actual use of imagery in cognitive processing.

Assessment methods of task-specific metamemory need to be improved in future studies. For example, children's knowledge of the effects of different instructions should also be investigated. More importantly, metacognitive strategies must be taken into account. They can be regarded as the link between statable knowledge about memory and memory performance. In order to influence memory performance, knowledge must evoke certain metacognitive strategies. In our study, reflection-impulsivity of cognitive style was assessed as an indicator of general information processing strategies. We assumed that the metamemory-memory connection should be stronger for reflective children. However, this assumption could not be supported.

Last but not least, longitudinal studies are needed in order to draw conclusions on the development, durability, and generalizability of the metamemory-memory link. Imagery training studies in which explicit metamemorial information is provided, can be regarded as short-term longitudinal studies. Carrying out such studies holds promise too. For example, existing evidence supports the assumption that a strategy transfer task may provide a more favorable context for the appearance of a connection between metamemory and memory (cf. Borkowski & Cavanaugh, 1980).

ACKNOWLEDGEMENTS
This research was supported by grant # AZ II/37 028 from the Volkswagen Foundation to Jürgen Bredenkamp, Werner Wippich, and to Silvia Mecklenbräuker.

REFERENCES

1. Borkowski, J.G., & Cavanaugh, J.C. (1980). Metacognition and intelligence theory. In M. Friedman, J.P. Das, & N. O'Connor (Eds.), Intelligence and learning. New York: Plenum Press.
2. Cavanaugh, J.C., & Perlmutter, M. (1982). Metamemory: A critical examination. Child Development, 53, 11-28.
3. Denis, M., & Carfantan, M. (in press). What people know

about visual images: A metacognitive approach to imagery. In D.G. Russell & D.F. Marks (Eds.), Imagery 2. Dunedin, New Zealand: Human Performance Associates.

4. Dunham, T.C., & Levin, J.R. (1979). Imagery instructions and young children's prose learning: No evidence of "support". Contemporary Educational Psychology, 4, 107-113.

5. Flavell, J.H. (1978). Metacognitive development. In J.M. Scandura & C.J. Brainerd (Eds.), Structural/process theories of complex human behavior. Alphen a.d. Rijn: Sijthoff & Noordhoff.

6. Kreutzer, M.A., Leonard, C., & Flavell, J.H. (1975). An interview study of children's knowledge about memory. Monographs of the Society for Research in Child Development, 40 (1, Serial No. 159).

7. Levin, J.R. (1981). On functions of pictures in prose. In F.J. Pirozzolo & M.C. Wittrock (Eds.), Neuropsychological and cognitive processes in reading. New York: Academic Press.

8. Levin, J.R. (1982). Pictures as prose-learning devices. In A. Flammer & W. Kintsch (Eds.), Discourse processing. Amsterdam: North-Holland.

9. Levin, J.R. (1983). Pictorial strategies for school learning: Practical illustrations. In M. Pressley & J.R. Levin (Eds.), Cognitive strategy research: Educational applications. New York: Springer.

10. Levin, J.R., & Lesgold, A.M. (1978). On pictures in prose. Educational Communication and Technology Journal, 26, 233-243.

11. Marschark, M., Richman, C.L., Yuille, J.C., & Hunt, R.R. (in press). The role of imagery in memory: On shared and distinctive information. Psychological Bulletin.

12. Paivio, A. (1971). Imagery and verbal processes. New York: Holt, Rinehart, & Winston.

13. Pressley, M. (1977). Imagery and children's learning: Putting the picture in developmental perspective. Review of Educational Research, 47, 585-622.

14. Reese, H.W. (1970). Imagery and contextual meaning. In H.W. Reese (Chm.), Imagery in children's learning: A symposium. Psychological Bulletin, 73, 404-414.

15. Richardson, J.T.E. (1985). Integration versus decomposition in the retention of complex ideas. Memory & Cognition, 13, 112-127.

16. Schneider, W. (1985). Developmental trends in the metamemory - memory behavior relationship: An integrative review. In D.L. Forrest-Pressley, G.E. MacKinnon & T.G. Waller (Eds.), Cognition, metacognition, and human performance. New York: Academic Press.

17. Stein, N.L., & Glenn, C.G. (1979). An analysis of story comprehension in elementary school children. In R.O. Freedle (Ed.), Discourse processing: Multidisciplinary perspectives. Norwood: Ablex.

2.4. DISCUSSION OF PART 2

IMAGERY, MEMORY, AND PROSE PROCESSING

ALAIN DESROCHERS

UNIVERSITY OF OTTAWA, CANADA

ABSTRACT
    The main purpose of this chapter is to comment on selected issues
raised during the first day of the European Workshop on Imagery and
Cognition. These issues are all concerned with the relation between
imagery processes and the cognitive representation of information
transmitted by the medium of language. The chapter comprises three main
sections. First, various interpretations of the concept of word
imageability are discussed. The second section concerns the role of
imagery variables in the recall of isolated words. Finally, the third
section is devoted to the role of imagery variables in prose processing.

1. INTRODUCTION
    Visual imagery has been a central theme in the study of cognition for
the past two decades. Not only has it inspired many systematic
investigations but it has become more and more closely intertwined with
other important topics such as memory, language, motor control,
problem-solving, and brain mechanisms. These ramifications are well
illustrated in the program of this first European Workshop on Imagery and
Cognition. Most of the papers presented over the first day of the
conference, however, were concerned with the relation between imagery
processes and the cognitive representation of information transmitted by
the medium of language. In my discussion of these particular contributions
I have chosen to highlight selected issues of common interest. The
remainder of this paper is divided into three main sections. In the first
section I discuss the concept of word imageability. The second section is
devoted to the role of imagery in the recall of isolated words. Finally,
in the third section, I address the role of imagery in prose processing.

2. THE CONCEPT OF WORD IMAGEABILITY
    I assume that we all have noticed that words differ in their capacity
to arouse mental images of things or events. We do not seem to have much
difficulty in making judgments on the ease with which different words
evoke mental imagery and in expressing this judgment on a seven-point
scale. Ratings of word imageability or concreteness (e.g., Paivio,
Yuille, & Madigan, 1968) routinely serve in the selection of linguistic
items for experiments. Although an important portion of imagery research
relates to the effect of this variable on performance in memory and
reading tasks, some researchers have asked themselves why words actually
vary in imageability. Three related sorts of answers appear in the papers
presented by van Loon-Vervoorn, Peraita and Ferrandiz, and Jones (this
volume).
    Van Loon-Vervoorn suggested that imageability is related to the means
by which words are learned. She distinguished between lexical
representations that are based on sensori-motor interactions with their

155

M. Denis et al. (eds.), Cognitive and Neuropsychological Approaches to Mental Imagery, 155–164.
© 1988 by Martinus Nijhoff Publishers.

referents and those that are based on linguistic definition. Because many words are initially acquired in the context of sensori-motor activities and later elaborated in a linguistic context, and vice versa, these bases may be thought of as the poles of a continuum rather than as a simple dichotomy. This view is indeed similar to that of Piaget and Inhelder (1966) among others. More importantly, however, this perspective appears to have implications for understanding the nature of verbal deficits in aphasia and, possibly, deep dyslexia as well (Jones, 1985).

A different but related way of investigating the basis of word imageability consists of transposing the problem into the larger context of conceptual representations. Visual images are taken here as a special case of conceptual representation. Many researchers have chosen to view conceptual representations as a set of features that are stored in long-term memory by abstraction processes. Denis and his collaborators (Denis, 1982a; 1982b; 1983; Hoffmann, Denis, & Ziessler, 1983), followed by Peraita and Ferrandiz (this volume; Ferrandiz & Peraita, 1984), have proposed a distinction between features that reflect sensory properties of objects and features that reflect other properties (e.g., evaluative, functional, or relational). The first type has been dubbed figurative features and the second type non figurative features (for a different viewpoint, see Medina, this volume). They then hypothesized that people's estimates of the ease with which a word arouses a visual image is determined by the richness in figurative features of its corresponding concept. Denis (1983) has shown that the estimated imageability value of words and the number of reported figurative features are significantly correlated, while Peraita and Ferrandiz (this volume) provided only a partial replication of this finding. It is further assumed that figurative features are not accessed and used every time a concrete word is processed. In their 'resting state' they are assumed to be stored in a discrete and amodal format in long-term memory. A mental image then is said to result from the actualization of figurative features in the construction of a composite configuration (for a similar view, see Kosslyn, 1980, 1981). Thus, at some representational level, figurative features are indistinguishable from any other elements of a general-purpose knowledge base.

Jones (1985; this volume) also proposed that the rated imageability of a word is determined primarily by the richness of the knowledge base. Unlike Denis, however, he made no distinction among classes of elements in the knowledge base. His main concern was to develop and test a more satisfactory measure of knowledge than rated imageability of words. This alternative measure, called word predicability, was operationalized as a rating, on a seven-point scale, of the ease with which a word referent can be described by simple factual statements. This measure was shown to be highly correlated (r = .88 in a sample of 125 words) with rated imageability. For this reason alone, word predicability is likely to correlate also with performance in a variety of cognitive tasks.

To sum up, two general points may be made. Although all the authors cited above assume some relationship between rated imageability and people's knowledge base, their respective characterization of the pertinent knowledge base varies both in explicitness and details. I don't intend this remark as a criticism; the most serious challenge for cognitive psychologists surely is to characterize human knowledge and account for its actualization in overt and covert behavior. We must welcome new attempts to meet these objectives. However, we also must provide ourselves with criteria to assess our progress and, in the present context, to assess the usefulness of concepts like imageability, figurative features, and predicability. As Jones (this volume) pointed out, there are at least two criteria to be considered, namely, predictive value and explanatory value. By the first criterion, imageability and predicability may be indistinguishable, and it may be premature to make any strong claim about figurative features because of the relative paucity of empirical studies on this issue. How we wish to apply the second criterion depends on how we define the term 'explanation'. If we interpret this term in the light of the behaviorist epistemology, then it is a close synonym of predictive value. If by this term we mean a fully articulated theory of the structures and operations that underlie imagery, the issue presently is undecidable. These concepts were explicitly intended to relate to one or another large-scale theory of meaning or knowledge (e.g., Le Ny, 1979; Anderson & Bower, 1973; Paivio, 1971, 1986). For any progress to be made on this issue, these concepts should be defined or characterized within the same theoretical framework. If the meaning of these terms does not transcend the particular framework in which it was introduced, we have no common basis for comparing their explanatory value.

3. IMAGERY AND MEMORY FOR INDIVIDUAL WORDS

It has been shown on many occasions that memory performance is better for highly imageable words than for less imageable words. This general finding has been reported in studies of recognition, free recall, and cued recall (for reviews, see Denis, 1979; Paivio, 1971, 1986; Richardson, 1980). An interesting sort of asymmetry is observed in cued recall: The effect of word imageability is greater on the item that serves as a retrieval cue than on the one that serves as the response (Paivio, 1965). This finding also is obtained if subjects are unexpectedly provided with the nominal response item as a retrieval cue, and are asked to provide the nominal stimulus item (Bower, 1972; Lockhart, 1969; Yarmey & O'Neill, 1969).

The first account of this phenomenon was Paivio's conceptual peg hypothesis "according to which the stimulus word functions as a 'peg' to which its associate is hooked during learning trials and from which it can be retrieved on recall trials. The more concrete the stimulus, the more 'solid' it is as a conceptual peg, and the better the recall" (Paivio, 1971, p.248). Jones (this volume) has pointed out the vagueness of the concept of trace solidity. He also suggested that an explanation that emphasizes the role of links among memory traces may be more appropriate or viable than one that stresses the role of individual trace properties (e.g., variations in the encoding of nodes). However, it is unclear whether Jones' preference is intended to apply to all forms of remembrance or only to cued recall. In any case, I believe that this contrast closely relates to the distinction made by many authors between item-specific information and relational information in memory traces (cf. Begg, 1982; Desrochers & Begg, 1987; Einstein & Hunt, 1980; Humphreys, 1978; Hunt & Einstein, 1981; Marschark, this volume; Marschark, Richman, Yuille, & Hunt, in press; Wippich, this volume). In this section, I shall discuss the nature and the role of these two kinds of trace information in the recall of isolated words.

Memory theorists usually are concerned with a) the content of memory after some material has been perceived, and b) the way in which this content is recovered and used in different retrieval environments. I shall roughly characterize the units of memory as being memory traces, each of which is a set of information pertinent to one or more events; traces may be organized into higher order units or chunks (e.g., Mandler, 1967; Miller, 1956). Because the distinction between item-specific and relational information relates to their function rather than to their substrate, the discussion will be focused on what the trace does rather than on what it is. The information in memory traces is often assumed to serve two basic functions, namely, to identify items, and to relate items within traces. Accordingly, item-specific information is taken as the information that identifies items, and relational information as the information that binds items together. In this perspective, information is thus viewed as the result of an interpretation by the subject.

The main problem we face in assessing the quality of item-specific information is to secure an index that is independent from its effects on recall. Because this sort of information cannot be input "directly" into the subject's cognitive system, its inception has often been fostered by the use of orienting tasks. This tactic is problematic because it often is difficult to ensure that subjects follow the instructions rigorously (i.e., that they engage in the activities described by the instructions and in them only) and that these instructions, when they are rigorously followed, have exactly the intended cognitive consequences. Even the use of normative data on words does not provide an entirely satisfactory solution to this problem because the expected interpretation of the stimulus item is subject to variation. Thus, the difficulty arises from the lack of absolute control over interpretive processes and, thereby, over the input that actually is processed by the subject. Assessing the quality of relational information also poses the same problem, which is particularly salient in studies of interactive imagery and imagery-based mnemonics. The cognitive operations of interest again are triggered indirectly by instructing the subjects to engage in a particular mental activity. This procedure again introduces a great deal of ambiguity into the decision rules scientists use to test and refute theoretical ideas. Inferences appear valid when the manipulation of interest works as expected. It is when the manipulation does not work as expected that serious problems of interpretations become evident.

How then can we know the exact input a cognitive system is processing? I doubt that scientists will ever find the answer to this question by direct query into the cognitive system. How we wish to answer it depends on how we choose to work as scientists. If we choose to favor extensive a priori theoretical elaboration followed by critical tests, then the challenge consists of formulating powerful conjectures (cf. Popper, 1972, 1982) which often take the form of computational models of the processes and structures that underlie the behavior of interest (see Pinker, this volume; Slack, this volume). If we choose to favor extensive empirical investigations followed by theoretical elaboration, it then is imperative to contrive research tactics that permit defensible inferences. Although both approaches have merits, I presently am more familiar with the latter, and I now turn to a general research tactic that was intended to strengthen the inferences made about the relation between imagery and recall. This approach is not without its problems but I view its emergence as a sign of progress. More importantly, it directs us to reconsider seriously the temptation to favor a class of theoretical models that focuses exclusively on the role of individual trace properties or on the role of links that bind trace information together.

Memory performance requires that the remembered traces be accessed and used in some task environment. This implies that a theory of memory must entail more than propositions about memory structures and processes, it must also entail a theory of the retrieval environment. This concern directs us to consider the factors in the retrieval environment that govern whether or not existing traces can be recovered and used effectively (see Bransford, 1979; Tulving, 1983). A systematic attempt to characterize both the requirements of the retrieval environment and the potential value of the discriminations a trace enables should help us refine the predictions memory theories can make. For example, cognitive activities that enhance the encoding of item-specific information may be particularly useful in task environments that make strong demands on trace access (e.g., in free recall and recognition tests). By contrast, cognitive activities that enhance the encoding of relational information may serve primarily in task environments that require the use of inter-item associations (e.g., in cued recall tests).

I now briefly describe two experimental problems on which progress has been made by investigating the interaction between encoding processes and task environments. The first problem concerns the effects of bizarre images on recall. Bizarre images may be understood as coherent composite structures that involve an infrequent or a restricted set of relations among its elements. A relational set may be infrequent because it departs from our usual daily experiences (e.g., A mail man who sells toothbrushes from door to door); it may be restricted because some "real-world" constraints are removed from the thematic coherence of the structure (e.g., A dog who rides a motorcycle down the street). If this characterization is appropriate, instructions to construct a bizarre image from a carefully drafted sentence should not enhance the encoding of relational information any less than instructions to construct a nonbizarre or common image. However, they may differ in terms of item-specific information which would make bizarre images more distinctive and discriminable, particularly if they are generated from a mixed list of bizarre and common sentences. We then would expect bizarre imagery to improve free recall, but to have no effect on cued recall. These expectations appear to be confirmed by an extensive series of investigations (for a review, see Einstein & McDaniel, 1987). The second problem for which the interaction between encoding instructions and task environments was examined is the effect of common interactive imagery on associative memory. Interactive imagery, unlike separate imagery, is assumed to enhance the encoding of relational information and, thereby, increase the number of items represented in a unitary trace. Relational information per se should promote successful cued recall but have no effect on free recall. Again this is the general finding that is obtained in numerous studies (for reviews, see Begg, 1982, 1983).

Returning to the issue of word imageability or concreteness, Desrochers and Begg (1987) have suggested that, relative to abstract words, concrete words are characterized, among other things, by their capacity to evoke readily a wider range of context-specific interpretations. This versatility implies that two or more concrete items are more likely than abstract items to be represented in a composite memory trace that uniquely specifies their interrelations. Accordingly, we would expect word imageability to enhance cued recall of item pairs only if subjects process them as related pairs rather than as isolated items. This actually is the main result that was obtained by Marschark and Hunt (1985) in an incidental learning experiment. In the item-specific encoding condition the concreteness effect was neutralized both in cued recall and free recall tests, whereas in the relational encoding condition it was very pronounced in cued recall and considerably weaker in free recall. This study again illustrates very well the benefits of examining the effects of word characteristics in a variety of retrieval environments.

4. IMAGERY AND PROSE PROCESSING

Prose materials may serve many communicative functions. A text may describe characters, objects, or events. It may inform or instruct the readers. Or it may be intended to alter the readers' opinions, attitudes, or beliefs. In order to achieve any of these goals, a text usually must convey a large amount of information, and the degree of involvement and the role of imagery in processing different types of prose are likely to vary. In this section, I shall discuss the effects of imagery processes on the time course of on-line reading and on memory for prose.

Denis (this volume) pointed out that researchers may choose to study the concurrent manifestations of imagery processes on reading or to study its long-term effects on the cognitive system. In the context of the former approach, he reported that high imagers usually take more time to read concrete materials than low imagers do. However, their respective reading times do not differ significantly with a highly abstract, non imageable text, suggesting that high imagers are not also slow readers. Reading times are not entirely under the control of text characteristics since high imagers can increase their reading speed when instructed to do so, and low imagers do decrease theirs when they are instructed to construct concurrently visual images of characters and events. One may ask what their eyes do while they read concrete and abstract materials under various instructions. Do we observe systematic variations in fixation time? In the number of regressions? With concrete materials, one might expect high and low imagers to differ only in their respective fixation latency for content words but not for function words. I am not aware of any empirical investigations that addressed these issues. The investigation of eye movements in this research program would provide invaluable information about the "oculo-motor distribution" of reading time for concrete and abstract sentences.

A related but considerably more difficult question concerns the "cognitive distribution" of reading time: what do people do cognitively when they read concrete and abstract sentences? The most common research tactic employed to address this question is to study some aspect of memory for the presented prose materials. In prose processing, it appears that comprehension and memory are intrinsically linked. This is so because comprehension may evolve considerably in the course of reading a text. Comprehension is assumed to take place at many levels (see van Dijk & Kintsch, 1983), ranging from the individual word, clause, sentence, or paragraph, to even larger units formed by abstracting information from lower levels (e.g., macropropositions). It is precisely to characterize better the intuitive idea of "levels" that hierarchical models of text structure representation were developed. More importantly, interpretive processes related to each level appear to be interdependent. This can be shown in the interpretation of individual words within a sentence context as well as in the interpretation of individual sentences within a paragraph context.

A sentence context often serves to highlight a particular sense of a word or a particular subset of its semantic features. Consider the following examples: (1) Michel lifted the piano, and (2) Michel tuned the piano. The readers' attention likely is drawn to the object's heaviness in the first sentence but to its acoustic potential in the second. The effect of contextual information on the interpretation of individual words can even be more extreme, as in the following examples: (3) Michel broke a record, he accidently dropped one of his Chopin albums from the balcony, and (4) Michel broke a record, he ate two kilos of spaghetti in an hour. These sentences serve to actualize either a concrete or an abstract sense of the target noun. The interpretation of sentences also can be altered by contextual information. Consider the following example: (5) John took Johannes' wallet and put it into his suitcase. Contextual information here may serve to disambiguate John's intentions and the owner of the suitcase. This information may either precede or follow sentence (5) in a paragraph. Another common consequence of contextual information is to help readers determine the important ideas in a text (for illustrations, see Anderson & Pichert, 1978; Pichert & Anderson, 1977). Thus, contextual information appears to serve at least two basic functions: to add constraints on the possible interpretations of linguistic units at various prose levels, and to help readers bind units of information within and between levels.

The investigation of word imageability effects on memory for prose raises several important issues concerning a) the level(s) at which these effects are expected to be detected, and b) the possible interactions with different retrieval requirements. Wippich (this volume) described a particular approach in order to deal with the first issue. The approach consists of specifying performance measures that are sensitive to information available at various levels of prose processing, namely, at the surface level, the text-base level, and the situation model level. A recognition test was used to measure surface level information, a reconstruction test for text-base level information, and an inferential recognition test for situation model level information. He reported a strong advantage of concreteness at each level of processing, and further indicated that this advantage may be reduced or neutralized under some procedural conditions. I view this and other similar deliberate attempts to relate performance measures to explicit theoretical concepts as a sign of progress in the study of memory for prose. These attempts provide opportunities to elaborate meaningful interpretations of the effects of word characteristics (e.g., word imageability) and their possible interaction with other variables (e.g., order of sentence presentation and orienting instructions during sentence encoding).

The specification of the relation between performance measures and theory, however, is not easy. Indeed, difficult problems arise in the course of developing a psychological theory of text processing and in selecting interpretable performance measures. I shall discuss briefly a common problem associated with prose recall. Because recall protocols reflect, however imperfectly, the subjects' interpretation of the original sentences, it is difficult to define or capture every possible recall unit by an entirely theory-driven set of decision rules. The recall of prose materials often is broken into "idea" units. This implies that paraphrases are allowed to some degree and the scoring of recall often requires a number of subjective judgments on the actual content of paraphrases. Thus the scoring criteria are not completely specified and their reliability is neither perfect nor invariant. Furthermore, if the relation between recall units and text structure is not sufficiently spelled out, it becomes difficult to characterize the nature of the information represented in recall protocols and, therefore, to localize the levels of prose recall that are affected by word imageability.

Recall performance also is known to vary with the retrieval requirements of the experimental task. This point is particularly important in studies intended to compare prose memory in various age groups (see Mecklenbräuker, this volume). Young children's free recall is notoriously poor (e.g., Brown, 1975). Compared to recognition and cued recall indices, free recall measures typically underestimate their memory for details and higher-level information units. For this and other reasons introduced earlier, I stress again the importance of varying the retrieval requirements (as Mecklenbräuker did) in the measurement of prose recall.

5. CONCLUSION

By way of conclusion I wish to raise a final question: How do we know that some measured behavior is under the influence of imagery processes? A common answer to this question is by ruling out nonimagery accounts of the phenomenon. This answer, however, is meaningless unless we have a theory of what an imagery process is and is not. The most common form of nonimagery processes reported by researchers relate to verbal rehearsal and abstract propositional descriptions. The validity of these contrasts has been publicly endorsed by some authors (e.g., Pylyshyn, 1973) but questioned by others (e.g., Anderson, 1978). Although the issue is still in dispute, we must recognize that this controversy has forced theorists to refine their characterization of what an image is and is not. These refinements have directed researchers to verify the expected effects of the special properties of imagery (i.e., those not shared by other forms of representation or other processes) in a variety of task environments.

ACKNOWLEDGEMENTS

Preparation of this chapter was supported by a research grant from the Natural Sciences and Engineering Research Council of Canada to the author. I am grateful to Collette Gélinas and Linda Wieland for helpful comments on an earlier draft of this chapter.

REFERENCES

1. Anderson, J. R. (1978). Arguments concerning representation for mental imagery. Psychological Review, 85, 249-277.
2. Anderson, J. R., & Bower, G. H. (1973). Human associative memory. Washington, DC: Winston.
3. Anderson, R. C., & Pichert, J. W. (1978). Recall of previously unrecallable information following a shift in perspective. Journal of Verbal Learning and Verbal Behavior, 17, 1-12.
4. Begg, I. (1982). Imagery, organization, and discriminative processes. Canadian Journal of Psychology, 36, 273-290.
5. Begg, I. (1983). Imagery instructions and the organization of memory. In J.C. Yuille (Ed.), Imagery, memory, and cognition: Essays in honor of Allan Paivio (pp.91-115). Hillsdale, NJ: Erlbaum Associates.
6. Bower, G. H. (1972). Mental imagery and associative learning. In L. W.Gregg (Ed.), Cognition in learning and memory (pp.51-88). New York: Wiley.
7. Bransford, J. D. (1979). Human cognition. Belmont, CA: Wadsworth Publishing Company.
8. Brown, A. L. (1975). Recognition, reconstruction, and recall of narrative sequences by preoperative children. Child Development, 46, 156-166.
9. Denis, M. (1979). Les images mentales. Paris: Presses Universitaires de France.
10. Denis, M. (1982). Images and semantic representations. In J.-F. Le Ny & W. Kintsch (Eds.), Language and comprehension (pp.17-27).

Amsterdam: North-Holland. (a)

11. Denis, M. (1982). On figurative components of mental representations. In F. Klix, J. Hoffmann, & E. van der Meer (Eds.), Cognitive research in psychology (pp.65-71). Amsterdam: North-Holland. (b)

12. Denis, M. (1983). Valeur d'imagerie et composition sémantique: analyse de deux échantillons de substantifs. Cahiers de Psychologie Cognitive, 3, 175-202.

13. Desrochers, A., & Begg, I. (1987). A theoretical account of encoding and retrieval processes in the use of imagery-based mnemonic techniques: The special case of the Keyword method. In M. A. McDaniel & M. Pressley (Eds.), Imagery and related mnemonic processes: Theories, individual differences, and applications (pp.56-77). New York: Springer-Verlag.

14. Einstein, G. O., & Hunt, R. R. (1980). Additive effects of individual-item and relational processing. Journal of Experimental Psychology: Human Learning and Memory, 6, 588-598.

15. Einstein, G. O., & McDaniel, M. A. (1987). Distinctiveness and the mnemonic benefits of bizarre imagery. In M. A. McDaniel & M. Pressley (Eds.), Imagery and related mnemonic processes: Theories, individual differences, and applications (pp.78-102). New York: Springer-Verlag.

16. Ferrandiz, P., & Peraita, H. (1984). Frecuencia, valor de imagen y tipos de rasgos, en categorias biologicas y no biologicas. Revista de Psicologia General y Applicada, 39, 1257-1278.

17. Hoffmann, J., Denis, M., & Ziessler, M. (1983). Figurative features and the construction of visual images. Psychological Research, 45, 39-54.

18. Humphreys, M. S. (1978). Item and relational information: A case for context independent retrieval. Journal of Verbal Learning and Verbal Behavior, 17, 175-187.

19. Hunt, R. R., & Einstein, G. O. (1981) Relational and item-specific information in memory. Journal of Verbal Learning and Verbal Learning, 20, 497-514.

20. Jones, G. V. (1985). Deep dyslexia, imageability, and ease of predication. Brain and Language, 24, 1-19.

21. Kosslyn, S. M. (1980). Image and mind. Cambridge, MA: Harvard University Press.

22. Kosslyn, S. M. (1981). The medium and the message in mental imagery: A theory. Psychological Review, 88, 46-66.

23. Le Ny, J.-F. (1979). La sémantique psychologique. Paris: Presses Universitaires de France.

24. Lockhart, R. S. (1969). Retrieval asymmetry in the recall of adjectives and nouns. Journal of Experimental Psychology, 79, 12-17.

25. Mandler, G. (1967). Organization and memory. In K. W. Spence & J. T. Spence (Eds.), The psychology of learning and motivation: Advances in research and theory (Vol. 1, pp. 327-372). New York: Academic Press.

26. Marschark, M., & Hunt, R. R. (1985). Imagery effects in paired associate learning: Now you see them, now you don't. Paper presented at the Canadian Psychological Association meetings, Halifax, Nova Scotia, Canada.

27. Marschark, M., Richman, C. L., Yuille, J. C., & Hunt, R. R. (in press). The role of imagery in memory: On shared and distinctive information. Psychological Bulletin.

28. Miller, G. A. (1956). The magical number seven, plus or minus two: Some limits on our capacity for processing information. Psychological

164

Review, 63, 81-97.
29. Piaget, J., & Inhelder, B. (1966). Les images mentales chez l'enfant. Paris: Presses Universitaires de France.
30. Paivio, A. (1965). Abstractness, imagery, and meaningfulness in paired-associate learning. Journal of Verbal Learning and Verbal Behavior, 4, 32-38.
31. Paivio, A. (1971). Imagery and verbal processes. New York: Holt, Rinehart and Winston.
32. Paivio, A. (1986). Mental representations: A dual coding approach. Oxford: Oxford University Press.
33. Paivio, A., Yuille, J. C., & Madigan, S. A. (1968). Concreteness, imagery, and meaningfulness values for 925 nouns. Journal of Experimental Psychology, 76 (1, part 2).
34. Pichert, J. W., & Anderson, R. C. (1977). Taking different perspectives on a story. Journal of Educational Psychology, 69, 309-315.
35. Popper, K. (1972). Conjectures and refutations: The growth of scientific knowledge. New York: Harper & Row.
36. Popper, K. (1982). The logic of scientific discovery. New York: Harper & Row.
37. Pylyshyn, Z. W. (1973). What the mind's eye tells the mind's brain: A critique of mental imagery. Psychological Bulletin, 80, 1-24.
38. Richardson, J. T. E. (1980). Mental imagery and human memory. New York: St. Martin's Press.
39. Tulving, E. (1983). Elements of episodic memory. Oxford: Oxford University Press.
40. Van Dijk, T. A., & Kintsch, W. (1983). Strategies of discourse comprehension. New York: Academic Press.
41. Yarmey, A. D., & O'Neill, B. J. (1969). S-R and R-S paired-associate learning as a function of concreteness, imagery, specificity, and association value. Journal of Psychology, 71, 95-109.

PART 3

IMAGERY PROCESSES IN
ADAPTIVE BEHAVIOR

3.1. IMAGERY PROCESSES AND WORKING MEMORY

IMAGERY AND WORKING MEMORY

ALAN D. BADDELEY

MRC APPLIED PSYCHOLOGY UNIT, CAMBRIDGE, ENGLAND

ABSTRACT

It is suggested that the concept of working memory offers a useful framework for discussing the phenomenon of imagery. The framework assumes a Central Executive aided by two slave systems, the Articulatory Loop and the Visuo-spatial Sketchpad. The Sketchpad is assumed to be responsible for the setting up and manipulating of temporary visuo-spatial representations, and as such to be an important component in the utilisation of imagery. Experiments are described that demonstrate the separability of visuo-spatial and verbal coding effects. Furthermore, the system is shown to be important for tasks that involve manipulating visual images, such as that of using a visual imagery mnemonic, but is not responsible for the advantage enjoyed by highly imageable words in verbal memory. The paper concludes by speculating on unsolved problems and future developments.

1. INTRODUCTION

The term working memory refers to the system assumed to be responsible for the temporary storage and manipulation of information involved in the performance of a range of cognitive tasks. The concept was developed by Graham Hitch and I as a result of a series of experiments concerned with the function of short-term memory (Baddeley & Hitch, 1974). These persuaded us to abandon the idea of a single monolithic short-term memory (STM) system, replacing it by the assumption that working memory comprises an alliance of interacting subsystems. We postulated a supervisory system of limited processing capacity, the Central Executive, supported by at least two slave systems, the Articulatory Loop and the Visuo-spatial Scratchpad or Sketchpad.

The Articulatory Loop is assumed to comprise two subcomponents, a phonological memory store and an articulatory rehearsal process; utilising these two simple components it is possible to provide a plausible account of the rich accumulation of experimental data suggesting an involvement of speech coding in many short-term memory tasks (Baddeley, 1986).

The Sketchpad is assumed to be responsible for the setting up and manipulation of visual images, and as such is of particular relevance to the present workshop. While the Sketchpad is much less adequately explored than the Articulatory Loop, we believe that it is sufficiently developed to offer a useful component to a more complete model of visual imagery. It is presented in the hope that although incomplete,

169

M. Denis et al. (eds.), Cognitive and Neuropsychological Approaches to Mental Imagery, 169–180.
© 1988 by Martinus Nijhoff Publishers.

it has the advantage of linking research on imagery to other
areas of cognition addressed by the working memory model.

2. THE DEVELOPMENT OF THE SKETCHPAD CONCEPT

The attempt to incorporate a slave system responsible for
imagery into working memory stemmed from the coincidental fact
that at the same time as Graham Hitch and I were exploring the
effects of concurrent digit span on memory, Gerard Quinn and I
were attempting to replicate a study by Atwood (1971) that was
concerned with visual and verbal coding. Atwood presented his
subjects with phrases that were either highly imageable (e.g.
Nudist devouring bird) or abstract in nature (e.g. The
intellect of Einstein was a miracle). Each phrase was followed
by a simple processing task that was presented either visually
or auditorily; Atwood reported that auditory processing
disrupted memory for abstract phrases, while visually-presented
material disrupted the retention of imageable items.

Unfortunately we were unable to replicate this effect,
and moved on to another imagery technique, that developed by
Lee Brooks (1968) in which a subject is given an immediate
verbal memory task where performance can be enhanced in one
condition by the use of visuo-spatial coding. It is perhaps
worth describing in more detail since the technique will
feature in several of the experiments I shall describe
subsequently. The subject is first shown a 4 x 4 matrix in
which one cell is designated the starting square. In the
imagery condition, he is required to remember and repeat back a
series of instructions regarding the placement of digits 1-8.
The instructions can be remembered by mapping them onto a route
through the matrix. Hence an example might be In the starting
square put a '1'; in the next square to the right put a '2'; in
the next square beneath put a '3'; in the next square beneath
put a '4' etc. This condition may be contrasted with a
formally equivalent set of phrases in which the spatial
adjectives are replaced by the non-spatial polar adjectives,
good-bad and weak-strong. For example In the starting square
put a '1'; in the next square to the good put a '2'; in the
next square to the weak put a '3'; in the next square to the
weak put a '4' etc. While such sequences could logically be
recoded spatially, at the rates of presentation normally used,
subjects find this impractical and rely on rote verbal memory.

We began our studies by exploring the effect of a visuo-
spatial concurrent task on subjects performing both conditions
of the Brooks procedure. Our secondary task involved pursuit
rotor performance with the subject required to keep a stylus in
contact with a spot of light following a circular track;
difficulty level was adjusted by varying the rotation speed,
and performance measured in terms of time-on-target. The
results were very clear, concurrent tracking produced a marked
disruption of performance on the imagery version of the Brooks
task, while having no effect on the non-imageable condition. A
second experiment showed that when subjects were instructed to
hold memory performance constant, then an imagery task
disrupted tracking more than a verbal task. In both cases the
effects were quite clear, suggesting the operation of some

system that was separable from that responsible for immediate memory for verbally-coded material (Baddeley, Grant, Wight & Thomson, 1975).

Is the system visual or spatial?

We initially began to refer to our system as being one responsible for <u>visual</u> imagery. It was however the case that our results were equally explicable in terms of a system that was spatial rather than visual in nature. We set out to test this as follows; the pursuit rotor is a task that places both visual and spatial demands on the subject. We therefore selected two potential disrupting tasks, one which was assumed to be spatial but not visual, while the second was assumed to be visual but not spatial.

Our spatial task involved auditory tracking; the subject was blindfolded and asked to keep a flashlight trained on the bob of a swinging pendulum. This was possible since the bob emitted a tone that changed in character whenever the flashlight was in contact with it. This task is clearly spatial, but not visual in the peripheral sense, since the subjects were blindfolded. Our visual task involved seating the subject in front of a large screen and requiring him to make yes/no judgements on whether successive stimuli were bright or dim. This is clearly a visual task, but one in which spatial factors were minimal.

When we combined these two secondary tasks with the Brooks matrix procedure, the results were clear. The visuo-spatial condition was maximally disrupted when combined with the spatially-based auditory tracking task, while the verbally-based Brooks condition showed the opposite pattern of results. It appears then that the system concerned is a spatial one rather than one reflecting peripheral visual input. This suggests that it may perform an important function in integrating information from different modalities. This raised the further question of whether our hypothetical Sketchpad system might play an important role in the use of visual imagery in verbal learning. We therefore carried out a number of experiments concerned with answering two questions, first whether the advantage enjoyed in verbal memory by imageable material is mediated by the system, and secondly whether the system is involved in setting up and using visual imagery mnemonics.

Imageability effects and the Sketchpad

Much of the revival of scientific interest in imagery probably stems from Allan Paivio's many demonstrations that the ease with which words can be remembered is well predicted by their rated imageability and concreteness (Paivio, 1971). One possible explanation of this phenomenon is as follows; a highly imageable word might be one having visuo-spatial characteristics that can readily be represented within the Sketchpad. This would allow two codes to be set up in parallel, a visuo-spatial code and a verbal or semantic code, with such dual coding facilitating later recall. This version of the dual coding hypothesis differs from earlier versions in making a specific suggestion as to the means whereby the visuo-spatial code is set up, a suggestion that we then went on to test directly by means of our secondary task procedure (Baddeley & Lieberman, 1980).

We presented our subjects with noun-adjective pairs that were either highly concrete and imageable such as <u>bullet-grey</u>, <u>strawberry-ripe</u>, or were abstract low imageability pairs such as <u>gratitude-infinite</u> and <u>idea-original</u>. On each trial, the subject would see five such pairs, and immediately afterwards be tested by being given the stimuli and asked to provide the responses; after a single trial, another quite separate list would be presented and tested. On half the trials, subjects were concurrently required to perform the pursuit tracking task, while in the remainder no secondary activity was required. Once again our results were clear in showing a massive effect of imageability, a small but significant effect of concurrent task, but no trace of an interaction. Concurrent tracking had no greater effect on the imageable items than on the abstract pairs, clearly arguing strongly against our earlier proposal, that the Sketchpad was an important mediator of the effects of imageability. Our results are much more consistent with the idea that imageability and concreteness reflect the way in which items are registered in long-term semantic memory, and as such our results are consistent with the view presented by Jones in the present workshop.

Imagery mnemonics and the Sketchpad

Our previous result suggests that the imagability effect does not depend on the operation of the Sketchpad, but it does not of course necessarily imply that the advantage gained from using imagery <u>mnemonics</u> is not Sketchpad-dependent. It could be argued for example that a subject who is using a visuo-spatial imagery mnemonic must manipulate the visuo-spatial images using the Sketchpad for temporary storage purposes. One might contrast this with an alternative view that might suggest that the Sketchpad was used only for performing short-term visual memory tasks, and played no role in the long-term learning of verbal material, even when imagery is involved. This was tested in a series of experiments (Baddeley & Lieberman, 1980).

In one study, subjects attempted to remember sequences of 10 unrelated words using either imagery or verbal coding. The imagery coding involved teaching the subjects a route through the campus of the University of Stirling which contained 10 landmarks, each of which could be used to help encode and store one of the items in the list. In order to recall, the subject imagined walking through the campus, reporting the item placed at each of the 10 locations. Rote verbal memory was encouraged by presenting the list too rapidly to allow visuo-spatial encoding, using a number of separate presentations so as to equate total time between the two conditions. When subjects were allowed to perform the task unimpeded by any secondary task, there was a clear advantage for the imagery mnemonic; concurrent tracking however completely abolished this advantage, suggesting that the Sketchpad does indeed play an important role in the manipulation of visual images necessary for the efficient use of a spatial location mnemonic.

At this point then the Visuo-spatial Sketchpad appeared to have the following characteristics: (1) It is a system for the temporary storage of visuo-spatial information. (2) It can be disrupted by concurrent visuo-spatial tasks. (3) The disruption appears to be spatial rather than visual in nature. (4) The enhanced memorability of imageable words does not appear to depend on the Sketchpad, but (5) The use of visuo-spatial imagery mnemonics does appear to depend on the Sketchpad.

3. SUBSEQUENT DEVELOPMENTS: GROWING POINTS AND PROBLEMS

After a relatively quiet period, there appears to be a resurgence of research concerning the characteristics of the Sketchpad; this work suggests that the system is almost certainly considerably more complex than the initial research indicated. Some of these developments will be described below.

Visual coding in immediate memory for letters

The Articulatory Loop system is assumed to be principally responsible for remembering sequences of unrelated digits or letters. The use of this system can be inhibited if the material is presented visually, and the subject required to suppress articulation through some irrelevant vocal task such as repeating the word "the". Under these circumstances, memory span is reduced, but by no means abolished (Baddeley, Lewis & Vallar, 1984). What system therefore stores the successfully recalled digits in this paradigm?

One possibility is that they are stored visually; this was explored in an unpublished study carried out jointly by Sergio Della Sala, Michel Deboek, Bob Logie and I. We selected letters that either had many features in common or were visually dissimilar. The items were presented sequentially and visually at a rate of one letter per second, after which subjects wrote their responses on a prepared answer sheet. In one condition, our subjects suppressed articulation during presentation and recall, while in the control condition no secondary task was used. While earlier results suggest that the visual similarity is not a significant factor when subjects are allowed to subvocalize in the normal way, the visual coding hypothesis would predict that a visual similarity effect would appear when phonological coding is prevented by articulatory suppression. The results showed that under control conditions, we obtained no effect of visual similarity, the expected result. Under articulatory suppression however, visual similarity did impair performance to a significant though small extent ($p < .05$). This result suggests that visual coding does occur, but the magnitude of the effect does not encourage an interpretation in purely visual terms. It seems much more likely that some more abstract visual code is used. The possibility of some form of abstract letter coding has of course been suggested on other grounds (McConkie & Zola, 1981). We have made a number of attempts to find a method of identifying and possibly disrupting this code, but so far without success.

Imagery and the unattended picture effect

Baddeley and Lieberman (1980) found that concurrent tracking caused a much clearer disruption of a location mnemonic than it did the one-is-a-bun pegword mnemonic. They interpreted this result on the assumption that the system was spatial rather than visual in nature. This and earlier results are however open to an alternative explanation. The disrupting task that was normally used was pursuit tracking, a task that itself has a very strong spatial component. It is entirely conceivable that different results would have been obtained had a less spatial and more visual disrupting task been used. This line of argument was explored in an ingenious series of studies by Logie (1986).

Logie chose to use the pegword mnemonic and attempted to explore conditions under which disruption could be enhanced. In a series of experiments, he showed that requiring the subject to classify pictures, or even patches of colour was sufficient to disrupt performance. Perhaps the most convincing piece of evidence however comes from a study in which the subject was not even required to actively process the secondary task, a phenomenon analogous to the effect of unattended speech in verbal memory.

Salame and Baddeley (1982) had showed that memory for visually presented digits could be disrupted by the concurrent presentation of irrelevant spoken material. Logie showed an exactly comparable effect for unattended visual material. Subjects were presented with the task of remembering sequences of words, being encouraged to use rote memory in one condition, and the one-is-a-bun pegword mnemonic in the other. On half the trials, pictures of objects were presented to the subject, while on the other half, no such concurrent stimuli were presented. The subject was instructed to look at the screen but ignore the pictures. In a second study, instead of unattended pictures, unattended verbal material was used, with the procedure otherwise being equivalent. The results of these two experiments are summarised in Figure 1.

It is very clear from these results that visually presented items cause substantial disruption of the use of the imagery mnemonic, while unattended speech disrupts rote verbal memory. This visual disruption occurs despite the fact that the spatial demands of the secondary task are minimal, and that the mnemonic in question is one that does not place heavy demands on spatial coding. These results suggest that our previous conclusion that the system is spatial rather than visual may have been premature. It seems likely that the Sketchpad is sensitive to both visual and spatial characteristics, with the point of maximum vulnerability depending on the characteristics of the memory task involved. Memory tasks that load heavily on spatial coding will be most sensitive to spatial disruption, while those involving a heavy visual component may be more sensitive to visual concurrent disruption. This does not necessarily however imply that these two aspects of coding will subsequently prove inseparable. It is equally likely that the Sketchpad system may prove to have more than one subcomponent, possibly depending on the relative contribution of visual and spatial coding. The evidence presented by Farah and her colleagues at this Workshop is broadly consistent with such a view.

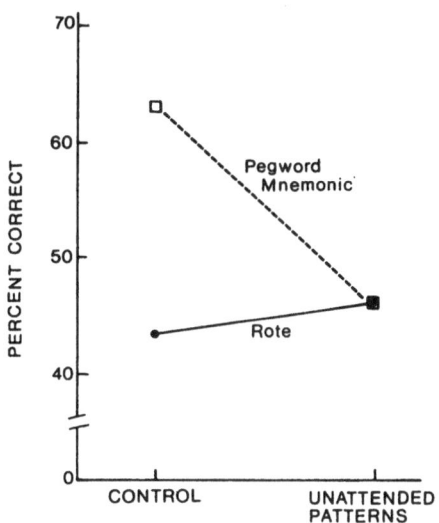

FIGURE 1. The influence of unattended input on the utilisation of a visual imagery mnemonic. Data from Logie (1986).

Sketchpad or Central Executive?

One of the most powerful methods of arguing for two separate systems is that of the double dissociation. A double dissociation occurs when one can demonstrate the presence of a phenomenon associated with hypothetical system A together with the absence of a phenomenon associated with B, coupled with a parallel demonstration of the reverse pattern, namely B without A. One of the best examples of this comes from arguments for the separability of long- and short-term memory systems, where classic amnesic patients can be shown to have normal immediate memory coupled with grossly impaired long-term learning, while STM patients may show the reverse, with grossly impaired memory span coupled with normal long-term learning (Shallice, 1979).

Using a broadly similar logic, Hitch and I argued for separate slave systems, the verbal Articulatory Loop system and the Visuo-spatial Sketchpad (Baddeley & Hitch, 1974). Interpretation was complicated however by the fact that we assumed a third component, namely the Central Executive, a system that is assumed to operate and control the slave systems. As Phillips and Christie (1977) have pointed out, this leaves our results open to alternative explanations. They argue for example that our results could be explained by assuming only two components, the Articulatory Loop and the Central Executive, with there being no necessity to assume a visuo-spatial system. They support their argument using data based on a task involving immediate memory for matrix patterns.

The Phillips and Christie paradigm involves presenting the subjects with a succession of matrix patterns, subsequently probing memory for the patterns in reverse order. Under these conditions, the very last item presented is tested first, and is assumed to reflect the content of a short-term visual memory system, while earlier items which show a much lower level of performance are assumed to reflect the operation of some more durable memory trace. The result that was most problematic for the Sketchpad interpretation of visual memory stemmed from an experiment in which they manipulated the intervening activity required between presenting the last pattern and testing its retention. During the interval, the subject was required either to perform a purely visual task, or to perform a more demanding arithmetic task. They found that the more demanding task caused greater forgetting, a result that they interpreted as suggesting that retention of the pattern was principally dependent on the operation of the Central Executive system rather than the Visuo-spatial Sketchpad.

How could we explain this result within the existing working memory framework? One possibility might be to argue that this task reflects the operation of some other aspect of the Sketchpad, different in nature from that involved in performing the Brooks tasks. This would certainly be possible, though somewhat unsatisfactory. Another possibility however stemmed from the fact that Phillips and Christie had in fact performed an incomplete experiment. One could argue that their study did indeed show the involvement of the Central Executive in a task that was likely to depend at least in part on the operation of the Visuo-spatial Sketchpad. This is indeed what would be predicted by the working memory interpretation. Such an interpretation would however make a further prediction, namely that in addition to any Central Executive demand, visual interference would be particularly harmful to performance on this type of task, whereas the reverse should occur when subjects were required to perform a task involving verbal coding. In short, a full design would require two tasks, the Phillips matrix task and a verbal equivalent, combined with two interfering tasks, one of which would be expected to interfere with visuo-spatial coding while the other would be expected to interfere with phonological processing. An explanation that assumed that the Central Executive and the Visuo-spatial Sketchpad were one and the same, would predict an interaction, but not a cross-over interaction, whereas the tripartite assumption of the current working memory model would predict a cross-over interaction.

This was explored in a study by Logie, Zucco and myself. The tasks used in this study are illustrated in Figure 2. As a visual memory test, we used the original Phillips task as modified by his colleague Lindsay Wilson to provide a visual memory span. In this modification, the subject is first of all shown a matrix comprising only four cells of which two are randomly filled. This is followed after a five-second gap with a re-presentation of the matrix in a form that is identical except that one of the filled cells is now empty. The subject's task is to point to the cell that has changed. After each successful response, the matrix is enlarged by adding two further cells. The procedure stops at the point at which the subject fails on three occasions. Span is represented as the mean size of the three largest matrix patterns for which the subject gives a correct response.

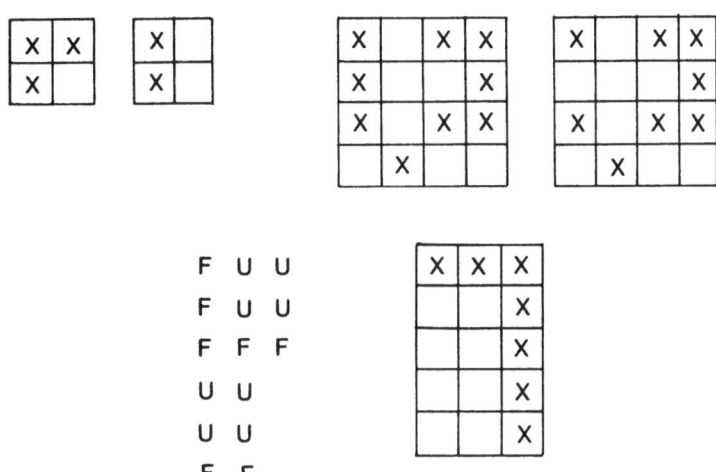

FIGURE 2. Examples of material used in the visual memory span, and in the visual interference task used by Logie, Zucco and Baddeley.

The verbal analogue of this task involved first visually presenting the subject with a sequence of consonants followed by a further sequence which differs from the first by one letter (e.g. X T - X L). The subject responds by pointing to the item that has changed. Each time the subject is successful, sequence length is incremented by one letter up to a point at which he makes three successive errors.

The visual interfering task involved requiring the subject to imagine a 3 x 5 matrix of cells. The experimenter then indicated which cells were filled and which unfilled in a systematic left-to-right and top-to-bottom order. The total pattern could then be interpreted as representing a digit; the subject's task was to identify that digit. Hence the digit 7 would be indicated as follows, where F = filled and U = unfilled: F F F U U F U U F U U F U U F.

Finally, as a task that would involve verbal coding we used simple cumulative addition. Hence the subject might be

given a sequence such as 5 + 2 (to which he should respond 7) +
3 (10) + 5 (15) + 9 (24). There is evidence from a recent
series of studies (Logie & Baddeley, 1987) that counting
involves the Articulatory Loop component of working memory.

The two memory tasks were each combined with the two
secondary tasks to produce the results shown in Figure 3. This
shows first of all that we are able to replicate the
observations of Phillips and Christie (1977) who showed that a
concurrent mental arithmetic task interfered with visuo-spatial
memory performance. Note however that the amount of
interference is very much less than that obtained from the
concurrent visuo-spatial task, suggesting an important visual
contribution to performance on this task. Given only these two
conditions however, it could reasonably be argued that the
visuo-spatial interference task simply took more of the Central
Executive than did mental arithmetic. This seems unlikely in
view of the results of performance on the verbal memory task,
where interference from visuo-spatial processing leads to much
less disruption than does concurrent mental arithmetic. In
short, the clear cross-over interaction is exactly what would
be predicted on the assumption of separate visuo-spatial and
verbal slave systems.

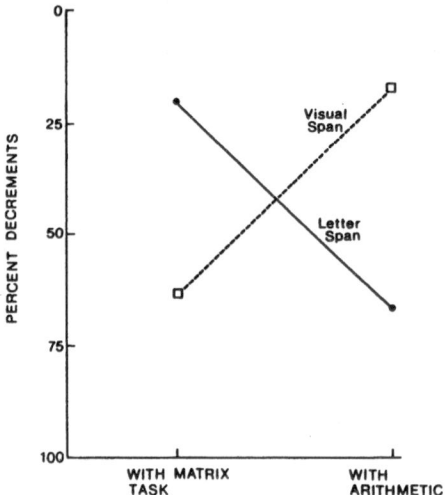

FIGURE 3.   Influence of a concurrent imagery or counting task
on visual and verbal memory. Data from a study by Logie, Zucco
and Baddeley.

While the results shown in Figure 3 do appear to be very
striking, it is important to point out that they are still not
logically compelling. In principle, a study involving a 2 x 2
design is not sufficient to prove conclusively the necessity to

assume a tripartite system. Logically, this requires a triple dissociation and an experimental design involving nine separate conditions. Since I would assume that working memory is likely to have more than three subcomponents, then this in turn is likely to be inadequate producing the need for designs involving 16, 25 and ever-increasing numbers of conditions if one is to pursue the dissociation logic to its conclusion. I would not regard this as a practicable development, and hence suggest that we revert to using a slightly less formal combination of sources of evidence to argue for the presence or absence of separate subcomponents. That being so, I would suggest that anyone wishing to argue that our data are less than convincing comes up with a plausible alternative explanation of the results reviewed in the present discussion.

4. CONCLUSION

I would like to suggest that the working memory model provides a useful framework for considering the mechanisms and processes underlying the utilisation of visual imagery. In particular, the dual-task interference procedure has provided good evidence for the importance of a temporary visual code that can be utilised in a range of tasks. It seems unlikely however that the Visuo-spatial Sketchpad itself will prove to be a unitary system, and the question of whether the more visual and more spatial aspects of imagery operate within a single process or represent the contribution of different subcomponents is an important current concern.

A second area of considerable uncertainty concerns the role of visual coding in remembering lexical material such as visually-presented letters. It seems likely that this takes advantage of codes that have been developed in the process of learning to read, whose relationship to the Sketchpad as a whole remains unclear. Another relatively unexplored aspect of the Sketchpad is the nature of the process underlying rehearsal; the mechanism whereby an image is refreshed is still far from clear.

Finally, we still know relatively little about the role played by the Sketchpad in performance of non-laboratory tasks; our own work indicates its importance in the use of visuo-spatial imagery mnemonics, while that of Farmer, Berman and Fletcher (1986) indicates that it is used in the Mannikin test, a measure of speed of visuo-spatial processing. An obvious further question is the role of the Sketchpad in reading, both at the level of comprehending texts that convey visuo-spatial information, and in terms of its possible role in the important but neglected question of how we maintain our place on the page while reading text. Finally, the role of imagery in complex multi-component tasks remains an interesting and important one, as is indicated by the work described at this workshop by my colleague Bob Logie.

REFERENCES

1. Atwood, G.E. (1971). An experimental study of visual imagination and memory. Cognitive Psychology, 2, 290-299.

2. Baddeley, A.D. (1986). <u>Working memory</u>. Oxford: Oxford University Press.
3. Baddeley, A.D., & Hitch, G.J. (1974). Working memory. In G. Bower (Ed.), <u>Recent advances in learning and motivation Vol. VIII</u>. New York: Academic Press.
4. Baddeley, A.D., Grant, S., Wight, E., & Thomson, N. (1975). Imagery and visual working memory. In P.M.A. Rabbitt., & S. Dornic (Eds.), <u>Attention and Performance V</u>. London: Academic Press.
5. Baddeley, A.D., Lewis, V., & Vallar, G. (1984). Exploring the articulatory loop. <u>Quarterly Journal of Experimental Psychology</u>, <u>36</u>, 233-252.
6. Baddeley, A.D., & Lieberman, K. (1980). Spatial working memory. In R. Nickerson (Ed.), <u>Attention and performance VIII</u>. Hillsdale, N.J.: Erlbaum.
7. Brooks, L.R. (1968). Spatial and verbal components in the act of recall. <u>Canadian Journal of Psychology</u>, <u>22</u>, 349-368.
8. Farmer, E.W., Berman, J.V.F.., & Fletcher, Y.L. (1986). Evidence for a visuo-spatial scratchpad in working memory. <u>Quarterly Journal of Experimental Psychology</u>, <u>38A</u>, 675-688.
9. Logie, R.H. (1986). Visuo-spatial processing in working memory. <u>Quarterly Journal of Experimental Psychology</u>, <u>38A</u>, 229-248.
10. Logie, R.H., & Baddeley, A.D. (1987). Cognitive processes in counting. <u>Journal of Experimental Psychology: Learning, Memory, and Cognition</u>, <u>13</u>, 310-326.
11. McConkie, G., & Zola, D. (1981). Language constraints and the functional stimulus in reading. In A.M. Lesgold., & C.A. Perfetti (Eds.), <u>Interactive processes in reading</u>. Hillsdale, N.J.: Erlbaum.
12. Paivio, A. (1971). <u>Imagery and verbal processes</u>. New York: Holt Rinehart and Winston
13. Phillips, W.A., & Christie, D.F.M. (1977). Interference with visualization. <u>Quarterly Journal of Experimental Psychology</u>, <u>29</u>, 637-650.
14. Salame, P., & Baddeley, A.D. (1982). Disruption of short-term memory by unattended speech: Implications for the structure of working memory. <u>Journal of Verbal Learning and Verbal Behavior</u>, <u>21</u>, 150-164.
15. Shallice, T. (1979). Neuropsychological research and the fractionation of memory systems. In L.-G. Nilsson (Ed.), <u>Perspectives on memory research</u>. Hillsdale, N.J.: Erlbaum.

INTERFERENCE EFFECTS IN THE VISUO-SPATIAL SKETCHPAD

GERARD QUINN

DEPARTMENT OF PSYCHOLOGY, THE UNIVERSITY, ST. ANDREWS, U.K.

ABSTRACT
    An experiment that uses an interference paradigm is used to investigate coding processes in the visuo-spatial sketchpad. The results confirm that a spatial interference task involving movement is more disruptive than a visual interference task. In addition, it is shown that the sketchpad is particularly susceptible to interference during the encoding of information while interference has little effect on the maintenance of information.

1.   INTRODUCTION

The working memory model put forward by Baddeley and Hitch (1974) is currently composed of three components: a central executive (CE), an articulatory loop (AL) and a visuo-spatial sketchpad (VSSP). These components have been subject to unequal development with the AL the most theoretically advanced while relatively little is known about the CE or the VSSP.

Most damaging from the viewpoint of theoretical development is the lack of sufficient information about the CE. This gap in our understanding is damaging because of the pivotal role the CE plays within the WM formulation. It controls the other components though the mechanisms by which control is exercised remain largely unexplored. Moreover, it shares some of the attributes of the AL; for example, when the loop's capacity is exceeded the CE can be brought in to provide additional storage space (Baddeley and Hitch, 1974). Because of the importance of the CE and because of the mobility of information within the working memory system, it is crucial to develop the necessary constraints which will permit assessment of the contribution of the individual components.

Fortunately, constraints are beginning to emerge. For example, the mechanisms of attention are plausibly located within the CE (Baddeley, 1983) and recognition of this casts light on the relationship between the CE and the AL (Baddeley, Eldridge and Lewis, 1981; Besner, Davies and Daniels, 1981). In addition, Richardson (1984) has shown that the contribution of the AL may vary depending on the extent to which the order of information presented to the subject has to be retained. Such results lead to the development of tractable indices which can be used to develop further the model.

Research on the VSSP has been less intense than on the

181

M. Denis et al. (eds.), Cognitive and Neuropsychological Approaches to Mental Imagery, 181–189.
© *1988 by Martinus Nijhoff Publishers.*

AL. Consequently, tractable indices are fewer and more uncertain. However, useful distinctions are beginning to emerge. As the name suggests, the VSSP deals with the representation of visuo-spatial information. Several authors, notably Baddeley and Lieberman (1980), have drawn a distinction between a visual and spatial representation. The distinction is not finely tuned and will rarely be absolute, nonetheless, judging from the tasks that have been used to investigate the VSSP movement has a role to play in spatial coding and spatial rather than visual interfering tasks cause greater disruption of the VSSP (Baddeley and Lieberman, 1980; Idzikowski, Baddeley, Dimbleby and Park, 1983; Quinn and Ralston, 1986).

Research has also shown that disruption of visuo-spatial memory is evident when the interference tasks are presented during presentation or retrieval of the spatial material (Brooks, 1967, 1968; Byrne, 1974). Little information is available on the susceptibility to disruption of a visuo-spatial representation during maintenance of the representation. This is of some theoretical significance since it is not clear that the cognitive processes which are used during the construction and reconstruction of the information in the sketchpad are the same as those used during the maintenance of the information.

The experiment to be reported here, which uses an interference paradigm to explore the coding processes used in visuo-spatial processing, has two aims. First, it seeks to provide further evidence that an interference task involving movements will cause more disruption in the VSSP than will a visual task. To this end, two types of sentences from Brooks (1967) are used: matrix sentences which refer to a spatial array and are assumed to be processed using the VSSP and control sentences which would not gain access to the VSSP but are likely to be processed using the AL. Second, it investigates the effect of interference tasks when they are presented either during presentation or maintenance of the to-be-remembered material.

2.   METHOD
2.1 Materials
The two types of the to-be-remembered sentences were derived from Brooks (1967). The matrix sentences consisted of 18 sets of eight sentences describing the placement of digits in a 5x5 mental matrix. Each set began with the sentence "In the starting square put a 1" with the following sentences having the form "In the next square up (to the right/to the left/down) put a 2" and so on up to 8. The digits were presented in ascending numerical order and each sentence within a set designated an empty square in the mental matrix. The first sentence always designated the second column of the second row. The control sentences had the same form as the matrix sentences and substituted the terms "to the good/bad/quick/slow" for the terms "up/down/to the left/to the right" used in the matrix sentences. The

first sentence of the control sentence set was always "In the starting square put a 1". In keeping with other researchers who have used this technique (e.g. Brooks, 1967; Baddeley, Grant, Wight and Thomson, 1975) the number of sentences in the control set had to be reduced to equate performance levels across the two conditions; in this experiment, the control sentences were reduced to six in each set.

Eighteen sets of matrix and of control sentences were produced. In no set were the same "directions " given more than three times in sequence. During sentence presentation the experimenter read the sentences to the subjects at a rate of 2.5 seconds per sentence. The matrix sets were presented in 20 seconds while the control sets were presented in 15 seconds. The subject's task was to repeat verbatim the sentence set at recall.

There were three interference conditions: no interference, spatial interference and visual interference. In the no interference condition, subjects were given no interference instruction. In the spatial interference condition, the subject was seated in front of a 5x4 array of buttons. The buttons were placed 4.7cm apart within the array and the whole array was covered by a cardboard box which was open at the end facing the subject. This end was covered by a black cloth which ensured that the subject could place his preferred hand on the array without thereafter being able to see the array or his hand. The task was to press the buttons in a horizontal-boustrophedal sequence starting with the top left button and reaching the bottom left button before retracing the sequence of presses, ending with the top left. The 40 presses were made within 20 seconds. The array was connected to an Apple II microcomputer which registered both the sequence and latency of presses so allowing both the correctness and the timing of the pushes to be monitored. In the visual interference task the subject had to watch the monitor of the Apple II which was located approximately 50cm in front of where he was seated. At the centre of the monitor a sequence of 20 rectangular patches of light measuring 1cm x 0.5cm were presented at a rate of one per second with an "off" and "on" time of 0.5 seconds. The patches were either bright or dim with a probability of 0.5. The subject held a single response button which had to be pressed whenever the patch was dim. Each response was recorded by the microcomputer. Pilot studies indicated that the rates shown for the two tasks encouraged comparable performances.

2.2 Subjects

Eighteen postgraduate students served as subjects in a split plot design. Nine served in the concurrent condition where the interference tasks were presented at the same time as the sentences and nine served in the sequential condition where the interference tasks were presented after the sentences. Subjects were tested individually.

2.3 Design

The experiment was a 2 (matrix or control sentences) x 3 (interference tasks) x 2 (concurrent or sequential interference) design. The six possible orders of the three interference tasks were presented to the first six subjects according to a Latin square design. The remaining three subjects were presented with orders which ensured that over the nine subjects, no one interference task held predominant position in the sequence of three. In the concurrent condition, 4 subjects started with the matrix sentences and five with the control sentences. These numbers were reversed in the sequential condition.

2.4 Procedure

Before the experimental trials began, subjects were given extensive training trials. Before the presentation of the matrix sentences they were shown a 5x5 matrix with the starting square marked. They were further shown how the sentence set related to the matrix and instructed to image the digits on a path round the matrix. They were then given four practice sets of the sentences alone and had to recall immediately after presentation. Similarly with the control sentences, the form of the sentence was illustrated and four practice trials were given. Subjects then practised the interference tasks. In the visual condition, the subjects practised responding to the lights until they made no more than two errors out of 20. In the spatial task, the subjects practised a pressing rate of one per 0.5 seconds ensuring that the task took 20 seconds to complete. Practice continued until subjects could complete the task within one second of the 20 seconds permitted. The rate was comfortable for the subjects, allowing a rhythm to be quickly established.

Before each of the six combinations of interference task x material, two practice trials of the combination were given before the six experimental trials.

Subjects in the concurrent condition received the interference task at the same time as the sentences were presented. With the control sentences where only 15 seconds were required for presentation, the interference tasks were started 5 seconds before the presentation of the sentences. After sentence presentation there was a delay of 20 seconds before recall. In the sequential condition, subjects received the interference tasks during the 20 second delay.

3. RESULTS

Recall data was scored in two ways. In the main analysis, one point was given for each set completely recalled in the correct sequence. This has the major advantage that the matrix and control sentences results can be directly compared. However, since each set contains 8 or 6 sentences, it has the disadvantage that a large amount of useful data is discarded with the possibility that the results will be distorted. For example, a subject scoring 7 correct sentences out of a set of 8 is given the same score of zero as a subject who scores 0 correct sentences out of a set of 8. To provide a check on any such distortion subsidiary analyses were separately run on the control and matrix sentences where one point was given for each correct sentence within the set.

For the main analysis, a 2x3x2 split plot design anova was run. The only main effect to reach significance was the interference tasks condition, $F(2,32)=36.25$, $p<0.001$. The no interference condition was significantly better than the visual interference condition which in turn led to superior performance than the spatial interference condition (Newman-Keuls, $p<0.01$ in both instances). Two interactions reached significance: the timing of interference x sentence material ($F(1,16)=24.1$, $p<0.001$) and, marginally, the interference tasks x sentence material ($F(2,32)=2.91$, $p=0.068$). The interference tasks x sentence material is theoretically important since it was hypothesised that the spatial interference tasks would cause more disruption to the matrix sentence than would the visual task. Further analysis of the interaction showed that while the no interference condition was superior to the visual interference condition which in turn was superior to the spatial interference condition with the matrix sentences, a different pattern emerged with the control sentences. With these sentences, the visual and spatial interference tasks performances were not different from one another although both differed from the no interference task condition ($p<0.01$ in all cases). In addition, visual interference caused a greater decrement in the control sentences (Newman-Keuls, $p<0.05$).

	No Interference	Visual Interference	Spatial Interference
Control Sentences	66.7	40.7	29.6
Matrix Sentences	72.2	52.7	33.3

TABLE I: Percent performance with the control and matrix sentences under the three levels of interference

Because this interaction was only marginally significant, the subsidiary analyses were consulted. Encouragingly, the same pattern emerged: with the matrix sentences the significant main effect of interference ($F(2,32)=29.23$, $p<0.01$) was further analysed to show the significant difference among the three levels (Newman-Keuls, $p<0.01$ in both cases) while with the control sentences the main effect ($F(2,32)=14.1$, $p<0.001$) was further analysed and showed that the spatial and visual interference tasks did not differ from one another but were both different from the no interference condition (Newman-Keuls, $p<0.01$). Scores derived from the main analysis are illustrated in Table I. The sentences x timing of interference interaction showed clearly that matrix sentence recall improved significantly when interference was after sentence presentation while control sentence recall fell significantly (Newman-Keuls, p<0.01 in both cases). Table II illustrates the performance levels.

	Matrix sentences	Control sentences
Concurrent	40.1	56.1
Sequential	62.3	37.65

TABLE II: Percent performance with the control and matrix sentences under concurrent and sequential interference

Any interpretation of these results requires analyses of the interference tasks. Without such analyses, it can be argued that there is a trade-off between performances on the sentences and interfering tasks such that more effort was devoted to the interfering task after the control sentences had been presented and less effort after the matrix sentences had been presented.

	Visual Interference	Spatial Interference
Concurrent	12.3	8.7
Sequential	0.2	3.3

TABLE IIIa: Percent errors under the two levels of interference and timing of interference in the matrix sentences

	Visual Interference	Spatial Interference
Concurrent	13.9	8.5
Sequential	2.4	3.8

TABLE IIIb: Percent errors under the two levels of interference and timing of interference in the control sentences

The visual and spatial tasks were analysed separately as they were essentially different types of tasks requiring a different number of responses. However, to ensure that matrix and control sentences did not have to be analysed separately, the first five seconds of the interference task responses in the matrix sentences condition were ignored as

were the first five seconds in the control sentences
condition which did not coincide with sentence presentation.
In the visual interference condition, one point was given
for each correct response or non-response, while, in the
spatial condition, one point was deducted for each button
pressed out of sequence. However, if one such press led to
an incorrect sequence being followed, for example, by
failing to go down to the next row and so retracing the
same row, no further points were deducted. Tables IIIa and
b show the percent errors in each of the conditions.

Two separate 2 (concurrent or sequential) x 2 (matrix
or control sentences) x 18 (subjects) anovas were carried
out with subjects nested within timing of interference.
Only the main effect of timing reached significance (visual
interference: $F(1,16)=11.68$, $p<0.01$; spatial interference:
$F(1,16)=8.26$, $p<0.025$). In both cases, interference after
presentation led to a better performance than interference
during presentation. Clearly, while it <u>could</u> be argued that
the fall in the recall of the control sentences with
sequential interference was due to more effort being
invested in the interference tasks, the same argument cannot
be applied to the matrix sentences where both recall
performance and interference task performance improve with
sequential presentation of the interference.

4. DISCUSSION
The most theoretically compelling interpretation of the
effects of the different interference tasks with the matrix
and control sentences is that the matrix sentences, being
encoded in the VSSP, are particularly vulnerable to spatial
interference. This task, involving movement which is
incompatible with the placing of the digits-in-position is
particularly disruptive. In contrast, a visual task
involving no movement is much less disruptive. The
disruption caused to the matrix sentences by the visual task
is most plausibly explained by its being a general
attentional effect acting through the CE. Such an
explanation is in keeping with the work of Besner et al
(1981) and with Logie (1986) who found a general deficit
caused by an attention-demanding visual interference task.
The same interpretation can be applied to the interference
effects with the control sentences. Theoretically neither
the visual nor the spatial tasks should have gained access
to the AL used in processing and rehearsing these sentences.
Any deficit would have been caused by interfering with the
attentional activity of the CE. The finding that the visual
and spatial tasks were equally disruptive here is consistent
with this interpretation, although the greater interference
caused by the visual task in the control than in the matrix
sentences further suggests that the dependency of the
control sentences processing on the CE may be greater than
the dependency on the CE of spatial processing.

The clear difference in the effects of concurrent and
sequential interference has two plausible interpretations
which may not be independent of one another. First, after
the encoding phase the form of the representation within the

VSSP may be sufficiently different to preclude any interference from the visual or spatial tasks used. The spatial code may be heavily involved only during actual processing of information, be it at encoding or retrieval (Idzikowski et al, 1983). At other times, such as during maintenance of the information, the processes used may be of a different nature. Second, during maintenance the involvement of the CE may be lessened. As has been noted above, some of the interference effects have their locus in the CE. It follows that whenever the dependency of the VSSP on the CE is reduced, interference will also be reduced.

In conclusion, these results confirm that spatial and visual encoding can be separately conceptualised with movement playing a part in the former. They also illustrate that the VSSP is susceptible to interference mainly during encoding (and retrieval (Idzikowski et al, 1983)) of information.

REFERENCES

1. Baddeley, A.D. (1983). Working memory. _Philosophical Transactions of the Royal Society of London B_, _302_, 311-324.
2. Baddeley, A.D., Eldridge, M. & Lewis, V. (1981). The role of subvocalisation in reading. _Quarterly Journal of Experimental Psychology_, _33A_, 439-454.
3. Baddeley, A.D., Grant, W., Wight, E. & Thomson, N. (1975). Imagery and visual working memory. In P.M.A. Rabbitt & S. Dornic (Eds) _Attention and Performance 5_. London:Academic Press.
4. Baddeley, A.D. & Hitch, G.J. (1974). Working memory. In G.H. Bower (Ed) _The Psychology of Learning and Motivation_, 8, 47-49.
5. Baddeley, A.D. & Lieberman, K. (1980). Spatial working memory. In R.S. Nickerson (Ed) _Attention and Performance 8_. Hillsdale, New York:Lawrence Erlbaum Assoc.
6. Besner, D., Davies, J. & Daniels, S. (1981). Reading for meaning: the effects of concurrent articulation. _Quarterly Journal of Experimental Psychology_, _33A_, 415-437.
7. Brooks, L.R. (1967). The suppression of visualisation by reading. _Quarterly Journal of Experimental Psychology_, _19_, 289-299.
8. Brooks, L.R. (1968). Spatial and verbal components in the act of recall. _Canadian Journal of Psychology_, _22_, 349-378.
9. Byrne, B. (1974). Item concreteness vs spatial organization as predictors of visual imagery. _Memory and Cognition_, _2_, 53-59.
10. Idzikowski, C., Baddeley, A.D., Dimbleby, R.D. & Park, S. (1983). Eye movements and imagery. Paper presented to the _Experimental Psychology Society_, April.
11. Logie, R.H. (1986). Visuo-spatial processing in working memory. _Quarterly Journal of Experimental_

Psychology, 38A, 229-247.

12. Quinn, J.G. & Ralston, G.E. (1986). Movement and attention in visual working memory. Quarterly Journal of Experimental Psychology, 38A, 689-702.

13. Richardson, J.T.E. (1984). Developing the theory of working memory. Memory and Cognition, 12(1), 71-83.

VISUAL WORKING MEMORY IN THE ACQUISITION OF COMPLEX COGNITIVE SKILLS

ROBERT H. LOGIE, UNIVERSITY OF ABERDEEN, UK

ALAN D. BADDELEY, MRC APPLIED PSYCHOLOGY UNIT, CAMBRIDGE, UK

AMIR MANE, EMANUEL DONCHIN and RUSSEL SHEPTAK, UNIVERSITY OF ILLINOIS AT URBANA-CHAMPAIGN, USA

ABSTRACT
Traditionally, visual working memory has been studied using laboratory tasks whose components are relatively clear, and where relatively little practice is involved. Few researchers have studied the role of visual working memory in complex tasks involving several components or whether this role changes with increased expertise on the tasks under study. This paper reports two experiments using secondary task methodology to study the role of visual working memory in learning a complex computer game "SPACE FORTRESS". Unlike earlier studies of working memory, the primary task relies on perceptuo-motor skills and accurate timing of responses as well as short and long term strategic decisions. Results showed that during early stages of training important components of the game were disrupted by secondary visuo-spatial tasks more than by secondary verbal tasks. With increased practice, this differential disruption by visuo-spatial tasks seemed to change. These results are interpreted in terms of a visual working memory system that plays an important but changing role during learning of complex skills. Theoretical implications of these results for the characteristics of a visual working memory system within the context of the Baddeley and Hitch (1974) working memory framework will be discussed.

1. INTRODUCTION

In the papers by Alan Baddeley and Gerry Quinn, the concept of working memory is described as a set of functional mechanisms for short term storage and processing of information. Baddeley reviews the evidence that one component of this system deals specifically with visuo-spatial material (Baddeley & Lieberman, 1980; Logie, 1986). Traditionally, visual working memory has been studied using laboratory tasks whose components are relatively clear, and where relatively little practice is involved.

The potential scope of this concept is, in principle, sufficiently wide to provide insight into an enormous number of tasks of widely varying complexity. Some studies have shown verbal working memory to be useful in the study of counting (Logie & Baddeley, 1987), and reading (Baddeley, Logie, Nimmo-Smith & Brereton, 1985). However, most of the 'ecologically valid' tasks so far chosen for study have been

M. Denis et al. (eds.), Cognitive and Neuropsychological Approaches to Mental Imagery, 191-201.
© 1988 by Martinus Nijhoff Publishers.

relatively simple and few have involved a substantive visuo-spatial component. Also there has been virtually no study of the effects of extensive practice on the role of the various working memory components.

Alan Baddeley and I were given the opportunity to become involved in a fairly large scale project concerned with training of complex cognitive skills. The project involved a number of subcontractors worldwide, all of whom studied training and learning of a complex computer game, SPACE FORTRESS, that was especially developed for this purpose. A theme underlying the general approach of this project taken by a number of subcontractors was that performance on SPACE FORTRESS may be fruitfully subdivided into a number of subcomponent skills. Our own approach aimed to test this directly by means of a secondary task procedure which has proved fruitful in the development of the concept of working memory. We were particularly interested in whether secondary task procedures would be appropriate in this context. We were also very keen to find out whether the working memory concept could be applied successfully and in turn the concept itself developed by this sort of task. Of particular interest to this meeting was the role of visuo-spatial working memory in the process of acquiring the skills necessary for learning the game.

2. PROCEDURE
2.1 Space Fortress

The computer game SPACE FORTRESS involves controlling the movement of a spaceship by means of a joystick control. A diagram of the layout of the computer screen and the controls is shown in Figure 1. The spaceship moves in a frictionless environment, and the joystick controls the forward acceleration only. A button inset into the top of the joystick controls the firing of missiles from the spaceship. In the centre of the screen is a space fortress. This can also fire missiles which the spaceship has to avoid. The fortress pivots around a central point, attempting to track the spaceship and destroy it with missiles. The spaceship in its turn attempts to destroy the fortress.

From time to time a space mine appears from a random position at the edge of the screen. This tracks the spaceship, and can damage the ship if they meet. The mines are of two types; a friend mine or a foe mine. If the mine is a friend, a successful hit by a missile from the ship causes the mine to crash into and damage the fortress. If the mine is a foe, the subject must change the status of the weapon system on his ship and then destroy the mine with a successful shot. The weapon system is changed by pressing a button on a separate control with the left hand. The mine is identified as a foe or a friend mine by letters which appear above the fortress.

One further complication is that from time to time, a variety of non alphabetic symbols appear below the fortress. The appearance of two dollar signs ($) one after the other signifies the availability of bonus points or a new supply of missiles for the ship. The subject may choose which is most appropriate at that stage in the game.

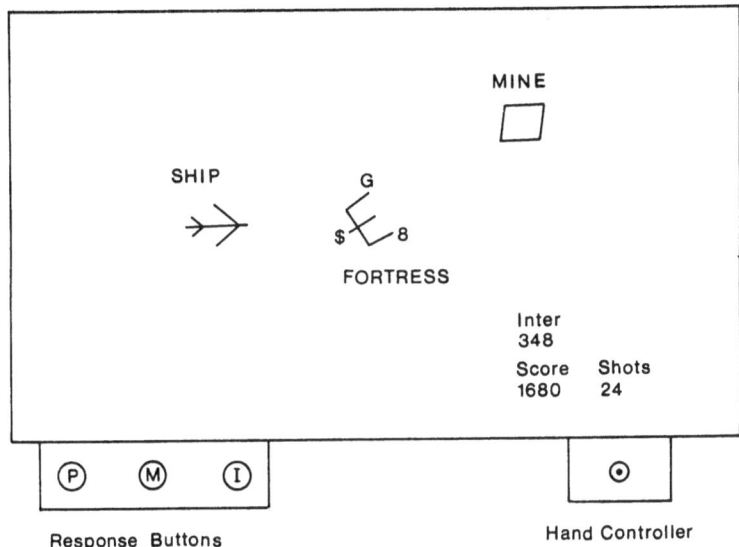

FIGURE 1. Computer display for Space Fortress.

An overall measure of performance is given by a points total. Points are gained by successful hits or destructions of the fortress or mines, as well as choice of bonus points when these are available. Points are lost when the ship is hit or destroyed either by a mine or the fortress. Points are also lost if the ship fires missiles 'in the red'. The ship has an initial supply of 100 missiles. Once this supply is exhausted, the ship may continue to fire missiles, but at a cost of points being deducted from the score. The selection of a missile bonus when this is available helps avoid this problem. Given the possibility of points being subtracted as well as added, it is common for a novice player to have a very large negative score.

In addition to this rather arbitrary measure of performance, a large number of individual measures of aspects of game performance were recorded. Over fifty parameters were measured, including efficiency of firing the missiles, the time taken to destroy a fortress or mine, the general movement of the ship around the screen and choice of missiles or bonus points when the dollar sign appears.

The task is obviously complex with a number of component perceptuo-motor and cognitive tasks involved. Our main approach was to provide a fairly complete analysis of the components of working memory which might be involved in learning and performing this task. However a complete analysis of this sort is beyond the scope of the present paper. A more complete account of these data can be found in Logie, Baddeley,

Mane, Donchin and Sheptak (in press).

Of particular interest to this conference is the role of visuo-spatial short term memory in this process. In order to study this aspect of performance, we chose a number of secondary tasks which it would be physically possible for the subject to carry out at the same time as playing SPACE FORTRESS. Under such dual task conditions, the assumption is that where tasks mutually interfere, this suggests that at least some of the cognitive mechanisms required for each task overlap to some extent. Where there is no significant disruption in performance of either task when the tasks are performed together, the assumption is that there is no overlap in the cognitive or other resources required and that the mechanisms involved are functionally independent. The papers by Baddeley and by Quinn both describe the application of this strategy to the study of visuo-spatial working memory.

We shall describe two experiments involving SPACE FORTRESS, performed concurrently with each of a number of secondary tasks. Experiment 1 involved subjects who had a basic training and knowledge of the game.

Experiment 2 studied these same subjects after a further period of practice on the game. This design allowed us to examine the possibly changing role of visuo-spatial processing with increasing levels of expertise.

2.2 Secondary Tasks

Two of the secondary tasks were designed to study the role of visuo-spatial coding in working memory. A further two tasks were chosen to involve equivalent verbal processing. This allowed a comparison of the extent to which the verbal and visuo-spatial components could be distinguished in this context. Other secondary tasks were involved in the main study, but these are not relevant to the present paper. Details are given in Logie et al. (in press).

2.2.1 Brooks visuo-spatial task. This was based on a task originally devised by Brooks (1967) that involved the subject retaining a sequence of movements through an imagined 4 x 4 matrix pattern. Details of this task are given in the paper by Baddeley. When combined with the game, subjects were presented with the secondary task continuously. Performance on this task is typically disrupted by visual and non-visual tracking tasks, suggesting some overlap between perceptuo-motor control and the visuo-spatial content of the main task (eg. Baddeley, this volume; Baddeley, Grant, Wight & Thomson, 1975). Tracking tasks interfere much less with the verbal equivalent described below.

2.2.2 Brooks verbal task. The subject again hears a set of sentences, but with the words 'GOOD', 'BAD', 'QUICK' and 'SLOW' substituted for directions in the visuo-spatial version.

While these tasks have been used fairly extensively in previous studies, there is a suggestion that the general cognitive load that they impose is fairly high, in addition to any specifically verbal or visuo-spatial component of the tasks. SPACE FORTRESS itself is quite a complex task, and we were concerned that the general cognitive load imposed by performing either of the Brook's tasks concurrently with the game would be so high as to swamp any differential interference effects. We therefore chose two further tasks designed to contrast visuo-spatial and verbal processing but with a lighter general processing load.

2.2.3 <u>Map task</u>. This involved presenting subjects with a map of an island on which were marked six locations. An example map is shown in Figure 2. On a given map the names of the locations were chosen from a particular category. For example one map contained the names of United States Presidents such as Washington Gulch or Reagan Airport. Subjects were given one minute to study the map and were then asked questions concerned with the relative direction between pairs of locations, for example: Is Washington Gulch Northwest of Reagan Airport?

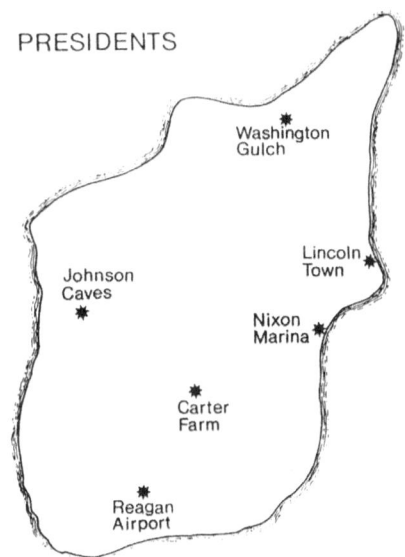

FIGURE 2. Example of a map used in the map task.

2.2.4 <u>Limerick task</u>. This was designed as a verbal equivalent of the map task, and involved the subject learning a short poem in the form of a limerick, for example:

There was a young thief of repute,
Whose ideas were surprisingly cute.
He built a balloon,
By the light of the moon,
And used it to gather his loot.

The subject was then given a number of questions concerned with the relative position of various words in the poem, for example:

Does thief come before surprisingly?
Does light come after gather?

The limerick was repeated four times from a tape recorder and the questions were presented through headphones. For both tasks responses were timed, and error responses were recorded.

2.3 General Procedure

The general procedure was designed to examine effects on performance at two different stages in training. A group of nine subjects were first given three hours of practice on the game. Next, they were given one session consisting of practice on each of the secondary tasks. There then followed two sessions where each secondary task was performed alone or with the game. Next, subjects were given a further five hours practice on the game alone, followed by a further two sessions involving the secondary tasks as before. Subjects were also asked to indicate the difficulty of performing each task on a ten-point rating scale. A rating of '1' indicated that the task was extremely easy. A rating of '10' indicated that the task was virtually impossible. Subjects were all students at the University of Illinois at Urbana-Champaign.

3. RESULTS

Space limitations reduce the scope for reporting details of statistical analysis. These are reported in Logie et al. (in press). In the present text, where a difference is reported, it is a statistically significant difference.

3.1 Three hours training

Game scores as a percentage of control game performance after three hours of training are shown in Figure 3. It is clear from the figure that the two Brooks' tasks produced substantial impairments in game score, but with no differential disruption by one or other of these tasks. The map task shows a similar level of disruption. However, the limerick task produced substantially less disruption in game score showing a contrast between limerick and map tasks.

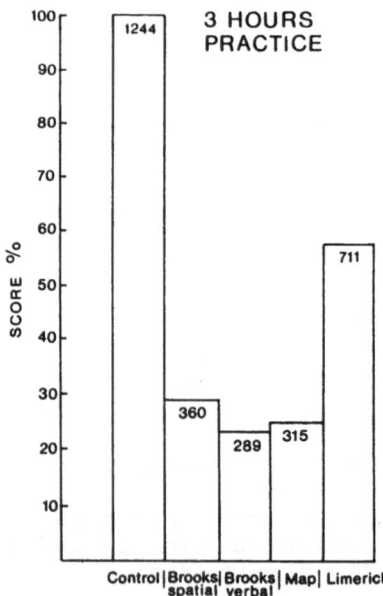

FIGURE 3.   Game scores after 3 hours of training.

Table 1 shows performance for each of the secondary tasks
in terms of the percentage decrements in these tasks when they
were performed concurrently with SPACE FORTRESS.   In contrast
to the effects on game score, the Brooks' spatial task was
somewhat more affected than was the Brooks' verbal task.
Similarly, the map task appeared to show a larger decrement in
performance when performed with the game than did the limerick
task.
     The mean ratings of difficulty are also shown in Table 1.
The Brooks' spatial task, when performed alone was rated as
being somewhat easier than the Brooks' verbal task.   The map
task was rated as not significantly more difficult than the
limerick task.

TABLE 1.   Percentage decrements in secondary task performance
in dual task conditions and mean ratings of difficulty for
secondary tasks performed alone.

	Brooks' Spatial	Brooks' Verbal	Map	Limerick
3 hours training				
Secondary task decrement	42.1	30.9	11.8	7.8
Secondary task difficulty	4.33	5.50	4.28	3.94
8 hours training				
Secondary task decrement	32.2	31.8	4.5	7.7
Secondary task difficulty	3.39	4.50	3.83	3.00

3.2 Eight hours training

     Game scores for each experimental condition are shown in
Figure 4 for subjects after a total of eight hours training. As
you might expect, the overall level of performance is higher
than that found earlier in training.   The overall score was
significantly affected by each of our secondary tasks.
However, the pattern of decrement appears to have changed. Game
score is most affected by the two Brooks' tasks with about the
same disruption from each. There remains a tendency for the map
task to produce a slightly larger decrement in game score than
does the limerick task.   However, the difference is much
reduced when compared with performance earlier in training.
Also, in contrast to previous results the map task is
associated with significantly better scores than are either of
the Brooks' tasks.
     Performance on the secondary tasks and difficulty ratings
are shown in Table 1. The decrements in the Brooks' verbal and
spatial tasks are equivalent at this level of training,
although the spatial task was rated as the easier of the two
tasks. The map task was rated as a little more difficult than
was the limerick task. However, the degree of decrement in
these two secondary tasks was statistically equivalent.

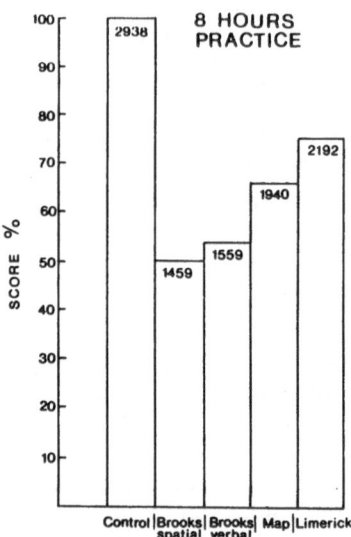

FIGURE 4. Game scores after 8 hours of training.

4. DISCUSSION

The results based on game score and secondary task performance early in training show a tendency for a rather larger degree of mutual impairment associated with the visuo-spatial than with the verbal tasks. This differential disruption is much reduced by further training and it cannot easily be explained in terms of trade-offs in performance between the primary and secondary tasks. For example, early in training the map task produced a larger decrement in game score than did the limerick task. However, these tasks were equally affected by concurrent game performance.

A complementary result was obtained with the Brooks' tasks. They produced equivalent amounts of disruption in game score, but the spatial task was clearly more affected by concurrent game performance than was the verbal task.

The results are also difficult to explain in terms of the relative difficulty of the tasks involved. The map and limerick tasks were rated as equally difficult at the early stage of training.

These results point to an importance of visuo-spatial processing during the early stages of training, on this complex perceptuo-motor task. The importance of visuo-spatial processing appears to diminish with increased experience in playing SPACE FORTRESS.

These results are of course based largely on an arbitrary measure of game performance, namely game score. Could our results be an artifact of the way the score was made up? In order to examine this possibility we also investigated a large number of measures of components of the main task. In addition to game score, a total of 56 parameters of different aspects of the game were recorded, for example the number of successful hits on the fortress, the amount of movement around the screen, time to respond to a friend or a foe mine and so on.

We examined 15 of these parameters in terms of how they were affected by each of our secondary tasks and the results are shown in Table 2. We do not have space here to describe each of the measures or our findings in detail (Logie et al., in press). However it is clear from the Table that at the early stages of training, the map task and the two Brooks' tasks affected substantially more game components than did the limerick task. This is in line with the results for game score.

However after further training, it is clear that a much wider range of components was affected by our secondary tasks. This is in contrast to the results for game score where the apparent effect of our secondary tasks grew less with training. This points to a changing rather than a diminishing role for visuo-spatial processing with increased experience on the primary task.

TABLE 2. Game components affected by each secondary task at different levels of training.

	3 hours training	8 hours training
Brooks Spatial	Fort Hits Fort Destructions RT to Friend Bonus % Total Shots	Fort Hits Fort Destructions RT to Friend Bonus % Total Shots RT to 'IFF' RT to Foe Inter-key RT
Brooks Verbal	Fort Hits Fort Destructions Bonus % Total Shots	Fort Hits Fort Destructions Bonus % Total Shots RT to 'IFF'
Map Task	Ship Damage Fort Destructions RT to 'IFF' Bonus % Inter-key RT	Fort Destructions RT to 'IFF' Bonus % Inter-key RT Fort Hits Total Shots
Limerick Task	Bonus %	Fort Hits Fort Destructions Total Shots

This aspect of the results is particularly interesting as the effects of extensive practice on the role of different working memory components has hitherto been largely unexplored. These results are consistent with the involvement in learning this task of the specialised visuo-spatial mechanism as described by Baddeley and by Quinn. If we view working memory as a set of mechanisms for the temporary storage and processing of information, it is entirely reasonable that the role of its different components would change with differing task characteristics. The characteristics of the demands of any given task are as likely to change with increasing expertise. This in itself is not surprising. What this particular approach has to offer is a technique for specifying the importance of component cognitive skills at different levels of expertise and for a wide range of complex tasks.

Is this approach any more useful than alternative approaches? A traditional approach to the study of cognitive workload in complex tasks relies on subjective assessments given by the trainee. However these judgements should be treated with caution. For example, a requirement to give a subjective assessment about the task may well change the way in which the task is carried out. Also, subjects may not have available to conscious inspection many aspects of skilled performance (Ericsson & Simon, 1980; Nisbett & Wilson, 1977). Our own data support these reservations since the subjective measure of difficulty was not a good predictor of the degree of performance decrement obtained.

A more theoretical approach is to adopt the view that different components of the task compete for general purpose resources. As expertise is gained, some of the processes involved become relatively automatic and demand less of the available resources (Shiffrin & Schneider, 1977). This approach could provide an explanation for why our secondary tasks appear to be associated with less of a decrement in game score with increasing practice. However it does not deal with for example the differential disruption produced by the map task as opposed to the limerick, despite a subjective assessment that these tasks were equivalent in difficulty. Neither can it easily cope with the increase in the range of game components affected with increasing expertise.

Our results have therefore provided evidence that is consistent with the importance in learning a complex perceptuo-motor task of a mechanism that is specialised in the temporary storage of visuo-spatial information. This in turn has shown the notion of a working memory to be useful for the study of considerably more complex tasks than has been common in the literature. The potential scope of this approach is threefold. It could provide a possible new methodology for the study of cognitive workload. It could provide insight into the rather more general question as to the processes which underlie skill acquisition. Finally, it could act as a basis for significant theoretical advances in the development of working memory as an increasingly influential and fruitful explanatory framework.

REFERENCES

1. Baddeley, A.D., Grant, S., Wight, E., & Thomson, N. (1975). Imagery and visual working memory. In P.M.A. Rabbitt and S. Dornic (eds.), Attention and Performance V, pp. 205-217. London: Academic Press.

2. Baddeley, A.D. & Hitch, G.J. (1974). Working memory. In G. Bower (ed.), The Psychology of Learning and Motivation, Vol. VIII, pp. 47-89. New York: Academic Press.

3. Baddeley, A.D. & Lieberman, K. (1980). Spatial working Memory. In R.S. Nickerson (ed.), Attention and Performance VIII, pp. 521-539. Hillsdale, N.J.: Lawrence Erlbaum Associates.

4. Baddeley, A.D., Logie, R.H., Nimmo-Smith, I., & Brereton, N. (1985). Components of fluent reading. Journal of Memory and Language, 24, 119-131.

5. Brooks, L.R. (1967). The suppression of visualisation by reading. Quarterly Journal of Experimental Psychology, 19, 289-299.

6. Ericsson, K.A. & Simon, H.A. (1980). Verbal reports as data. Psychological Review, 87 215-251.

7. Logie, R.H. (1986). Visuo-spatial processing in working memory. Quarterly Journal of Experimental Psychology, 38A, 229-247.

8. Logie, R.H. & Baddeley, A.D. (1987). Cognitive processes in counting. Journal of Experimental Psychology: Learning, Memory and Cognition, 13 (2) 310-326.

9. Logie, R.H., Baddeley, A.D., Mane, A., Donchin, E., & Sheptak, R. (in press). Working memory and the analysis of a complex skill by secondary task methodology. Acta Psychologica.

10. Nisbett, R.E. & Wilson, T.D. (1977). Telling more than you know: Verbal reports on mental processes. Psychological Review, 84, 231-259.

11. Shiffrin, R.M. & Schneider, W. (1977). Controlled and automatic human information processing: II. Perceptual learning, automatic attending and a general theory. Psychological Review, 84, 127-190.

THE EFFECTS OF CENTRAL VERSUS PERIPHERAL DISTRACTION ON VISUAL AND
VERBAL LEARNING

KLAUS BISCHOF

INSTITUTE OF PSYCHOLOGY, UNIVERSITY OF BASEL, SWITZERLAND

ABSTRACT
    The main objective of this work was to investigate the exis-
tence of specific visual and spatial aspects of visual imagery.
Using Brooks' (1967) interference paradigm, subjects had to form
visual images (size: 2, 4 or 8 degrees) and at the same time watch
visual distractor films. Results yielded only tendential evidence
for specific visual and spatial aspects in visual imagery. However
vivid visualisers were better at the visual imagery task and
non-vivid visualisers better at the verbal task. An increase in
size of the image improved performance, particularly of the vivid
visualisers.

1. INTRODUCTION
    The main objective of this work was to investigate the exis-
tence of specific visual and spatial aspects of visual imagery. It
is possible that imagery in general, and visual imagery in particular is epiphenomenal, as suggested by Pylyshyn (1973, 1981).
Pylyshyn (1981) argues that in imagery experiments subjects do not
really use imagery, but consider their task as being to simulate the
witnessing of certain real events mentally and therefore to use
their tacit knowledge to cause the simulation to proceed as they believe it would have in reality. Pylyshyn (1981) would claim that
during the actual experience of visual imagery, people do nothing
other than think very strongly about the object, and do not actually
experience something like a seen image.
    A second purpose of this experiment was to establish a method
whereby one problem of imagery experiments would be avoided:
namely, the confounding of experimental results by subject-generated
hypotheses. To avoid this, performance must be measured directly.
This and other problems with imagery experiments have been pointed
out by Intons-Peterson (1983).
    One way to measure performance directly was first implemented
by Brooks (1967) who modified a classic signal detection paradigm by
Segal (1908). Segal (1908) let subjects generate visual images
while simultaneously trying to discover pictures on a screen.
Brooks (1967) modified this task such that the generation of images
was interfered with by having subjects read text. The visual stimuli distracted and thus decreased generation of the visual image
being formed within a matrix. Under a text reading condition recall
of visual images produced more errors than under a condition of simply hearing the same text.
    It could be argued that Brooks (1967) has already measured both

M. Denis et al. (eds.), Cognitive and Neuropsychological Approaches to Mental Imagery, 203–212.
© 1988 by Martinus Nijhoff Publishers.

visual and spatial aspects, by having the subjects both construct the matrix visually and recall the ordered spatial organisation, however this paradigm had its problems, the elimination of the most important one of which is discussed here. Since reading itself is a demanding task, involving a lot of cognitive processing such as analysing and categorising, it may itself confound the actual visual distraction by letters. In the present work the distracting task was modified to reduce the amount of thinking to a minimum, subjects merely watched the distractors. According to Brooks' (1967) results it is hypothesised that the passive attending of visual information should cause interference in solving the imagery task, compared with a task that requires the learning of a series of sentences, equivalent in length to those of the Brooks visualising task, but differing in that they could only be learned by rote. A further hypothesis is that these "verbal learning sentences" would not show much interference from the visual distractors.

Another aspect that the writer considers important is individual differences. Suppose the hypotheses in imagery experiments were tested separating vivid from non-vivid visualisers. Should it not then be the case that the two groups perform differently, since imagery tasks particularly demand the ability to visualise? Why then not use this important information in experiments? Although the differential method is used occasionally in the literature, it is neither used consequentially nor stringently enough. In some experiments (e.g. Finke and Kosslyn, 1980) authors use differential methods such as imagery vividness questionnaires, yet for no obvious reason abstain from using them in others (e.g. Kosslyn et al., 1983; Finke and Kurtzman, 1981). Taking into account individual differences, it was hypothesised that interference with visual images would be stronger in the group of vivid visualisers, but there should be no difference across groups in the case of the verbal task with visual distractions. The individual differences thus support a differentiated hypothesis, as previously suggested by Underwood (1975) who even suggests they be taken as a crucible in theory construction. In my own theoretical account (Bischof, 1987) an attempt was made to show how these individual differences can be integrated into imagery theory.

One problem remains unclear, namely how large to make the distraction relative to the visual field. One might expect a lot of distraction if the whole visual perceptual field is distracted, however there appears to be a need to have the visual image field the same size as that of the distracting visual field. Taking an analogy with perception, one could postulate a central field of visual imagery (where one would expect a clear and vivid image), and a peripheral field where it is less clear and vivid. Continuing this analogy, Steiner, Bischof and Fröschl (1984) split the size of the distraction at 2 degrees of visual angle (the size of the fovea). Central distraction was thus 2 degrees wide and peripheral distraction was the whole field around this.

Steiner, Bischof and Fröschl (1984) attempted to test whether vivid and non-vivid visualisers show different imagery performance under central versus peripheral distraction. Using three sets of 15 word pairs with the same high imagery value (Bredenkamp and Wippich, 1977), the pairs were presented at 5 second intervals with an ISI of 11 seconds. During visualisation of these word pairs, different

films were shown on a screen. One showed white geometrical forms
moving randomly on a dark background either in the central area, or
in the periphery. The other film was still and showed only the dark
background. The moving forms resembled snowflakes in the wind.
Cued recall measured performance after each distraction condition.
This experiment yielded important results: 1) The separation of
vivid from non-vivid visualisers produced differentiated results;
2) Vivid visualisers tended to be impaired more with central distraction, while non-vivid visualisers were more impaired during
peripheral distraction. Another experiment confirmed this finding
(Bischof and Steiner, 1985).

What size is the central field of visual imagery, i.e. that
field in which the image is experienced sharply? There are tentative suggestions, but no research directly addresses this topic.
One important piece of evidence for the size of the central field of
visual imagery comes from Kosslyn (1980). He let subjects visualise
different objects such as rectangles, line drawings of animals, or
animals drawn from memory and then visualise the objects coming
nearer until they overflowed at the edges. This meant that the process of the visual image overflowing was " ... not an all-or-none
thing, such as happens when a picture runs over the edge of a
cathode-ray tube. Instead, images may fade progressively toward the
edges until they are not evident; the point at which one decides
that an imaged object is not apparent is not sharply defined"
(Kosslyn, 1980, p. 84). The angle at which this overflowing occurred in these experiments was around 20 degrees. Thus a first ap-
proximation of the size of the central field was determined. What
was puzzling however was that other angles were determined in other
experiments.

Finke and Kosslyn (1980) and Finke and Kurtzman (1981) performed experiments in which they tried to determine how far an analogy could be taken between a perceptual phenomenon and the same
phenomenon experienced in imagery. Without going into the details
of all these studies the common basis was firstly to find that angle
where different figures were seen as different but indiscriminable
(i.e. seen as one figure) and then made more peripheral by moving
the fixation point away from the center. Here the relevant result
was that the central field of imagery was anything up to 100 degrees. The vivid imagers usually have a larger central field of
visual imagery.

Clearly there is a large difference between the size found by
Kosslyn and by Finke. The putative central field does not seem to
be easily determinable. Possibly this is due to differing methodologies, and the criteria that subjects use to make the decisions
might differ across the two experimental methods. In the present
experiment there remained some doubt as to what size to make the
visual images. Anything up to 100 degrees seemed justifiable.
Since controlling the size of the central field was necessary
however, it was decided to restrict the size of the image (and consequently the size of the central distraction field) to 2, 4 and 8
degrees under different conditions. No hypothesis concerning the
performance under the three different imagery size could thus
be formulated: Performance under three combinations of imagery and
distraction field (where the relative size of the two fields was
bigger, equal or smaller) was compared.

2. PROCEDURE

The interference paradigm (Brooks, 1967) was used to measure performance of visual imagery under visual distraction conditions.

2.1. MATERIALS AND METHODS

2.1.1. SUBJECTS

108 subjects (47 males, 61 females) were recruited from university courses. The mean age was 21 years, ranging from 15 to 52, s.d.= 7.4.

2.1.2. DESIGN

Each experiment consisted of two sessions so that half the tasks were done in each session. Each session lasted one hour. In each session 30 tasks (15 verbal and 15 imaginal) were performed. At the end of the second session individual imagery ability was measured using imagery questionnaires. At the end of the experiments subjects received a small token sum to cover travel expenses.

The independent variables in the experiment were type of task (visual or verbal), location of distraction, size of distraction (2, 4, or 8 degrees), and size of the visual image to be generated (2, 4, or 8 degrees). A further independent variable was the individual imagery ability, i.e., whether subjects classified themselves as vivid or non-vivid visualisers. The designation was made using Marks' (1973) VVIQ, and Gordon's (Richardson, 1969) test of visual imagery control (GTVIC). The two scores were summed, and the median taken, subjects in the upper 50% being designated as vivid (or good) imagers and the others as non-vivid (or poor) imagers.

The dependent variables were the number of mistakes made in the visual imagery task and in the verbal task. A mistake was a deviation in sequence from the visualised or learned sequence. The possible influence of the experimental variables described was to be controlled for by the verbal task.

Each subject had to solve ten visual imagery and ten verbal tasks under central and peripheral distraction. A verbal task always preceded a visual one. No subject was tested in more than one imagery or distraction size condition, but each group was split into half who had to solve the tasks under central distraction first and half who had to solve it under peripheral distraction first. This procedure was reversed in the second session.

The design of the experiment was planned such that one subject would be tested under exactly one combination of the different sizes of distraction and imagery.

2.1.3. MATERIALS

The materials can be grouped by characteristics as follows:

1) Primary tasks: These are visual imagery tasks and verbal learning tasks. They were a modified version of Brooks (1967) such that the numbers to be visualised in the original were replaced with white squares and these were increased in number to 10 squares in a 4 x 4 matrix. Since the squares had to be visualised consecutively, a certain form was produced. The subject's task was to generate that form and describe it to the experimenter. The verbal learning task consisted of 10 sentences, but spatial adjectives in each sentence were replaced by other adjectives so that the whole row had to be learned by rote.

2) Secondary tasks: These were the distracting films. The entire visual field was divided into microfields of small squares the same size as those to be visualised. Squares blinked individually either in a central or peripheral field. In the central distraction condition the peripheral field was kept black; and vice versa for the peripheral distraction condition. The stimuli were generated by a computer program and presented on a TV screen.

3) Imagery questionnaires:

a) Marks' Vividness of Visual Imagery Questionaire (VVIQ): Marks' (1973) VVIQ seems to be one of the best questionnaires so far on the vividness of visual imagery.

b) Gordon's Test of Visual Imagery Control (GTVIC): The most commonly used test of the control of visual images is that of Gordon (see Richardson, 1969). The GTVIC measures how easily visual images can be generated and manipulated (Ernest, 1977). The test contains 12 questions (Richardson, 1969), rated in a similar fashion to the VVIQ.

The validities of the questionnaires are indicated in the reviews by Sheehan, Ahston & White (1983). Both questionnaires were previously translated into German and tested for reliability. The results were comparable to the English versions (Bischof, 1984).

2.1.4. APPARATUS

For visual distraction an Electrohome Monitor and an Apple II europlus, programed with TGS (1982) was used.

3. RESULTS
3.1. RESULTS: MAIN EFFECTS

Visual imagery tasks are solved better than verbal tasks. This was the first significant result of the experiment (F=149.9; df=1,90; p=0.000) and confirmed the results of earlier work.

Central distraction has a greater effect than peripheral distraction (F=14.8; df=1,90; p=0.000). This result is true taking both tasks together. More importantly, we will see this comparison later across verbal and visual tasks.

All subjects are not equally good in solving all tasks. The vivid visualisers were not significantly better in general (F=0.02; df=1,90; p=0.88) across tasks. Later this result will be broken down into its components.

Different distractor size did not affect performance in general. Whether distractor field size was 2, 4, or 8 degrees did not matter (F=0.15; df=2,90; p=0.86). This result was confirmed by multiple t-tests on the individual combinations.

The result of varying imagery field size is irrelevant so far, since it could not be varied in the verbal task. In the next section we move from the main factors to consideration of the emergent interactions.

3.2. RESULTS: INTERACTIONS

The interaction between task and imagery ability surprisingly reflects the influence of different imagery ability on performance on both tasks. The significant interaction (F=6.16; df=1,90; p=0.015) indicates that the visual tasks are performed better by the vivid visualisers than by non-vivid visualisers, while the verbal tasks are performed better by the non-vivid visualisers.

This result has important implications for further use of the questionnaires. Obviously both Marks' and Gordon's questionnaires not only measure individual imagery ability, but also imply ability to perform on the two tasks under central and peripheral distracting conditions. The vivid visualisers identified by the questionnaires are also the better visualisers in the visual imagery tasks. Whether non-vivid visualisers are also better verbalisers remains speculative.

The differential interaction also provides a strong indication for the use of imagery questionnaires in visual imagery experiments. Had they not been used this result would have gone unnoticed!

Interaction between task and site of distraction: It was hypothesised that central visual distraction ought to interfere more with the visual than with the verbal task. This was not shown to be the case (F=0.51; df=2,90; p=0.48). This is less important in general, since the more specific prediction concerns only the group of vivid visualisers.

Interaction of imagery ability and size of visual image: In this analysis, a tendency towards the interaction of these emerged (F=2.69; df=2,90; p=0.073).

It might have been expected that the vivid visualisers' performance decreases with the increasing size of central distraction. However distraction seemed relatively unimportant in this interaction. Instead it appeared that it was the size of the visual image that was important.

One puzzling effect emerges in this interaction, namely that non-vivid visualisers show good performance on the 4 degree condition. This is possibly due to the number of subjects in each of the three conditions of relative size. In the 4 degree conditions there was an equal number of subjects for the three relative size conditions, while in both the 2 degree and 8 degree conditions, there was a disproportionate number of subjects in the condition where distraction field size exceeded imagery field size.

EXAMINATION OF INDIVIDUAL DIFFERENCES

All differences in the results section which follows were tested for significance using t-tests.

Differential hypotheses: Vivid visualisers make more mistakes during central distraction than during peripheral distraction in the visual task.

For this analysis all 108 subjects were used, divided into vivid and non-vivid visualisers using the median as cutoff. The hypothesis was confirmed: Vivid visualisers were significantly more distracted in the central condition (t=2.61; df=54; p=0.012) of the visual imagery task while non-vivid visualisers were not significantly distracted on the visual task (t=1.05; df=52; p=0.3). In the verbal learning task however, a surprising result emerged: Vivid visualisers scores also showed greater interference during central than peripheral distraction (t=2.67; df=54; p=0.01) as compared to non-vivid visualisers' scores (t=1.86; df=52; p=0.07). Thus vivid visualisers are affected by distraction in both the visual and the verbal learning task, compared to the non-vivid visualisers.

THE PARTICULAR EFFECT OF INCREASING IMAGE FIELD SIZE

During the course of analysis it became apparent that the contribution of visual image size had been underestimated. First the indications for this finding are presented and then some consequences.

1) The first indication that visual image size was important came from the tendency of visual image size to interact with imagery ability. This interaction signalled an increase in performance for vivid visualisers when image size increased. Since this result came from an analysis that did not differentiate the visual from the verbal task, a further analysis was done.

2) A further indication came from comparing the relative size of image with distraction field size. When the central visual image was bigger than the distractor field then fewer errors were made than when relative size was reversed. In the former case subjects had to make their image become bigger than the size of the central distraction.

Summarising the data, it can be claimed that central visual distraction affects performance in good imagers. This is true for both the pure visual imagery task and the verbal control task. The distraction however showed less effect on the non-vivid visualisers. Thus it appears that the differential hypothesis is partially verified - a difference does exist between vivid and non-vivid visualisers. However it also appears that the specific visual aspects in the distraction task also have an effect on the verbal task. This is discussed later.

3) Although the peripheral distraction intrudes into the larger imagery field, compared with central distraction this does not seem to have a strong effect on the imagery task. The result appears then to be caused not entirely by distraction, but by the size of the visual image.

To consolidate these speculations relating image size to the differential hypothesis, the difference in performance was tested on two extreme groups. The vivid visualisers on 2 degrees both in the distraction and the visual task were compared with the 2 degrees of distraction group again, but this time with an image size of 8 degrees. The groups differed significantly (t=2.03; df=102; p=0.05) but since multiple t-tests were used, this can only be described as a tendency, since the significance requirement would have to be p=0.0034 (Bonferroni). Thus all we can say is that vivid visualisers show a tendency to be more distracted by central rather than peripheral distraction. There is no strong proof that size of image is an important factor in solving the visual task under visual distraction. An important consequence, however, comes from looking more closely at the role size of visual image plays. Implicit in this work is the question of the ability of individuals to vary image size. Rather than answer this by experiments which measure performance by visualising and deciding introspectively the size of the image, we need tasks that measure performance on different image sizes in a controlled and indirect way.

FINAL REMARKS ON RESULTS

Other analyses which considered the reproduction of the image as a whole instead of errors only gave ceiling effects, in that the forms appeared to be represented and reproduced quite well. The difficulty appeared to be in the actual stepwise nature of the reproduction. Analysis of covariance and scatterplots with the sociodemographic data did not reveal any relevance for these factors.

4. DISCUSSION

1) In the introduction, the main task was designed in order to verify the existence of specific visual and spatial aspects of visual imagery. According to Brooks' (1967) results, it was hypothesised that passive attending to visual information would result in interference on the imagery task. However it was also hypothesised that, compared with a task that requires the rote learning of a series of sentences of equivalent length to the visually descriptive ones, more interference would be shown by visual distractors on the visual task. Since there was no interaction of task and distraction this hypothesis had to be rejected. Both task conditions, however, were formulated so as to differentiate between two subject groups. Vivid visualisers were expected to make more mistakes in the central distracting conditions of the visual task than in the peripheral conditions. As a control to ensure that results of distraction could not be simply explained away by another factor (e.g., attention) the verbal task was introduced. Performance on this task was expected to be similar across central and peripheral distracting conditions. The results confirmed all these hypotheses with one exception, namely that the vivid visualisers were not only distracted when trying to visualise, but also during the verbal tasks. Thus it would seem that the specific visual and spatial aspects of imagery could not be shown, since obviously a task supposed to be solved purely by rote learning ought not to have been affected by centrally distracting visual information. However it might be claimed that the imagery questionnaires were measuring a factor that had nothing to do with imagery, but instead measured a factor related to attention. Perhaps vivid visualisers' attention is somehow more disturbed by central distraction than that of non-vivid visualisers. This connection is not evident from the literature, so more work is required to solve this problem. The difficulty is in the performance of the non-vivid visualisers. They performed exactly as expected, with no significant interference shown in either the verbal or visual tasks. In the case of the vivid visualisers the experimenter realised that the subjects were trying to develop strategies to solve the verbal task better, since it was found to be more difficult to solve. Future experiments should ensure that the two tasks are made equally difficult. It appeared that subjects occasionally discovered that they could recode the verbal task visually by replacing the word with spatial arrangements, and possibly the responses in the verbal task have been confounded by visual imagery strategies. This would explain the above result.

Another result indicating the existence of actually experienced visual-spatial aspects of the imagery task is the significant interaction of task and imagery ability. Subjects who claim to have been experiencing vivid images do better in solving the imagery task. Likewise non-vivid subjects show better performance on the verbal task. This result partially validates the imagery questionnaires. Performance in a purely visual task is reflected in individual subjects' imagery ability.

A further phenomenon, related to the interference paradigm, is that increasing the quantity of visual stimuli blinking in the centre (by increasing the angle from 2 to 8 degrees) did not cause a general decrease in performance. This suggests that quantity of distracting information may not be important in the interference paradigm. It seemed that, particularly with vivid visualisers, the distraction had no effect, and was excluded from the image. Some subjects even commented that they ignored the distraction, looking right through it when they formed an image.

One unanticipated result is due to the possible effect image size has on its regeneration. Larger images appear to be more easily generated than smaller ones. Kosslyn and Alper (1977) found evidence for increased difficulty with decreased image size. They experimented with word pairs, with one word group to be visualised smaller than its usual and natural size, while another word group had to be visualised in its normal size. The words that were visualised smaller than normal size were recalled more poorly than the control group. Although this might be criticised on methodological grounds, the result as it stands supports our finding. We consider the experienced image size to be a very important part of visual imagery, and this is the topic of our current research effort.

2) The conclusion of this study is that there are some lines of evidence indicating actually experienced visual and spatial aspects of imagery. However these are not strong, and more experimentation is required to establish the replicability of these findings. A further important aspect of visual imagery is the size of the experienced image, but this must be established using actual performance measures rather than subjective reports.

ACKNOWLEDGEMENTS
The author wants to thank G. Steiner and J. Gammack for comments on this work and the Swiss Research Foundation (Project Nr. 1.768.0.83 and 1.122.0.85) for financial support.

REFERENCES

1. Bischof, K. (1984). Reliabilitätsstudie zweier Vorstellungsfragebögen. Unveröffentlichtes Manuskript. Basel: Institut für Psychologie.
2. Bischof, K. (1987). Individuelle Unterschiede beim visuellen Vorstellen. Bern: Peter Lang Verlag.
3. Bischof, K. & Steiner, G. (1985). Is there a central and a peripheral field during visual imagery? International Imagery Bulletin, 2, 15.
4. Bredenkamp, J. & Wippich, W. (1977). Lern- und Gedächtnispsychologie. Stuttgart: Klett.
5. Brooks, L.R. (1967). The suppression of visualization by reading. Quarterly Jounal of Experimental Psychology, 19, 289–299.
6. Dixon, W.J. (1981). BMDP Statistical Software. Berkeley: University of California Press.
7. Ernest, C. H. (1977). Imagery ability and cognition: A critical review. Journal of Mental Imagery, 2, 181–216.
8. Finke, R.A. & Kosslyn, S.M. (1980). Mental imagery acuity in the peripheral visual field. Journal of Experimental Psy-

212

        chology: Human Perception and Performance, 6, 126-139.

9. Finke, R.A. & Kurtzman, H.W. (1981). Area and contrast effects upon perceptual and imagery acuity. Journal of Experimental Psychology: Human Perception and Performance, 7, 825-832.

10. Intons-Peterson, M. J. (1983). Imagery paradigms: How vulnerable are they to experimenters' expectations? Journal of Experimental Psychology: Human Perception and Performance, 9, 394-412.

11. Kosslyn, S.M. (1980). Image and mind. Cambridge, Mass.: Harvard University Press.

12. Kosslyn, S.M. & Alper, S.N. (1977). On the pictorial properties of images: Effects of image size on memory for words. Canadian Journal of Psychology, 31, 32-40.

13. Kosslyn, S.M., Reiser, B.J., Farah, M.J. & Fliegel, S.L. (1983). Generating visual images: Units and relations. Journal of Experimental Psychology: General, 112, 278-303.

14. Marks, D.F. (1973). Visual imagery differences in the recall of pictures. British Journal of Psychology, 64, 17-24.

15. Pylyshyn, Z.W. (1973). What the mind's eye tells the mind's brain: A critique of mental imagery. Psychological Bulletin, 80, 1-24.

16. Pylyshyn, Z.W. (1981). The imagery debate: Analogue media versus tacit knowledge. Psychological Review, 88, 16-45.

17. Richardson, A. (1969). Mental imagery. London: Routledge and Kegan Paul.

18. Segal, S. (1908). Ueber den Reproducktionstypus und das Reproduzieren von Vorstellungen. Archiv für die gesamte Psychologie, Vol. xii, 124.

19. Sheehan, P.W., Ashton, R. & White, K. (1983). Assessment of mental imagery. In: Sheikh, A.A. (Ed.), Imagery: Current theory, research, and application. Chichester: John Wiley and Sons.

20. Steiner, G., Bischof, K. & Fröschl, Th. (1984). Do good imagers differ from bad ones in central vs. peripheral imagery processing? Paper read at the 25th Annual Meeting of the Psychonomic Society, San Antonio (Texas).

21. TGS (1982). The Graphic Solution. Palo Alto: Accent Software.

22. Underwood, B.J. (1975). Individual differences as a crucible in theory construction. American Psychologist, 30, 128-134.

GENERATING AND MAINTAINING VISUAL IMAGES :
THE INCIDENCE OF INDIVIDUAL AND STIMULUS CHARACTERISTICS

MARGUERITE COCUDE

CENTRE D'ETUDES DE PSYCHOLOGIE COGNITIVE
UNIVERSITE DE PARIS-SUD, ORSAY, FRANCE

ABSTRACT
Experiments were conducted to investigate the temporal characteristics (latency and duration) of visual images in response to verbal stimuli. The results show that these two parameters are not influenced by the same factors. Latency is sensitive to imagery value and emotional tonality of stimuli, whereas duration increases with emotional intensity and dynamic content of stimuli. In addition, latency is affected by self-report imagery vividness, and duration by individual mental concentration abilities. These findings strengthen the hypothesis of a functional distinction between generation and maintenance processes in visual imagery.

1. INTRODUCTION

Three issues related to the temporal characteristics of visual imagery will be discussed in this paper : First, what are the intrinsic characteristics of conscious, voluntary, and controllable visual images generated in response to verbal stimuli ? Secondly, what factors have an influence on the generation and the duration of visual images ? And thirdly, what strategies do subjects use to elaborate images ?

The hypothesis underlying our research is that the formation of a visual image corresponds to the temporary activation, in a specialized processor, of representational units stored in long-term memory. The activation of these units elicits psychological events having a figural content. Activated representations are accessible to conscious inspection. To study the temporal characteristics of mental images, two parameters have to be taken into account, namely, latency of image generation and duration of image while it persists in subject's mind.

Generation latency can be operationally defined as the time that elapses between the experimenter's presentation of some stimulus and the subject's declaration that an image has been formed and is actually present in his or her mind. Duration is the period during which a subject who has just generated an image can testify that it is still present in his or her mind. This period corresponds to the involvement of "refreshing" processes acting upon the image (Kosslyn, 1980). Every image vanishes sooner or later, but as long as it is accessible to consciousness, the subject can explore it (Kosslyn, Reiser, Farah, & Fliegel, 1983), transform it

213

M. Denis et al. (eds.), Cognitive and Neuropsychological Approaches to Mental Imagery, 213–222.

(Shepard & Cooper, 1982), and so on. The subject can also keep it in mind passively and indicate when the image formed is changing. We opted for a definition of duration in terms of the persistence of an unmodified image. The extreme case of a modification observed by subjects is the cessation of this image.

The first period, generation latency, has been widely investigated, either in its own right (Paivio, 1966) or in research focusing on learning and memory (Morris & Reid, 1973 ; Richardson, 1977). Amongst the most significant factors affecting latency, one must include concreteness as regards the stimulus, and imagery abilities as regards the subject (Denis, 1982). By contrast, there is almost no information available in the literature about image duration, except the Simpson and Bergin data (1971).

The first series of experiments I conducted in collaboration with Michel Denis served to develop the procedural and methodological groundwork for the investigation of the generation latency of visual images as well as their duration, in response to verbal stimuli.

The reaction times were obtained by the classical method of button-pressing. Recently, Kosslyn, Cave, Provost, and von Gierke (1986), by using a new, more objective method, have confirmed the validity of this classical method. The presentation of stimuli was always auditory to avoid visual interference. We asked the subjects to devote their entire attention to the first visual image they produced in response to the verbal stimulus. They indicated the moment when the image had in any way been modified, by pushing the button again. Then subjects were required to describe verbally the image they had generated and state how it had been modified. Subjects were allowed to keep their eyes closed or open, given the evidence that image generation is not influenced by this factor (Weber & Castleman, 1970). Instructions referred to the clarity and the vividness with which the image was formed, but not to its rapidity.

2. IMAGERY VALUE OF STIMULUS WORDS

In the first experiment, we attempted to assess variations of image generation and image duration as a function of the imagery value of the verbal stimuli (Cocude & Denis, in press). These stimuli were nouns without emotional connotations. They were assigned to three categories according to their rated imagery value (Table 1). Subjects were undergraduates in psychology, 16 female and 5 male (mean age : 28.1 years).

Our study replicated the classical findings on image latency : The higher the noun imagery value, the shorter the latency. Furthermore, as far as concrete words were concerned, the generation latencies were affected by individual imagery vividness as measured by Marks' (1973) Vividness of Visual Imagery Questionnaire (VVIQ) : High imagers had shorter latencies for concrete words, but they were not more skillful than low imagers in generating visual images in response to abstract noun stimuli. On the other hand, noun

Categories	Mean Imagery Value (max. = 6)	Mean Emotional Value (max. = + 3)
HI words	5.31	+ 0.41
MI words	3.91	+ 0.17
LI words	1.83	- 0.39

Table 1
Imagery value of stimulus words

HI words : bouteille (bottle), canard (duck), montre (watch), oreille (ear), rocher (rock), soulier (shoe), tapis (carpet), taxi (taxicab).

MI words : croquis (sketch), distance (distance), éclipse (eclipse), empreinte (imprint), géant (giant), peuple (people), plombier (plumber), sculpteur (sculptor).

LI words : effet (effect), fonction (function), instant (instant), méthode (method), notion (notion), principe (principle), prudence (caution), système (system).

imagery value did not influence image duration. In addition, individual imagery vividness, as assessed by the VVIQ, did not affect the persistence of images.

3. MENTAL CONCENTRATION

Some of the subjects showed special ability in maintaining images for all the verbal stimuli. Through informal discussions, we learnt that most of them regularly did judo, archery, or yoga. These techniques are all known for developing mental concentration (Murphy & Donavan, 1983). Therefore we decided to use the same paradigm in a new experiment comparing hatha-yoga adepts and psychology students unfamiliar with mental concentration techniques as a control group (Cocude & Denis, 1986).

The two groups did not differ in their ability to generate visual images : Mean generation times were quite similar in hatha-yoga and in control students. However, mean durations were different between both groups. The hatha-yoga subjects maintained their images significantly longer than control students (Figure 1).

An analysis based on the number of years of hatha-yoga training revealed that, while generation latencies did not differ in experts (12 years training) and novices (2 years training), the longer the time of regular exposure, the longer the duration of visual images. Experts evidenced much longer image durations than novices (Figure 2).

This experiment showed clearly that some individual factors strongly influence the duration of images, in particular, mental concentration, as is acquired through yoga techniques. Furthermore, the data suggest that the ability to maintain mental images may be enhanced by training.

These two experiments led us to make assumptions about the strategies developed by subjects, in particular for

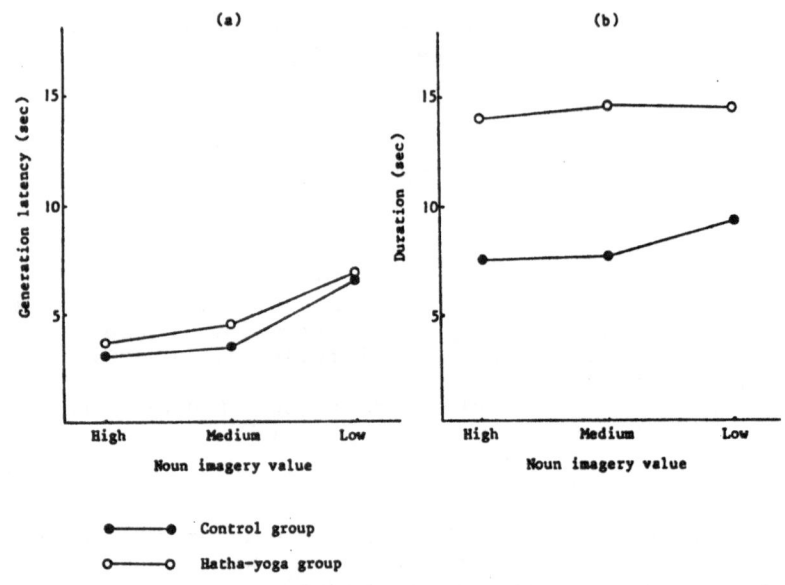

Figure 1
Mean generation latencies (a) and mean durations (b)
of images as a function of noun imagery value,
for hatha-yoga and control groups.

abstract nouns : In order to form an image in response to a
low imagery item, such as "principle" or "notion", subjects
need increased cognitive resources, such as inner verbal
association, metonymies, or codified symbols. They also use
clever strategies, for example, projecting a written word
onto their "mental screen". Such strategies take time. But,
once generated, images for low imagery words are maintained
as easily, and sometimes more easily, than for high imagery
words.
   The results lend support to the assumption of a functional distinction between those processes governing the
generation of visual images and those involved in the temporary maintenance of these images, since both parameters -
latency and duration of images - are not sensitive to the
same factors.

4. EMOTION
   We frequently observed modifications of response times
at certain points in the experimental session which may have
been related to emotional factors. In order to test the influence of emotional factors, a new experiment was conducted
on the effects of the emotional value of words on temporal
characteristics of visual images (Cocude, in preparation).
   Nouns with high imagery value were selected. They were
assigned to three categories according to their emotional
intensity values rated on a scale by independent judges, as
in the previous experiments (Table 2).

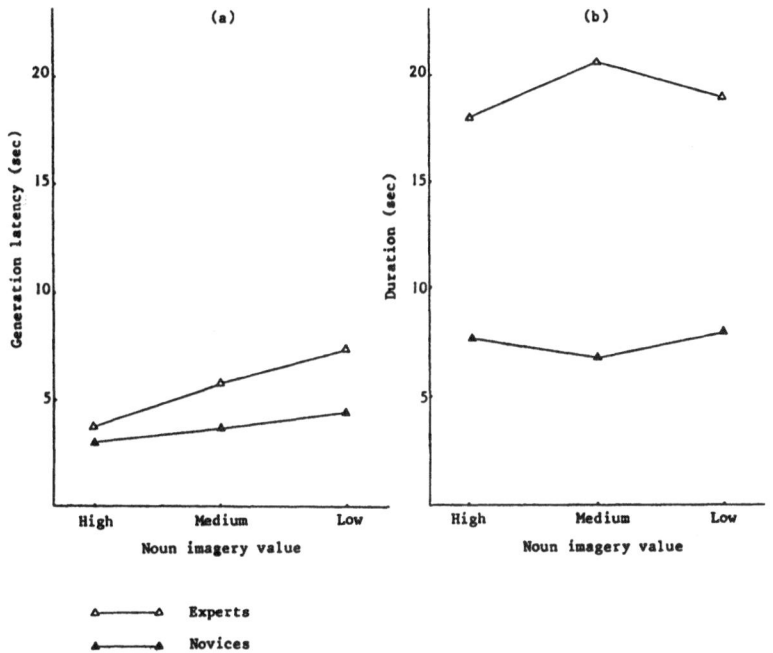

Figure 2
Mean generation latencies (a) and mean durations (b)
of images as a function of noun imagery value,
for experts and novices in hatha-yoga.

Categories	Mean Emotional Value (max. = ± 3)	Mean Imagery Value (max. = 6)
e+	+ 2.09	5.13
eo	+ 0.35	5.15
e-	- 2.06	4.76

Table 2
Emotional value of stimulus words

Subjects were psychology students, without any previous yoga or clinical training, or emotional therapies histories. They were randomly divided in two groups : an experimental group (11 female and 9 male, mean age : 29.2) and a control group (15 female and 15 male, mean age : 28.1).

In the experimental group, subjects, received the imagery task with the same design as previously. Immediately after the end of the imagery task, they were asked to rate the verbal stimuli they had been exposed to for emotional intensity on a scale. The control group was simply requested to rate the emotional intensity of the same stimuli.

The results concerning the generation latencies and the durations of visual images are illustrated in Figure 3. Emotional value of verbal stimuli clearly influenced both temporal parameters. First, positive and neutral stimuli elicited significantly more rapid visual images than negative stimuli (Figure 3a). Secondly, image duration was significantly shorter for neutral than for high emotionally connotated stimuli. On the other hand, positive and negative stimuli did not differ significantly (Figure 3b).

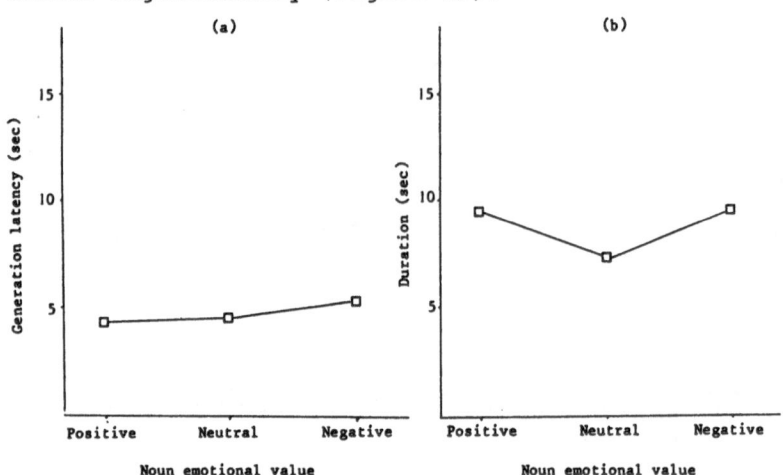

Figure 3
Mean generation latencies (a) and mean durations (b)
of images as a function of noun emotional value.

These findings imply that a single factor can differentially affect the two parameters. Generation latency is mainly concerned with the quality of emotion : Positive (or even neutral) concrete verbal stimuli facilitate image generation, while negative stimuli apparently inhibit it and require more time. Duration is more affected by another component of emotion, its intensity : The more emotional the verbal stimulus, the longer the duration of the image.

We also analyzed the data with the emotional value of the stimuli estimated by the subjects themselves, and not by independent judges as previously (Figure 4). The results become more sharply contrasted when the subjects' own estimation of the emotional value of the stimuli is taken into account : Latency is much longer for highly negative stimuli when estimated by the subjects themselves (Figure 4a). Duration is also lengthened for both highly positive and negative stimuli, but remains unchanged for neutral words (Figure 4b).

Finally, we compared rated emotional intensity of verbal stimuli in the experimental group and the control group. On the average, subjects in the experimental group gave highly emotional (positive and negative) stimuli less extreme ratings than did subjects in the control group, while there was no difference among groups in their ratings of neutral stimuli. This result suggests that recourse to visual imagery alters the emotional connotation of concrete words in the period of time immediately following the imagery task, when

these words carry a high emotional value. Our assumption is
that the difference consists in a sort of emotional "neutra-
lization" of the words. While this result may seem
surprising, it is consistent with the verbal descriptions the
subjects provided of their images. Subjects tended to
"waterdown" the content of negative images as well as
positive ones. For instance, the stimulus word "corpse" was
imaged as wax dummy ; a caress was imaged in relation to a
pet rather than to a person.

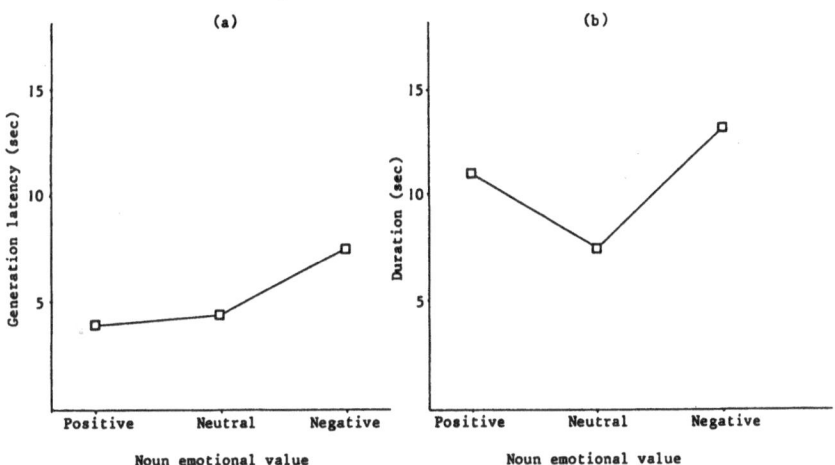

Figure 4
Mean generation latencies (a) and mean durations (b)
of images as a function of noun emotional value
as rated by subjects themselves.

It is naturally impossible to restrict the influence of
emotional variables on visual images to the stimuli alone.
The influence also derives from the individuals themselves. A
stimulus rated on the average as neutral may, of course, have
highly emotional connotations for a subject because of
personal reasons, due to powerful memories. These individual
factors have their repercussions upon the temporal parameters
of the images.
A further line of explorations would be to investigate
whether inhibition of emotional imagery remains active when
the psychophysiological state of the subject is different :
It is reasonable to assume that the psychophysiological state
in which the stimulus is received by the subject (whether the
subject is relaxed or under stress for example) affects the
nature and the content of the image generated. This should
also be discernable in its temporal characteristics. New
experiments are being planned to test this hypothesis, first
using the same sort of subjects who were used previously but
whose psychophysiological state has been modified ; secondly,
testing subjects known to have psychic disorders such as
depression. This research should contribute to more accurate
knowledge of the theoretical foundations of psychotherapeu-

tical methods involving mental imagery (cf. Strosahl & Ascough, 1981).

5. DYNAMIC/STATIC CONTEXT EFFECTS

The persistence of visual images is apparently affected by their internal dynamics. Visualizing scenes either like films or like still photographs in response to verbal stimuli may be expected to influence image duration differentially.

In a preliminary set of studies, Michel Denis and I investigated the duration of images elicited by the verbal descriptions with high image-evoking value and without emotional connotation. The same object-noun was inserted either into a dynamic or a static context (Table 3).

Object-noun	Static context	Dynamic context
Dog	A dog halted in front of a hare	A dog chasing a hare
Hoop	A hoop leaning against a wall	A hoop rolling down a hill
Skater	A skater resting on a bench	A skater skating on the ice
Car	A broken down car on the side of a road	A racing car clocking rounds on a circuit

Table 3
Examples of dynamic/static stimulus material

Results showed that the visual image of an object with repetitive movement was maintained longer than that of a static object. If this finding is confirmed, it will suggest that dynamicity is a factor favoring the "refreshment" of images. We are extending investigations in this way by taking into account movements involving the body, for instance gym exercises. The main question is how and to what extent the temporal parameters of the actual movement itself are involved (Denis, 1985 ; Johnson, 1982). We hope to define the associations - if any - between duration of imagined movements and of actual movements. This study is part of a research program on motor learning and its implications in sports activities.

6. CONCLUSION : SPECIFIC FACTORS INFLUENCE LATENCY AND DURATION OF IMAGES DIFFERENTIALLY

Generating and maintaining visual images are not influenced by the same factors, as summarized in Table 4. These findings strengthen the hypothesis of a functional distinction between generation and maintenance processes in visual imagery. According to this hypothesis, generation processes consist of finding, in memory, the representational units necessary for image formation and activating these units in a specialized processor. These operations involve mechanisms controlling the emotions of the individual. If the filters are efficient, a visual image becomes available in the processor. Another family of processes then relays the

	Type of Factor		Generation	Duration
Factors Related to Stimuli	Imagery Value		+	
	Emotion	Tonality	+	
		Intensity		+
	Dynamics			+
Factors Related to Individuals	Mental Concentration			+
	Imagery Abilities		+	

Table 4
Overview of factors affecting image generation
and image duration

generation processes in order to maintain the activation of
the image above a certain threshold. When the available
resources have been depleted, the image ceases, but the
duration of the image can be lengthened if the stimulus has
special arousing value, for instance, high emotional
intensity, or repetitive dynamics.

Another feature which is made clear is that one can
maintain images longer by regular practice of certain
techniques. By developing mental concentration and mental
control, individuals are able to increase the duration of
their visual images.

REFERENCES

1. Cocude, M. (in preparation). L'influence de la variable
   émotionnelle sur les images visuelles. Université de
   Paris-Sud, Orsay, Manuscript in preparation.
2. Cocude, M. & Denis, M. (1986). The time course of
   imagery: Latency and duration of visual images. In D.
   G. Russell, D. F. Marks, & J.T.E. Richardson (Eds.),
   Imagery 2, (pp. 57-62). Dunedin, New Zealand : Human
   Performance Associates.
3. Cocude, M. & Denis, M. (in press). Measuring the temporal
   characteristics of visual images. Journal of Mental
   Imagery.
4. Denis, M. (1982). Les aspects temporels de l'activité
   d'imagerie. Psychologie Française, 27, 134-145.   -—
5. Denis, M. (1985). Visual imagery and the use of mental

practice in the development of motor skills. <u>Canadian Journal of Applied Sport Sciences</u>, <u>10</u>, 4S-16S.

6. Johnson, P. (1982). The functional equivalence of imagery and movement. <u>Quarterly Journal of Experimental Psychology</u>, <u>34A</u>, 349-365.

7. Kosslyn, S. M. (1980). <u>Image and mind</u>. Cambridge, MA : Harvard University Press.

8. Kosslyn, S. M., Cave, C. B., Provost, D. A., & von Gierke, S. M. (1986). Sequential processes in image generation : Evidence from an objective measure. Harvard University manuscript.

9. Kosslyn, S. M., Reiser, B. J., Farah, M. J., & Fliegel, S. L. (1983). Generating visual images : Units and relations. <u>Journal of Experimental Psychology : General</u>, <u>112</u>, 278-303.

10. Marks, D. F. (1973). Visual imagery differences in the recall of pictures. <u>British Journal of Psychology</u>, <u>64</u>, 17-24.

11. Morris, P. E., & Reid, R. L. (1973). Recognition and recall : Latency and recurrence of images. <u>British Journal of Psychology</u>, <u>64</u>, 161-167.

12. Murphy, M., & Donavan, S. (1983). A bibliography of meditation theory and research : 1931-1983. <u>Journal of Transpersonal Psychology</u>, <u>15</u>, 181-227.

13. Paivio, A. (1966). Latency of verbal associations and imagery to noun stimuli as a function of abstractness and generality. <u>Canadian Journal of Psychology</u>, <u>20</u>, 378-387.

14. Paivio, A. (1971). <u>Imagery and verbal processes</u>. New York : Holt, Rinehart & Winston.

15. Richardson, A. (1977). The meaning and the measurement of memory imagery. <u>British Journal of Psychology</u>, <u>68</u>, 29-43.

16. Shepard, R. N., & Cooper, L. A. (1982). <u>Mental images and their transformations</u>. Cambridge, MA : The MIT Press.

17. Simpson, H. M., & Bergin, J. C. (1971, June). Imagery latency and duration. Paper presented at the meetings of the Canadian Psychological Association, St John's, Newfoundland.

18. Strosahl, K. D., & Ascough, J. C. (1981). Clinical uses of mental imagery : Experimental foundations, theoretical misconceptions, and research issues. <u>Psychological Bulletin</u>, <u>89</u>, 422-438.

19. Weber, R. J., & Castleman, J. (1970). The time it takes to imagine. <u>Perception and Psychophysics</u>, <u>8</u>, 165-168.

PROCESSING OF ORDER WITH PICTURES

ALAIN LIEURY

UNIVERSITE DE HAUTE-BRETAGNE, RENNES, FRANCE

ABSTRACT
Memory for pictures is often described as being under a non-sequential processing system. The three experiments reported here show that serial memory for words is superior to that for pictures only in the case of standard instructions. In contrast, serial memory for pictures is better when either overt verbalization or articulatory suppression are imposed. It is argued that processing of order is possible in imaginal coding and that the lexical component of verbal coding of words may explain the superiority of words over pictures in standard instruction conditions.

The superiority of pictures over words in memory tasks is generally reversed when serial recall and reconstruction are used. There is a general agreement that this result indicates that image coding is handled by a non-sequential processing system contrary to verbal coding. The non-sequential nature of this processing might be due to the holistic nature of retinal or visual processing. But the problem is probably more complex than may be assumed, as empirical and logical arguments show.

1) Empirical evidence :
- Using a reconstruction of serial order, Nelson, Reed, and McEvoy (1977) showed that pictures are superior to words.
- The efficiency of the loci method, as a mnemonic, is also an indication that image coding may be efficient in coding order (Crovitz, 1969).

2) Logical obstacles :
- First, it is difficult to think of a genuine system of processing of order for words because sequential memory tasks are often very difficult with words and involve various strategies, except for short sequences (Oléron, 1978, 1980).
- Secondly, in most experiments comparing pictures and words, words are presented in a graphic form, which is a subcategory of pictures. Therefore, why is sequential processing possible for the graphic forms of words and not for pictures ? Obviously, it is not because of peripheric mechanisms like retinal functioning or visual processing. In addition, visual processing is not holistic but frequently sequential, due to exploratory saccadic movements. Noton and Stark (1971), for example, assumed that there is a memory for

223

M. Denis et al. (eds.), Cognitive and Neuropsychological Approaches to Mental Imagery, 223–227.

order of exploratory saccadic movements.
  - Thirdly, why are pictures not superior to words when
presentation time enables dual coding ? When there is dual
coding of pictures, pictures are coded verbally. As the
verbal code enables sequential memory, why doesn't the verbal
coding of pictures enable sequential coding ? Paivio and
Csapo's (1969, 1971) ingenious assumption was that the recall
of pictures is equal to the recall of words for long presentation times due to the verbal component of picture processing, but that pictures should be inferior to words for short
presentation times, when implicit labelling is not possible.
However, experimental results have not always gone in this
direction.
  Three experiments were conducted to reexamine the problem of image coding and sequential processing. Experiment I
partly replicated the classical results of Paivio and Csapo
(1969), with presentation times from 120 to 1920 ms (Table
1). The lists included 9 items and we used a video technique
(for details on the method, see Lieury & Calvez, 1986 b).

	Presentation time (ms)				
	120	240	480	960	1920
Pictures	1.41	1.50	2.16	3.08	4.25
Words	1.25	1.83	2.41	3.16	3.75

Table 1 : Mean verbal recall of order for pictures and words
           as a function of presentation time.

  Pictures were not better recalled in order than words,
as in the Paivio and Csapo study (1969). Nevertheless,
pictures were not less well recalled than words for shorter
times as predicted by Paivio and Csapo's hypothesis (1971).
Moreover, liberal scoring (correct responses in any order)
showed that pictures were not better recalled than words with
time presentations superior to 480 ms as with free recall
instructions and the same material (Lieury & Calvez, 1986 a).
  Experiment II was conducted to test the hypothesis that
some specific strategies are involved when recall is serial.
With verbal material, several experiments have shown the importance of lexical component (Levy, 1975 ; Lieury &
Choukroun, 1985). In this experiment, verbalization conditions during memorization were controlled. Three conditions
were examined : a) a standard, control condition, where the
subjects were only asked to memorize and were given no other
explicit instructions as to verbalization ; b) an overt
verbalization condition, where the subjects were asked to

either name pictures or read words aloud ; (c) an articulatory suppression condition, where the subjects were asked to repeat "la, la, la..." during the presentation of pictures or words. Three presentation times were used : 240, 480, and 720 ms.

Results yielded the same result for recall in order as in Experiment I (similar to Paivio and Csapo, except for short presentation times) in the standard condition (Figure 1). But in the overt verbalization and the articulatory suppression conditions, pictures were better recalled in order than words at 480 and 720 ms. These results do not support the hypothesis of a non-sequential system for the processing of pictures. On the other hand, sequential processing for words seemed to be related to lexical coding in the standard condition since pictures are superior to words in the articulatory suppression condition. We can assume that a lexical code is responsible for the superiority of words in the standard condition.

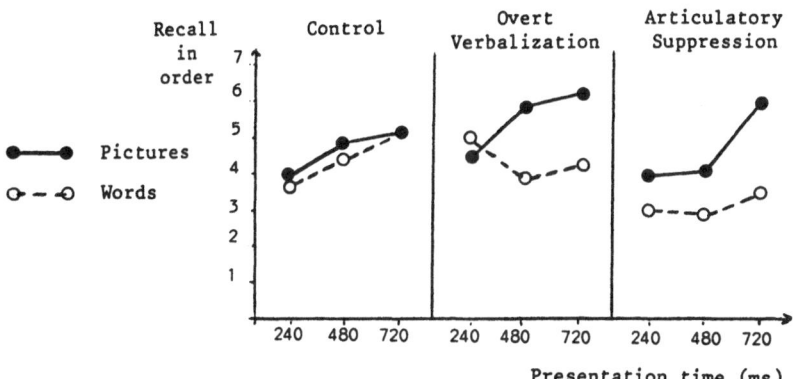

Figure 1 : Mean recall of pictures and words as a function of presentation time in the three conditions

In Experiment III, conducted with Régine Poirot, lists of 3 to 8 items (pictures or words) were compared in two sequential memory tasks in overt verbalization and articulatory suppression conditions. The verbal recall of order and the reconstruction of order were better for pictures than for words, expecially in the articulatory suppression condition (Table 2).

To conclude, the image code can integrate certain sequential information better than the verbal code, and the hypothesis of a non-sequential processing system for pictures seems to be invalidated. The differential results in standard conditions and in overt verbalization and articulatory suppression conditions can be explained by the composite nature of the verbal component of dual coding (Lieury & Calvez, 1986 a) : the verbal component is composed of an obligatory seman-

	% Serial Recall		% Reconstruction	
	Overt Verbalization	Articulatory Suppression	Overt Verbalization	Articulatory Suppression
Pictures	67.78	55.60	77.27	75.45
Words	63.78	45.15	65.66	57.12

Table 2 : Percentage of serial recall and reconstruction of order for pictures and words as a function of conditions.

tic coding (interpretation of the picture) and an optional lexical coding (Table 3).

	Pictures			Words	
Codes	Imaginal	Semantic	Lexical	Semantic	Lexical
Standard	+	+		+	+
Overt Verbalization	+	+	+	+	+
Articulatory Suppression	+	+		+	

Table 3 : Schematic representation of hypothetical influence of lexical coding in the serial recall of pictures and words.

Lexical coding seems to be involved in memory of order for words but not for pictures only in the case of standard instructions, which masks a true possibility of processing order for imaginal coding.

REFERENCES

1. Crovitz, H.F. (1969). Memory loci in artificial memory. Psychonomic Science, 16, 82-83.
2. Levy, B.A. (1975). Vocalization and suppression effects in sentence memory. Journal of Verbal Learning and Verbal Behavior, 14, 304-316.
3. Lieury, A., & Calvez, F. (1986). Le double codage des dessins en fonction du temps de présentation et de l'ambiguïté. L'Année Psychologique, 86, 45-61. (a)

4. Lieury, A., & Calvez, F. (1986). Codage imagé et traitement séquentiel. L'Année Psychologique, 86, 329-347. (b)

5. Lieury, A., & Choukroun, J. (1985). Rôle du mode de présentation (visuel, auditif, audio-visuel) dans la mémorisation d'instructions. L'Année Psychologique, 85, 503-516.

6. Nelson, D.L., Reed, V.S., & McEvoy, C.L. (1977). Learning to order pictures and words : A model of sensory and semantic encoding. Journal of Experimental Psychology : Human Learning and Memory, 3, 485-497.

7. Noton, D., & Stark, L. (1971). Scanpaths in eye movements during pattern recognition. Science, 71, 308-311.

8. Oléron, G. (1978). Latence des réponses dans l'évocation immédiate de brèves séries de mots. L'Année Psychologique, 78, 61-78.

9. Oléron, G. (1980). Is there a span of sequential evocation ? International Journal of Psycholinguistics, 15, 5-26.

10. Paivio, A., & Csapo, K. (1969). Concrete image and verbal memory codes. Journal of Experimental Psychology, 80, 279-285.

11. Paivio, A., & Csapo, K. (1971). Short term sequential memory of pictures and words. Psychonomic Science, 24, 50-51.

3.2. IMAGERY PROCESSES IN PROBLEM SOLVING AND IN THE ACQUISITION OF MOTOR SKILLS

MENTAL IMAGERY AND PROBLEM SOLVING

GEIR KAUFMANN

DEPARTMENT OF COGNITIVE PSYCHOLOGY
UNIVERSITY OF BERGEN, NORWAY

ABSTRACT
The question of the functional role of imagery in problem solving is examined. A theory is presented which rests on the premise that translating a problem from a propositional to an analog format gives access to a set of simpler cognitive processes of a perceptual kind. Within this theoretical framework an inverse relation between the utility of imagery and degree of programming in the task is postulated. The implications of this hypothesis are analyzed, and evidence bearing on its validity is briefly discussed. It is concluded that available evidence supports the theory. Finally, the theory is used as a basis for explaining why concretization normally facilitates performance.

1. INTRODUCTION AND CONCEPTUAL ANALYSIS

As documented in several reviews of research (Kaufmann, 1979, 1980, 1984a; Richardson, 1983), a substantial body of research evidence deals with the potential role of imagery in human problem solving. This particular brand of imagery research has, however, a more fragile theoretical base than the research in the fields of memory and learning. There is,thus, a great need for a theoretical structure that can serve to integrate and give meaning to the empirical evidence presently available, and to give direction to future research. The aim of the present paper is to suggest a candidate for such a theory and test its validity against existing evidence in the field.

1.1. The scope of problem solving

In definitions of problem solving it is emphasized that the individual has a problem when he/she has a goal, but is uncertain as to what series of actions he/she should perform to reach it (Raaheim, 1974; Simon, 1978). The uncertainty experienced by the subject may be seen as resulting from a gap between the situation at hand and the desired result (Ray,1955). Major stimulus conditions responsible for the gap are complexity, novelty and ambiguity (e.g. Bourne et al.,1971; Raaheim,1961,1974). We have previously argued that a satisfactory definition is to regard a problem as a discrepancy between an existing situation and a desired state of affairs (Kaufmann, 1984b; Pounds,1969).This definition incorporates both "presented problems", where the individual is confronted with a difficulty that has to be handled, "anticipated problems", where a future difficulty is foreseen, and "constructed problems", where the individual "finds" a problem by comparing an existing situation with a future, hypothetical state of affairs.

1.2. Dimensions of problems

Problems may be classified in many ways. Here we will focus on two di-

231

M. Denis et al. (eds.), Cognitive and Neuropsychological Approaches to Mental Imagery, 231–240.
© 1988 by Martinus Nijhoff Publishers.

mensions that are particularly pertinent to the question of the role of imagery in problem solving.

The concrete-abstract dimension is clearly relevant to the present inquiry. The concept of concreteness-abstractness has been defined in different ways in the psychological literature (e.g. Paivio, 1971, pp. 16-18). It may refer to how directly the stimulus relates to particular objects and events, to dispositions or reaction-tendencies in the sense of reacting to specific details vs. general properties of the situation (Goldstein & Scheerer, 1941), or to the degree dimensions of space and time beyond the here-and-now are dealt with.

Sticking closely to the basic definition of a problem, Simon (1977) classifies problems in terms of varying degrees of programming. From this angle, problems are conceived as falling along a continuum from well-programmed to non-programmed tasks. A problem is programmed to the extent that the problem-solver has a definite procedure to handle it. Problems are nonprogrammed when they are novel for the subject, unstructured or unusually complex. The concept of level of programming in problems is an interesting one in the sense that it is sufficiently open to include all the major determinants of problem-difficulty (i.e. novelty, complexity and ambiguity).

1.3. Defining imagery

The term 'imagery' is rather ambiguous. It may be used to denote, in a general way, cognitive content, which is both of a sensory and nonsensory kind (see Kaufmann, 1979). More frequently, 'imagery' refers to representational processes of a specific quasi-sensory kind - usually to the visual modality. In the present context we will consequently use the term 'imagery' as equivalent to visuo-spatial representational processes.

1.4. Two kinds of imagery effects

An important prerequisite for addressing the question of the possible functional properties of imagery is to make a conceptual distinction between different conditions that may determine the usefulness of imagery as a symbolic tool in task performance. One set of conditions may be termed availability conditions. Here imagery may be used because it is easily available and highly appropriate for the type of information to be handled, such as concrete and visual-spatial information. However, the conditions where imagery is most readily available may not be the same as the conditions where it is most strongly needed. Imagery may be most readily available in concrete tasks, but conceivably is most highly needed in abstract task-environments. Such a distinction opens the avenue for exploring a second type of imagery effect related to what may be termed utility conditions.

2. THEORY AND PREDICTIONS

2.1. Imagery and concreteness-abstractness

In most theories of imagery, its intimate relationship to concreteness and a perceptual/spatial type of information is emphasized (e.g. Paivio, 1971). The idea here is, of course, that imagery is closely linked to perception (e.g.Finke,1985) and is easily available and appropriate as a mode of representation when the task is concrete, and the information to be processed is perceptual and spatial. The evidence in favor of this hypothesis seems quite strong in the area of learning and memory (Paivio, 1983). While the relationship between imagery and task concreteness has not been studied in the same systematic and comprehensive way in problem solving, it is a reasonable hypothesis that the link will hold in this domain too.

2.2 Imagery and level of programming

What about imagery in relation to level of programming in the task environment?

A rather firmly established conclusion reached in contemporary research on problem solving is that the individual has to resort to so-called weak methods when the task at hand is low in programming (Newell,1969; Simon, 1978). Weak methods are general, pragmatic strategies which may be applied over a wide range of problems. They are "weak" in the sense of lacking precision, and do not guarantee success, in contrast to strong methods which are precise, tailor-made to the situation and a safe and fast way to solution of the task. It is tempting to explore the possibility that the same general principle can be applied in the domain of representational methods.

From a developmental perspective, Bruner et al. (1966) argued that cognitive growth is characterized by the evolution of increasingly more powerful representational systems, with the concrete, perceptual-based imagery system preceding the abstract and propositional, linguistic symbolic system. Along similar lines, we have argued that learning a language gives rise to a new system of representation, fueling a new and more powerful way of thinking which is abstract, propositional, and computational in the general sense of involving rule governed inferences (Kaufmann, 1986).

These arguments suggest the following major hypothesis: A linguistic-propositional representational format is a strong one in the sense that great precision may be achieved in the form of explicit descriptions. It is easily and quickly manipulated and contains the full range of computational operations within its potential. In contrast, imagery is more ambiguous, sluggish and less easily manipulated and only realizes simple cognitive operations of a perceptual kind, like anticipations and comparisons. Taking this line of reasoning into the general theory of strong and weak methods, it follows that imagery may have the potential of giving access to a set of simpler, perceptual-like cognitive operations. This may be useful and even necessary under conditions of low programming in the task environment, where computational operations in the sense of rule-governed inferences are difficult or impossible to perform. More specifically, limitations of the possibility of using computational operations may be due to lack of experience with the task at hand (either factual or strategic), where computational processes break down due to lack of rule-based information to feed on (novelty). Limitations of computational operations may also result from strain on working memory capacity due to high information load (complexity). Finally, uncertainty as to which rule or procedure should be applied may lead to computational dysfunctions (ambiguity).

The basic elements and structure of the theory are presented in Table 1.

Table 1. Elements and structure of the theory

CONSCIOUS REPRESENTATIONS	VERBAL		IMAGINAL	
MODE OF OPERATION	COMPUTATIONAL Transformations (Rule governed inferences)		PERCEPTUAL Simulations (Mental modelling)	
Main information processing categories	Deductive reasoning	Inductive reasoning	Perceptual comparisons	Perceptual anticipations
UNDERLYING REPRESENTATIONS	PROPOSITIONAL		ANALOG	

Morris & Hampson (1983) have argued that consciousness has the functions of monitoring and regulating task performance when processing does not run automatically. Consequently, conscious representations will be used in non-routine tasks. We agree with this general thesis and distinguish consequently between conscious representations and underlying representations. However, the Morris & Hampson position is a highly general one and does not distinguish between the functional properties of different kinds of conscious representations with regard to the automatic-deliberate processing dimension. Conscious representations may either be verbal or imaginal and seen as the manifestations of underlying representations that are propositional and analog. Reasoning in a verbal-propositional format involves transformations in the sense of rule-governed inferences which fall into two main categories: Deductive inferences where certainty of reasoning may be attained, and inductive inferences which is related to hypothesis formation and hypothesis evaluation.

The mode of processing involved in imagery is perceptual and may be characterized as simulations rather than transformations (e.g. Rumelhart & Norman, 1985). This means that in imagery we try to imagine what will happen under actual or hypothetical perceptual conditions (rather than inferring it through logical transformations). An imagery-based representation may be isomorphically related to the object represented in the form of an analog. An example would be the images presumably involved in the mental rotation task contrived by Shepard (1978). Imagery based representations may, however, also be highly symbolic, as in the case of Einstein's exploration of the relativity of optical events, when he imagined himself riding alongside of a lightbeam exploring what he would see compared to a stationary observer (see Kaufmann, 1979).

Images thus may be best described as perceptual-like mental models (e.g. Johnson-Laird, 1983). The basic premise of the present theory is that imagery-based mental models are constructed for the purpose of accessing simpler cognitive operations of a perceptual kind. More specifically we will suggest that deductive operations may be translated into simple, quasi-perceptual comparisons, where certainty of judgment may be reached. The imagery parallel to inductive operations may be quasi-perceptual anticipations, where a future state of affairs may be imagined on the basis of a previous sequence of events. The theory proposed here links the functional utility of imagery specifically to a low level of programming in the task environment. Below, a brief excerpt of the empirical evidence specifically relevant to the imagery-level of programming link will be given.

3. EMPIRICAL EVIDENCE
3.1. Informal studies

In line with theoretical expectations, reports pertaining to the development of major inventions and scientific discoveries suggest that the inventors were visualizing complex situations when their revealing "flash of insight" took place (Kaufmann, 1979, 1980; Shepard, 1978). In his work with "Synectics-groups", Gordon (1961) also emphasizes the functional significance of imagery in the process of invention (see also Walkup, 1965). In several phase models of creative thinking, the same point is made: The initial discovery phase is seen to involve transformational activity in the imagery medium, while the second stage related to verification is presumed to involve the more "logical" and directed verbal symbolic system (McKellar, 1951; Rugg, 1963).

Such informal evidence and descriptive statements are suggestive of a link between imagery and a low level-of-programming. But firmer evidenc than this is needed. A summary will therefore be given of empirical research from earlier and more recent experimental work, which pertains to our general hypothesis concerning the functional usefulness of visual imagery and linguistic representation in regard to the level of programming dimension in problem solving (see Kaufmann, 1980, 1984a, for extensive discussions).

3.2. Excerpt from early imagery research

In the early literature on the role of imagery in cognition, it is interesting to note that several prominent workers in the field, such as Galton (1883), Titchener (1910), Bartlett (1927), and Pear (1927), all agree in assigning major importance to imagery in the processes of change and invention in thinking. Several experiments from the early period seem to confirm such points of view. Fox (1914) and Comstock (1921) both found that cognitive conflict was the most important condition for promoting imagery, while the contrary condition of "smooth" thinking was unfavorable for the production of imagery. Woods (1915) and Finkenbinder (1914) obtained evidence indicating that imagery is the more important mode of representation where the task contains a high degree of novelty.

These findings which relate imagery to "conflict", "change", and "novelty" all converge in attributing a potentially prominent role to imagery in low-programmed task environments. However, these early experiments are not particularly stringent in regard to design. Therefore, we must look to contemporary research for more precise evidence.

3.3. Imagery and language in relational inferences

Probably the most systematic and well-controlled experiments on the issue of symbolic representation in problem solving have been done in the field of deductive thinking. The particular tasks under scrutiny are known as "linear syllogisms" or "three-term series" problems. The following is an example:

        Anne is taller than Jean
        Mary is shorter than Jean
        Who is tallest?

Recent research on the solution of three-term series problems has focused on two competing theories: The Image theory and the Linguistic theory. According to the Image theory (Huttenlocher, 1968), the subject will attack the problem by combining the premises into a unitary representation in the form of a mental image, and then "read off" the answer. According to this interpretation, it will, for instance, be easier to place a premise in the representational array if its first item is an "end anchor", that is, occurring at one end of the final array, rather than as a middle item. The evidence supports the Image theory on this point.

The imagery interpretation has, however, been challenged by Clark (1969a, 1969b). Clark claims that the difficulties in solving three-term series problems may be explained by way of psycholinguistic principles, such as congruity (the individual will search for information that is congruent with the form of the question). In the course of the research that has been done, ad hoc assumptions have made it hard to distinguish the competing theories in terms of empirical implications (see Johnson-Laird, 1972). On one point, however, the evidence at hand indicates a clear and systematic difference in the functional properties of imaginal and linguistic representational strategies in the solution of linear syllogisms. In our own theory, it follows explicitly that imagery has its most important function in the initial phase of the problem solving process. Subsequently, with increasing familiarity, a purely linguistic representation will be the more economical one. Precisely this developmental pattern has been demonstrated in experiments performed by Wood (reported by Johnson-Laird, 1972). A similar developmental pattern as that observed by Wood has been demonstrated by Quinton and Fellows (1975). Clearly in line with the theoretical expectations raised above, the function of imagery is linked to the condition of high task novelty. From several experiments of the concept formation type, similar results are reported: In the "discovery-stage" a clear effect of the imagery variable is obtained. In a subsequent "transfer" phase, the imagery effect seems to disappear, for a purely linguistic representation to take over (Kaufmann, 1980, 1984a; see also Helstrup, 1977).

Potts & Scholz (1975) isolated the time required to encode the two premises of a three-term series problem from the time required to generate an answer to the test question. The results obtained indicated that the subjects tend to integrate the two premises into a single, unified representation in the way posited by the image theory. It is interesting to note that the effect is particularly pronounced under conditions of high incongruity. Also their evidence suggests that complexity is an important determinant of the usefulness of an imagery representation (e.g.stronger effect with larger number of premises).

3.4. Symbolic representation in ideational fluency performance

A promising task for testing the general hypothesis under consideration is the ideational fluency situation developed by Guilford (1967). The results from a series of experiments with ideational fluency tasks seem to show that the ideas given early in the production sequence tend to be rather conventional and stereotyped, whereas high quality and original ideas appear at a later stage (Parnes,1961). On the premise that amount of processing required for task performance increases systematically during the given production time, it follows from our theory that the utility of imagery will increase correspondingly.

In an experiment designed to test this hypothesis (Kaufmann, 1981), the imagery-construct was operationalized through scores on a spatial visualization test. When the predictor effect for the spatial visualization test was calculated in relation to performance at different time intervals in the production sequence, a remarkably systematic pattern emerged. The results showed a systematic increase in predictor efficiency with increasing production time, from non-significance in the 1-min. interval to strong significance in the 4-min. interval. No systematic relationship was obtained for a verbal control test.

3.5. Symbolic processes and the discovery of a rule

Processes involved in the induction and application of a rule in problem solving may be studied in water jar tasks involving volume measuring problems. In this kind of task, the subject is presented with a description of a certain number of empty jars and a given quantity of fluid. The jars contain a specified amount of volume, and the task of the subject is to figure out how to obtain a stipulated volume of fluid, given certain precise specifications. The task of the subject is to find the correct rule for performing the transformations, apply it to subsequent problems and switch to a different rule when required.

An experiment was designed to examine the role of imagery and linguistic strategies in this type of problem (Kaufmann,1984a). Imagery and linguistic strategies were operationalized through (a) variations in stimulus presentation, (b) subjects' report of use of strategies, and (c) scores on a spatial visualization test. There was no effect of variations in stimulus presentation. However, a systematic relationship between symbolic strategies measured by (b) and (c) and problem solving was observed. According to both subjects' reports and scores on the spatial visualization test, imagery seems to be used predominantly in the initial phase of the problem. Subsequently, the subjects switch to a linguistic strategy.

3.6 Imagery in chess

Imagery has often been pointed to as an important cognitive operation in chess playing (e.g. Milojkovic, 1982). The evidence is, however, largely anecdotal, and little in the way of systematic experimental research has been carried out. Recently, Milojkovic (1982) made an interesting attempt to improve upon this state of affairs. He examined the problem-solving performance of novices with that of chess masters, and investigated the role of imagery by making creative use of the "mental travel" experimental design devised by Kosslyn (1980). A major finding was the existence of a systematic effect for imagery among novices, but not for masters. Milojkovic argues that whereas novices are likely to use imagery during problem solving, masters base their judgments on more abstract representations of board positions. These findings fall nicely in line with much evidence suggesting that task novelty is a major determinant of the functional use of imagery in problem solving.

3.7. Mathematical problems

In mathematical problems the task often is to find efficient computational procedures for calculating a specified kind of answer using some precisely specified information. Largely from testimonial evidence, Skemp (1971) suggests that visual imagery has an important function in mathematical problem solving. Hadamard, the mathematician, emphasizes the general need for imagery under the condition of high task complexity (cited by Gordon, 1961, p. 114). Such testimonial evidence may be suggestive, but suffer from obvious limitations in interpretability.

On a more systematical level, Barabat (reported in Smith,1964) obtained some suggestive findings from a comprehensive investigation of mathematical aptitude with samples of boys and girls in grammar school. The geometry tests had a substantial loading on the spatial factor. This finding has been replicated in several other investigations (Smith, 1964). On the algebra test there was a significant loading on the spatial factor for girls, but not for boys. Wrigley (1958) obtained negative loading on the mathematical group factor for verbal tests, but positive for spatial visualization tests. This pattern was found with algebra as well as geometry tasks. Werdelin (1958) also obtained positive effects for the spatial factor in relation to mathematical aptitude. Again the verbal factor had the lowest correlations of all factors included. In a large-scale investigation,where Guilford-tests were used to predict mathematical performance, Hill (reported in Smith, 1964) found a positive relationship between scores on visualization tests and general mathematical aptitude. A low and insignificant correlation was obtained in the case of verbal ability (measured by a vocabulary test). Of considerable interest in the context of the hypotheses we have raised, is the conclusion drawn by Vernon (1950) from a study of the mathematical abilities of college students and army cadets. Vernon found that the effect of spatial ability was particularly pronounced at the high grade level - a finding that has been replicated in more recent research(Poole & Stanley, 1972; Sherman, 1979). These findings indicate that visualization may play an important role in abstract problem solving, particularly at the advanced level. However, more precise and experimentally based research is clearly needed in this area which involves issues of great importance both from a theoretical and applied point of view.

Tentative observations along experimental lines have been made by Paige and Simon(1966) on algebra word problems. Paige and Simon discovered that there were systematic individual differences in the kinds of strategies

238

used by the subjects. In the present context the most interesting difference was that between preference for a "verbal" vs. "physical" strategy. The "verbal" strategy consists in representing the problems mainly as sets of equations. In the "physical" strategy, the subjects report that they visualize physical or spatial representations (in the form of diagrams, graphs or models) as aids in solving the problem. An interesting consequence of using a spatial representation was that the subjects could more easily detect contradictions or impossible combinations of information – a finding that links imagery to the ambiguity determinant of task difficulty.

4. CONCLUSION

This outline of research from a wide assortment of different tasks suggests that imagery is called into play under conditions of low programming in the task environment. The results thus fall nicely in line with the central thesis of the present theory. It must be admitted, however, that most of the research in casu has not been explicitly guided by systematic theoretical considerations, and a more focused, systematic and detailed empirical testing program is clearly needed. At the present juncture the theoretical postulates set forth here should be regarded as forming a conceptually and empirically justified hypothesis.

The discussion above has focused on the functional properties of imagery relevant to the amount of processing required by a task with exclusive address to the postulated utility effects of the imagery variable. However, the theory is a two-dimensional one, where imagery is also related to the type of information to be processed. Availability effects for the imagery variable, where imagery is expected to be more readily used with concrete and perceptual information have not been studied on the same broad and systematic scale in the area of problem solving as in memory and learning tasks. The evidence does seem, however, to rule out the contention often expressed to the effect that imagery is exclusively tied to concrete and perceptual/spatial task information (e.g. Kosslyn, 1983; Paivio, 1971). As we have seen, there may be an important role for imagery in highly abstract tasks, particularly under low-programmed task conditions. When level of programming is controlled, however, there is tentative evidence of a facilitating effect of concreteness (Kaufmann, 1979). In the present theoretical formulation, such findings may be taken to mean that imagery is an appropriate representational medium for the processing of perceptual/spatial information. However, availability and utility effects may also be seen as intimately related. The present theory implies that concretization of a task (by way of visuals, graphs, diagrams etc.) may activate imagery and thus facilitate performance by giving access to a set of simpler cognitive operations.

REFERENCES

1. Bartlett, F.C.(1927). The relevance of visual imagery to thinking. British Journal of Psychology, 18, 23-29.
2. Bourne, L.E., Ekstrand, B.R., & Dominowski, R.L.(1971). The psychology of thinking. London: Prentice Hall.
3. Bruner, J.S., Olver, R.R., Greenfield, P.M. et al.(1966). Studies in cognitive growth. New York: Wiley.
4. Clark, H.H.(1969a). Linguistic processes in deductive reasoning. Psychological Review, 76, 387-404.
5. Clark, H.H.(1969b). The influence of language in solving three-term series problems. Journal of Experimental Psychology, 82, 205-215.

6. Comstock, C.(1921). On the relevancy of imagery to the process of thought. American Journal of Psychology, 32, 196-230.
7. Finke, R.A.(1985). Theories relating mental imagery to perception. Psychological Bulletin, 98, 236-259.
8. Finkenbinder, E.O.(1914). The remembrance of problems and of their solutions: A study in logical memory. American Journal of Psychology, 25, 32-81.
9. Fox, C.(1914). The conditions which arouse mental images in thought. British Journal of Psychology, 6, 420-431.
10. Galton, F.(1883). Inquiries into human faculty and its development. London: MacMillan.
11. Goldstein, K., & Scheerer, M.(1941). Abstract and concrete behavior: An experimental study with special tests. Psychological Monographs, 52, 491-510.
12. Gordon, W.J.J.(1961). Synectics: The development of creative capacity. New York: Harper & Row.
13. Guilford, J.P.(1967). The nature of human intelligence. New York: McGraw Hill.
14. Helstrup, T.(1977). The role of reference fields in learning of artificial language expressions. Scandinavian Journal of Psychology, 18, 196-300.
15. Huttenlocher, J.(1968). Constructing spatial images: A strategy in reasoning. Psychological Review, 75, 556-560.
16. Johnson-Laird, P.N.(1972). The three-term series problem. Cognition, 1, 57-82.
17. Johnson-Laird, P.N.(1983). Mental models. Cambridge: Harvard Universities Press.
18. Kaufmann, G.(1979). Visual imagery and its relation to problem solving: A theoretical and experimental inquiry. Oslo/Bergen/Tromsø: Universitetsforlaget.
19. Kaufmann, G.(1980). Imagery, language and cognition. Oslo/Bergen/Tromsø: Universitetsforlaget.
20. Kaufmann, G.(1981). The functional significance of visual imagery in ideational fluency performance. Journal of Mental Imagery, 5, 115-120.
21. Kaufmann, G.(1984a). Mental imagery in problem solving. International Review of Mental Imagery, 1, 23-25.
22. Kaufmann, G.(1984b). Can Skinner define a problem? The Behavioral and Brain Sciences, 7, 599.
23. Kaufmann, G.(1986). The conceptual basis of cognitive imagery models: A critique and a theory. In D.Marks(Ed.), Theories of image formation. New York: Brandon House.
24. Kosslyn, S.M.(1980). Image and mind. Cambridge: Harvard Universities Press.
25. Kosslyn, S.M.(1983). Ghosts in the mind's machine. New York: W.W. Norton.
26. McKellar, P.(1957). Imagination and thinking. New York: Basic Books.
27. Milojkovic, J.D.(1982). Chess imagery in novice and master. Journal of Mental Imagery, 6, 125-144.
28. Morris, P.E., & Hampson, P.J.(1983). Imagery and consciousness. New York: Academic Press.
29. Newell, A.(1969). Heuristic programming: Ill-structured problems. In J. Aronosky(Ed.), Progress in operations research, Vol.3. New York: Wiley.
30. Paige, J.M., and Simon, H.A. (1966). Cognitive processes in solving algebra problems. In B. Kleinmuntz (Ed.), Problem solving: Research, Method and Theory. New York: Wiley.

31. Paivio, A.(1971). Imagery and verbal processes. New York: Holt, Rinehart and Winston.
32. Paivio, A.(1983). The empirical case for dual coding. In J.C. Yuille (Ed.), Imagery, memory and cognition. London: Lawrence Erlbaum, 1983.
33. Parnes, S.J.(1961). Effects of extended effort in creative problem solving. Journal of Educational Psychology, 3, 117–122.
34. Pear, T.H.(1927). The relevance of visual imagery to the process of thought. British Journal of Psychology, 28, 1–14.
35. Poole, C., & Stanley, G.(1972). A factorial and predictive study of spatial abilities. Australian Journal of Psychology, 24(3),317–320.
36. Potts, G.R. & Scholz, K.W.(1975). The internal representation of a three term series problem. Journal of Verbal Learning and Verbal Behavior,14, 439–452.
37. Pounds, W.(1969). The process of problem finding. Industrial Management Review, 11, 1–19.
38. Quinton, G., & Fellows, B.J.(1975).'Perceptual' strategies in the solving of three-term series problems. British Journal of Psychology, 66, 69–78
39. Raaheim, K.(1961). Problem solving: A new approach. Oslo/Bergen/Tromsø: Universitetsforlaget.
40. Raaheim, K.(1974). Problem solving and intelligence. Oslo/Bergen/Tromsø: Universitetsforlaget.
41. Ray, W.S.(1955). Complex tasks for use in human problem solving research. Psychological Bulletin, 52, 134–149.
42. Richardson, J.T.E.(1983). Mental imagery in thinking and problem solving. In J.St B.T. Evans (Ed.), Thinking and reasoning Psychological approaches. London: Routledge & Kegan Paul.
43 Rugg, H.(1963). Imagination. New York: Harper & Row.
44. Rumelhart, D.E., & Norman, D.A.(1985). Representation of knowledge in memory. In R.C Atkinson,R.Herrnstein,G.Lindzey,& R.D.Luce(Eds.), Stevens' Handbook of Experimental Psychology. New York: Wiley.
45. Shepard, R.N.(1978). The mental image. American Psychologist, 33, 125–137.
46. Sherman, J.(1979). Predicting mathematics performance in high-school girls and boys. Journal of Educational Psychology, 71, 247–249.
47. Simon, H.A.(1977). The new science of management decision. Englewood Cliffs, N.J.: Prentice Hall.
48. Simon, H.A.(1978). Information-processing theory of human problem solving. In W.K. Estes(Ed.), Handbook of learning and cognitive processes.Vol.5. Human information processing. Hillsdale, N.J.: Lawrence Erlbaum.
49. Skemp, R.R.(1971). The psychology of learning mathematics. Penguin.
50. Smith, I.M.(1964). Spatial ability. London: University of London Press Ltd.
51. Titchener, E.B.(1910). A textbook of psychology. New York: Macmillan.
52. Vernon, P.E.(1950). The structure of human abilities. London: Methuen.
53. Walkup, L.E.(1965). Creativity in science through visualization. Perceptual and Motor Skills, 21, 35–41.
54. Werdelin, I.(1958). The mathematical ability: Experimental and factorial studies. Lund: Ohlsson.
55. Woods, E.L.(1915). An experimental study of the process of recognizing. American Journal of Psychology, 26, 313–387.
56. Wrigley, J.(1958). The factorial nature of ability in elementary mathematics. British Journal of Educational Psychology, 28, 61–78.

IMAGERY AS A COGNITIVE STRATEGY

TORE HELSTRUP

DEPARTMENT OF COGNITIVE PSYCHOLOGY
UNIVERSITY OF BERGEN, NORWAY

ABSTRACT
Imagery may alternatively be conceptualized as a representation system, or treated as cognitive operations. In our laboratory the function of imagery strategies has been examined from a problem solving point of view with the goal of relating performance to task variables such as novelty, complexity or difficulty. Experiments on memory and metaphors are discussed in terms of a strategy model of problem solving. A central point is the assumption that imagery operations may easily be brought under the subject's control, and used as optional elements of general problem solving strategies.

1. INTRODUCTION

A research program aiming to decide whether imagery is a representation system or a set of strategy operations would probably be futile. Much evidence indicates that it is both. However, the representation system interpretation has been the dominant one within this research area (Paivio, 1971, 1983). According to Paivio the verbal system operates temporally with information represented in sequential formats, whilst the imagery system operates with visuo-spatial information in a parallel format. The verbal system can be used with abstract as well as with concrete material, whereas the visual system is specifically suited for processing concrete material. Since the two systems are supposed to operate either independently or in interaction, concrete material may be processed in two representation media whereas abstract material must be handled by the verbal system alone.

Several versions of dual-code inspired theories have been developed. Engelkamp and Zimmer (1983, 1984, 1985) have extended the model to include a third system for motor meaning representations. They also argue that a superordinate abstract conceptual representation system spans over and integrates the three modal subsystems. Kaufmann (1986) on the other hand has suggested that the imagery system is a subordinated support system for the more general linguistic system.

Common to representation system theories is the assumption that mental processes have to take place within a limited number of specified code dimensions. This assumption is related to hypotheses about trace localization put forth in most information processing theories of memory. Memory events are here thought to be stored as point units at definite places in the memory system. Structural representation assumptions like these may be justified, but have certainly turned out to be hard to test. Existing evidence as concerns memory seems equally consistent with assumptions about non-localized distributed memories (cf. Anderson, 1973; Hinton & Anderson, 1981; Murdock, 1983).

In the same way that "system" has been a key word for structural

M. Denis et al. (eds.), Cognitive and Neuropsychological Approaches to Mental Imagery, 241-250.

theories, "strategy" is a corresponding catchword for functionalist approaches. Several strategy interpretations have been put forward since the pioneering work of Bruner et al.(1956) on concept formation. In the context of imagery, Katz (1983, 1987) has recently focused on the inter-action between problem solver and task situation. According to Katz, the performer needs to know, before carrying out a strategy, something about when to use the strategy (metamemory), about how the strategy has to be performed (skill),and about the person who is to utilize the strategy (the self as an agent). In other words, all round strategy systems do not exist. On the other hand there are a multitude of strategy operations to be used in individually different ways dependent on various task factors. Yet it would be wrong to characterize strategy behaviour as unpredictable. Precise predictions, however, require precise knowledge about the interaction of task and problem solver.

Strategies constitute what Tolman (1932) termed means-end relations. The subject, situated in a specific task situation, has a desired goal. Utili-zation of a suitable strategy may help the subject to reach this goal. Most strategies require the execution of a sequence of suboperations. These may be different or similar. To learn a list of nouns may accordingly be done by verbally rehearsing some items, by visually imaging others, or by constructing a story about still other items, and so on.

It may be of relevance to distinguish between the nature and the function of strategy operations. Differentiation, grouping, and repetition are functions which may be obtained by use of imagery or by verbal opera-tions. But grouping or repetition may alternatively be specified as types of operations - and left to be performed verbally or by means of imagery at the subject's discretion. Among the imagery operations a further division may be made between spatial and nonspatial operations. Several imagery operations only work with two-dimensional information (image inspection), whereas other imagery operations may handle depth and movement information (image manipulation).

To draw a sharp line between verbal and visual imagery operations is in many cases impossible. Presented with a series of words and being told to give free associations or to construct a story about the items, the indivi-dual will usually make use of mixed strategies (Helstrup, 1981). The method of loci serves as a good illustration of a mixed strategy task. Cornoldi and his collaborators have recently conducted several experiments making ingenious use of this memorizing technique (DeBeni & Cornoldi, 1985). Subjects are first instructed to establish vivid and stable visual images of a given selection of public places in their local environment. In the next stage the subjects are requested to memorize lists of items by mentally placing the information in the visualized localities. In our own use of the method of loci subjects have been told to visualize themselves at specified places in their local environment, and then to imagine that they perform different specified tasks at these spots - with instructions to memorize the acts. In this way imagery processes become mixed with verbal, motor, and associative processes, together constituting a sequence of operations qualifying as a memory strategy.

The Bergen group of cognitive psychologists have in various connections dealt with the familiarity dimension of problem situations (cf. Raaheim, 1961, 1974, 1984; Kaufmann, 1980, 1984, 1986; Helstrup, 1976, 1984a, 1986). Imagery operations seem for instance to be more useful with new and unfamiliar tasks than verbal operations which turn out to be relatively more successful with familiar information (e.g. Kaufmann, 1980). Routine situations are probably handled by mechanized operations, and whether verbal or visual operations have been automatized is of less concern. The positive relation between intelligence and problem solving found with intermediately difficult tasks (Raaheim, 1974), may perhaps reflect differential use of visual and verbal processes. Evidence indicates that imagery operations are conducive to transform new, unfamiliar information into formats more easily labelled by verbal tags. Memories can then be more readily addressed through verbal categorizations, thus leading to an intelligent utilization of previous experience. Evidence also suggests that imagery operations are particularly useful in completely unfamiliar situations demanding a mixture of trial-and-error and creative explorations (cf. Kaufmann & Helstrup, 1985). In sum the present argument is that a strategy interpretation of imagery may explain how visual imagery is integrated with other types of cognitive activities. In my own approach, strategy performance has been analysed as a type of problem solving behaviour. Here strategy operations are assumed to be selected and modified through hypothesis testing and informative feedback (Helstrup, 1976, 1985a).

In the strategy interpretation, imagery is not regarded as a separate representation system. Rather it is seen as a set of optional strategy operations to be used together with other mental operations. This interpretation is related to models where memories are considered as arrays, vectors, or attribute dimensions (Bower, 1967; Underwood, 1969). Memories and cognitive representations are not treated as localized units with definite strengths, but as being distributed over the cognitive space and characterized by the availability of search cues. In learning and memory imagery operations are used both in encoding and retrieval of information. In thinking and problem solving, imagery operations are used to transform information to a more suitable format. The strategy approach always focuses on the problem solver as the user of imagery, not on imagery as an isolated system.

2. EXPERIMENTS ON IMAGERY STRATEGIES

As elements of strategies, imagery operations are supposed to be controlled by the performing agent. It is not a question of switching on and off different representation systems, but of selecting the right imagery operations. The general usefulness of imagery with simple memory tasks has been richly documented (cf. Paivio, 1971; Richardson, 1980; Wippich, 1980; Wippich & Bredenkamp, 1979). In one of our own experiments (Helstrup, 1981), the point was not to examine the functional importance of imagery, but rather to inquire whether people know when to use different sorts of memory operations. If processing operations do not become automatically evoked by stimulus conditions, but are under strategic control, one should expect subjects to be able to state how they plan to undertake a memory task before the actual task performance. Anticipations of strategy uses could then be compared to strategies reported to have been used in real memory experiments.

To explore this metamemory question forty-six naive subjects were presented with descriptions of some standard memory tasks. They were then asked to describe how they would have handled the task of memorizing the items. The tasks included a list of visually presented CVC syllables, a list of auditorily presented digits, and visually presented block-design patterns. Illustrations of the list materials were provided, and information given about how memory would have been tested. The subjects, however, were told to abstain from efforts to memorize, only to explain how they would have proceeded if they were to participate in a "real" experiment. Another group of thirty subjects was then given the same memory tasks. Immediately after the completion of each memory test these subjects described what they actually had done in order to memorize the materials.

Both sets of strategy descriptions were then classified in four categories. The association category included operations which elaborated the presented information or which added new information not given in the stimulus material. Visualization included all kinds of imagery operations. Repetition referred to silent, rote rehearsal operations, whereas grouping comprised all attempts to select or to arrange items in smaller units than the whole list. Reported strategy descriptions often contained elements from several operation classes, and were therefore tallied under more than one category. Described operations that could not be classified in the four categories were ignored in this analysis.

Table 1. Percentage of subjects anticipating and performing four kinds of memory operations with CVC syllables, Figural Forms(FF), Digit Spans(DG), and Block Designs(BD).

| Operation | Task | | | |
	CVC	FF	DS	BD
Association				
anticipation	28	24	7	9
performance	40	33	20	10
Visualization				
anticipation	7	37	13	28
performance	3	17	3	37
Repetition				
anticipation	63	48	65	9
performance	47	23	53	3
Grouping				
anticipation	33	33	46	76
performance	53	57	40	90

Table 1 shows the percentages of subjects reporting use of that strategic operation. For instance twenty-eight percent of the subjects anticipated that they would employ associative operations, whereas forty percent of the subjects in the other group reported after task performance actually having made use of associative operations with that task, and so on.

Considering the great variation in use of strategies, the profiles over anticipation and performance conditions match rather well. It is evident that subjects know a good deal about how to handle such tasks. This observation is in line with results obtained by Denis and his collaborators, who have demonstrated that in several respects people's common sense opinions about the nature of imagery are in agreement with laboratory findings (Denis & Carfantan,1985). As regards mental imagery it should be noticed that serial lists, like the three first tasks reported in Table 1, are usually not processed by means of visual operations.When the same strategy-interview method is used with memory for pictures or concrete material, the reported frequencies of imagery operations are found to be much higher (Helstrup, 1981).

Another illustration of imagery strategies is provided by cue-competition tasks, where temporal order cues are pitted against spatial order cues (Helstrup, 1982, 1984b). Subjects are here given a frame containing empty slots, each slot being marked with different labels. Let the slots be numbered from 1 to n from left to right. Items can then be presented one by one in random order by asking subjects first to imagine the seventh slot filled with item x, then to imagine the third slot filled with item y, and so on. The items may be presented auditorily or visually according to standard procedures of list presentation.

One experiment of this kind used two lists, each with ten items (Helstrup, 1985b).In one list the items were a mixture of names of famous persons (politicians, movie stars) and familiar persons (your father, yourself). The second list consisted of the names of familiar cartoon figures. This second list thus was supposed to contain more impersonal material than the first list. Statistical analyses of the results showed significantly better recall for person items than for cartoon items, and that the cartoon list gave the usual primacy-recency curve, whereas no serial position effect was obtained for the person items. Along with other experimental evidence (Helstrup, 1985b), these results suggest that imagery is used differently when one is active and self-involved as compared to what is the case when a passive, noninvolved attitude is taken.

The observations referred to above were intended to illustrate how imagery is used as parts of strategies in handling simple memory tasks. The problem facing the subject is to select and to carry out the proper types of information processing operations. If a memory task is transformed to a situation containing more familiar and personal elements, problem solving is also facilitated when imagery is employed. Although imagery is often found to be relatively more useful than verbal operations with new as opposed to well-known material (cf.Kaufmann,1980; Morris & Hampson, 1983), imagery operations too may be more successful with familiar than with unfamiliar memory tasks. In the remainder of this paper, the focus will be on the role of mental imagery with more complex tasks. As an illustration, a study of visual and verbal strategies in metaphor processing will be discussed.

Figurative language is especially interesting because of the intersection of verbal and visual processes, and because in many instances it carries meaning in spite of syntactical anomalies. In metaphor processing purely linguistic operations may fail if not backed up by nonlinguistic cognitive processes. Metaphor research therefore is important since it indicates that modern linguistic theories are founded on all too narrow conceptions of language (cf.Ortony, Reynold & Arter, 1978; Ortony, 1979a; Honeck & Hoffman, 1980). Psychological research on metaphors has focused on the dynamics behind figurative expressions, how for instance different types of topic-vehicle similarity relations may help to convey the meaning hidden in the ground of the metaphor (e.g. Verbrugge & McCarrell, 1977; Tourangeau & Sternberg, 1981, 1982; Trick & Katz, in press). The experiment to be described below aimed at exploring the interaction between verbal and imagery processes by employing figurative phrases as task material. A metaphor may be defined as an expression with several interpretational levels, where at least one level carries a literal meaning and another level a figurative meaning. Metaphoric usage takes place when both levels are activated; but the expressions can, of course, also be used nonmetaphorically at each level separately (cf. Ortony, 1979b).

In the first experiment two tasks were constructed, intended to measure comprehension and production of metaphors. The comprehension test was an abridged version of a test developed by Kaufmann (1970, 1973a, 1973b). The present version contained ten subtasks. Each item presented a relatively simple metaphoric expression which the subjects were requested to explain.

The answers were then scored for adequacy on a three-point scale. Starting from scratch most people may well have a vague notion of what is meant by a metaphor. However, it was assumed that going through the metaphor comprehension test the subjects would be given a sufficient understanding about the nature of metaphors and figurative language. The results proved this assumption to be reasonable. After the comprehension test, the subjects succeeded fairly well with the production tasks, and did not ask questions about the meaning of the word "metaphor".

The production task contained five items which required literally described themes (e.g. ugly house) to be rewritten in a metaphorical form, along with five items where a target word (e.g. the ocean) was to be metaphorically described by making use of a given key word (e.g. clock). The same scoring procedures were used as those for the comprehension test. An inter-rater correlation of around 0.90 was obtained, suggesting sufficient reliability.

The metaphor tests were given together with several other tasks, including a vocabulary test, a mental rotation test, and two tests measuring comprehension and use of gestural language. The subjects were divided into two instruction groups. The imagery group was told that they were going to receive a number of different tasks, all demanding the use of communicational and linguistic skills and abilities, and that in order to solve the tasks it would be important to make active use of visual imagery and carefully consider the images evoked by the words to be tested. The verbal group was given similar instructions and informed that it would be important for task solutions to make active use of language and to carefully consider the linguistic meaning of each of the words to be tested.

These instructions do not specify any operation to be used, but might – if successful – create different processing attitudes. To the extent that strategies are subject controlled, the subjects were expected to be able on their own to select the relevant kinds of imagery and verbal operations when confronted with the task demands, without further experimenter specifications.

Results from the first experiment showed a statistically significant difference in number of produced metaphors in favour of the imagery instructions group (M = 14.8 vs. M = 8.3), but no difference in metaphor comprehension, or between the scores on any of the other tests. A second experiment was run in order to check the reliability of the observed difference. With enforced instructions the subjects were expected to form even more pronounced strategy attittudes than in the first experiment. The results, shown in Table 2, confirm this prediction.

Table 2. Mean metaphor comprehension and metaphor production.

Tasks	Instructions	
	Verbal	Imagery
Metaphor comprehension	13.7	16.6
Metaphor production	10.5	13.9
Concrete metaphors	2.9	4.8

Significantly higher comprehension scores as well as production scores were obtained with the imagery group. The experiment also included a new metaphor production task, in Table 2 referred to as "concrete metaphors".

This task contained five items where the targets and keys were presented as concrete objects, and no mention of their "names" was made. The rationale was to reduce possible verbal biases, thereby facilitating instructional effects. The results of the two experiments suggest that use of figurative language does not only depend on linguistic ability factors. Processing attitudes induced by instructions produce marked effects, without effortful or protracted training. Such processing attitudes are strategic because they can be controlled by the performing agent. The positive effect of imagery strategies is not surprising. But that metaphor effects are so easily obtained is noteworthy, and suggests interesting practical applications in educational contexts.

Whether visual imagery conditions facilitate what verbal conditions hamper might be discussed. A control group answering the same metaphor tests without attitude instructions obtained scores between those found with the visual and verbal groups. Correlational analyses also suggest a difference between visual and verbal factors. It seems safe, then, to conclude that the instructions induced a real processing difference.

Having established a process difference between imagery and verbal strategies for comprehension and production of metaphors, the next step was to examine whether similar strategy differences would also influence the acquisition and retention of metaphors. Lists of simple figurative expressions were constructed, and presented to groups receiving different processing instructions. The verbal instructions required the items to be memorized by means of verbal repetition (rehearsal), the visual instructions to memorize by imaging the meaning of the expressions. Goodness ratings and comprehension tests were also administered.

The lists were presented with repeated trials, and with free recall tests given immediately after each trial. The instructions emphasized that the answers on the memory tests ought to be reproduced with the same wordings as the originally presented expressions, and only literally reproduced items were accordingly counted as correct. Two experiments were conducted. Neither of them showed significant differences in learning rate or in recall as a function of strategy. Nor were there any significant correlations between recall and goodness ratings of the metaphors. High recall, however, was linked to high comprehension scores.

On the basis of the observed superiority of imagery operations with visual materials, and from the observations with the present comprehension-production studies, one should predict imagery strategies to facilitate memorization of metaphor materials. However, three points should be made. In the first place it may be incorrect to conceive of metaphors as concrete material, since they can be interpreted at both a literal and a figurative level. Secondly, there is a difference between instructions specifying the operations to be used, and instructions creating general, open processing attitudes. Thirdly, the learning-memory tasks could be handled by keeping all processing at the literal level – a solution which may have been encouraged by the demand for literal reproductions. Taken together, however, our studies indicate important differences between visual and verbal strategies in the comprehension and production of metaphors, but not when it comes to learning and retention of the same information.

3. CONCLUSION

Imagery strategies are regularly used with simple memory tasks, sometimes resulting in better memory than with verbal strategies. Imagery operations are, however, normally used in interaction with verbal processes. When imagery strategies do not lead to differences in amount of memory, they may

still produce other side effects than verbal operations, e.g. dissimilar
serial position curves. For more complex tasks like comprehension and
creation of metaphors imagery strategies may function as broad attitudes or
processing orientations with positive effects. But absence of observed
differences in recall between visual and verbal strategies may simply mean
that both strategies have been equally efficient, and does not necéssarily
imply that the experimental manipulations have been unsuccessful. Performance efficiency is in many domains a poor criterion to evaluate strategies.
Yet enough experimental findings exist demonstrating significant differences
between imagery treatments and other treatment conditions to convince even a
sceptic that this process difference is a "real" one.

In conclusion it is suggested that imagery operations work in two ways:
by holding operations, or by transformation operations. The holding function
requires the formation of images, with stability and vividness as important
imagery aspects. The transformation function concerns image manipulations
involving subtraction or addition of information compared to what is given
in the stimulus materials, i.e. a representation of the original information
in new formats.

In context of attention and short-term memory holding operations are of
great importance. To image a complex set of information as an integrated
visual image is an efficient way to keep information alive while selective
or elaborative processes are carried out. In the coding of information for
long-term storage transformation operations are likely to be used.

In the context of thinking and problem solving the first reactions are
frequently verbal operations, which may fail to solve the tasks. The problem
then is to find more adequate (verbal) responses. Here the transformational
functions of imagery come into focus. For imagery in connection with transformation functions the following predictions are set forth: (a) When the
performer has useful verbal labels for handling the information given in the
first format, imagery operations will not increase performance levels; (b)
If the second transformed format is associated with even less useful verbal
labels than the first format, imagery operations should result in impover-
ished achievements; (c) When useful verbal denotations are more easily found
for the transformed information, imagery should improve performance.

To point out that imagery and verbal operations are utilized in
conjunction is not by itself very provocative. Although multicode representation theories assume the independence of visual and verbal processes, they
also assume interaction to take place. However, a strategy interpretation
implies that interaction is the normal situation. Whereas a representation
system theory tends to divide cognition into compartments, a strategy
interpretation helps to integrate the different aspects of cognition – an
integration which is caused by the fact that strategies are controlled by
the performing individual.

REFERENCES

1. Anderson, J.A. (1973). A theory for the recognition of items from short
   memorized lists. Psychological Review, 80, 417-438.
2. Bower, G.H.(1967). A multicomponent theory of the memory trace. In K.W.
   Spence & J.T. Spence (Eds.), The psychology of learning and motivation.
   Vol.1. New York: Academic Press.
3. Bruner, J.S.,Goodnow, J.J. & Austin, G.A.(1956). A study of thinking. New
   York: Wiley.
4. DeBeni, R. & Cornoldi, C.(1985). Effects of the mnemotechnique of loci in
   the memorization of concrete words. Acta Psychologica, 60, 11-24.

5. Denis, M. & Carfantan, M.(1985). People's knowledge about images. Cognition, 20, 49-60.
6. Engelkamp, J. & Zimmer, H.D.(1983). Aktivationsprozesse im multimodalen Gedächtnis. Arbeiten der Fachrichtung Psychologie Nr. 83. Saarbrücken: Universität des Saarlandes.
7. Engelkamp, J. & Zimmer, H.D.(1984). Motor programme information as a separable memory unit. Psychological Research, 46, 283-299.
8. Engelkamp, J. & Zimmer, H.D.(1985). Motor programs and their relation to semantic memory. The German Journal of Psychology, 9, 239-254.
9. Helstrup, T.(1976). Hva er kognitiv psykologi? Bergen,Oslo,Tromsø: Universitetsforlaget.
10. Helstrup, T.(1981). Kognitive prosesser i kort-tids hukommelse. Bergen: Sigma.
11. Helstrup, T.(1982). Serial position effects: The influence of operation shift, ascribed position and spatial presentation order. Scandinavian Journal of Psychology, 23, 119-129.
12. Helstrup, T.(1984a). Serial position phenomena: Training and retrieval effects. Scandinavian Journal of Psychology, 25, 227-250.
13. Helstrup, T.(1984b) Serial position phenomena; memory for acts, contents and spatial position patterns. Scandinavian Journal of Psychology, 25, 131-146.
14. Helstrup, T.(1985a). Problem solving as a paradigm for cognitive psychology. Psykologisk rapportserie, Universitetet i Bergen, 6, No.5.
15. Helstrup, T.(1985b). Self, imagery and memory. Psykologisk rapportserie, Universitetet i Bergen, 6, No. 7.
16. Helstrup, T.(1986). Separate memory laws for recall of performed acts? Scandinavian Journal of Psychology, 27, 1-29.
17. Hinton, G.E. & Anderson, J.A.(1981). Parallel models of associative memory. Hillsdale,N.J.: Erlbaum.
18. Honeck, R.P. & Hoffman, R.R.(Eds.)(1980). Cognition and figurative language. Hillsdale, N.J.: Erlbaum.
19. Katz, A.N.(1983). What does it mean to be a high imager? In J.C.Yuille (Ed.), Imagery, memory and cognition. Hillsdale, N.J.: Erlbaum.
20. Katz, A.N.(1987). Individual differences in the control of imagery processing: Knowing how, knowing when, and knowing self. In M.A.Mc Daniel & M. Pressley (Eds.), Imagery and related mnemonic processes. New York: Springer-Verlag.
21. Kaufmann, G.(1970). Språk og problemløsning. Hovedoppgave i psykologi, Universitetet i Oslo.
22. Kaufmann, G.(1973a). Metaphors and creative thinking. I. A descriptive study. Reports from the Institute of Psychology, University of Bergen, No. 1.
23. Kaufmann, G.(1973b). Metaphors and creative thinking.II.The relationship to visual imagery. Reports from the Institute of Psychology, University of Bergen, No. 2.
24. Kaufmann, G.(1980). Imagery, language and cognition. Bergen,Oslo,Tromsø: Universitetsforlaget.
25. Kaufmann, G.(1984). Mental imagery in problem solving. International Review of Mental Imagery, 1, 23-25.
26. Kaufmann, G.(1986).On the conceptual basis of imagery models: A critique and a theory. In D.F.Marks (Ed.), Theories of imagery formation. New York: Brandon House.
27. Kaufmann, G. & Helstrup, T.(1985). Mental imagery and problem solving: Implications for the educational process. In A.A.Sheikh & K.S.Sheikh (Eds.), Imagery in education.Farmingdale,N.Y.: Baywood.

28. Morris, P.E. & Hampson, P.J.(1983). Imagery and consciousness. London: Academic Press.
29. Murdock, B.B., Jr.(1983). A distributed memory model for serial-order information. Psychological Review, 90, 316-338.
30. Ortony, A.(Ed.)(1979a). Metaphor and thought.Cambridge,England: Cambridge University Press.
31. Ortony, A.(1979b). Beyond literal similarity. Psychological Review, 86, 161-180.
32. Ortony, A., Reynolds, R.E. & Arter, J.A.(1978). Metaphor: Theoretical and empirical research. Psychological Bulletin, 85, 919-943.
33. Paivio, A.(1971). Imagery and verbal processes. New York: Holt,Rinehart & Winston.
34. Paivio, A.(1983).The empirical case for dual coding. In J.C.Yuille (Ed.) Imagery,memory and cognition. Hillsdale, N.J.: Erlbaum.
35. Raaheim, K.(1961). Problem solving: A new approach.Oslo,Bergen,Tromsø: Universitetsforlaget
36. Raaheim, K.(1974). Problem solving and intelligence. Oslo,Bergen,Tromsø: Universitetsforlaget.
37. Raaheim, K.(1984). Why intelligence is not enough. Bergen:Sigma.
38. Richardson, J.T.E.(1980). Mental imagery and human memory. London: MacMillan.
39. Tolman, E. C.(1932). Purposive behavior in animals and men. New York: Appleton Century-Crofts.
40. Tourangeau, R. & Sternberg, R.J.(1981). Aptness in metaphor. Cognitive Psychology, 13, 27-55.
41. Tourangeau, R. & Sternberg, R.J.(1982). Understanding and appreciating metaphors. Cognition, 11, 203-244.
42. Trick, L. & Katz, A.N. (in press). The domain interaction approach to metaphor processing: Relating individual differences and metaphor characteristics. Metaphor and Symbolic Activity.
43. Underwood, B. J.(1969). Attributes of memory. Psychological Review, 72, 89-104.
44. Verbrugge, R.R. & McCarrell, N.S.(1977). Metaphoric comprehension: Studies in reminding and resembling. Cognitive Psychology, 9, 494-533.
45. Wippich, W.(1980). Bildhaftigkeit und Organisation. Darmstadt: Steinkopff.
46. Wippich, W. & Bredenkamp, J.(1979). Bildhaftigkeit und Lernen. Darmstadt: Steinkoppf.

MENTAL PRACTICE :
IMAGE AND MENTAL REHEARSAL OF MOTOR ACTION

ALAIN SAVOYANT

COGNITION ET MOUVEMENT, UA CNRS 1166, MARSEILLE, FRANCE

ABSTRACT
    An overview of theoretical accounts of mental practice effects leads to two questions. First, it is emphasized that the relevant differentiation between mental and motor components in motor skills should not become a radical separation. Two cognitive intervention modes in motor skill are distinguished : on the one hand, planning and organizing of the motor sequence, and on the other hand, motor programming and control. Secondly, when mental practice is characterized by its relationship to physical practice, the evocation and triggering of the motor program are considered to be the same in both cases. A possible source of feedback in mental practice can be found not so much in the specific kinaesthetic information linked to the imagined movement as in the spatio-temporal structure of that information.

1. INTRODUCTION

    The idea that mental practice may have a positive effect on motor learning seems at best paradoxical : not only does it go against common sense ("Practice makes perfect", see also Denis & Carfantan, 1985), but also is in contradiction with the widely accepted arguments of motor control theorists such as Schmidt (1982) who points out the specific nature of mental practice while emphasizing the idea that "in order to learn a movement, one must experience active physical practice of it".
    Research on mental practice has been forced to come to grips with this paradox from its inception, as can be seen from the two well established data schematized below :
    - Mental practice is not purely mental, as has been shown by the existence of subliminal muscular activity in subjects who are asked to imagine that they are carrying out a motor action (Jacobson, 1932).
    - Actual physical practice is not purely physical, in which case the motor action has a symbolic component of varying importance (Sackett, 1934).
    These data have given rise to the two theories on mental practice. In the first theory, called the "psychoneuromuscular theory", the essential factor in the effectiveness of mental practice in learning is the kinaesthetic feedback resulting from the subliminal activity accompanying mental practice (Richardson, 1967). According to the other theory,

251

M. Denis et al. (eds.), Cognitive and Neuropsychological Approaches to Mental Imagery, 251–258.
© *1988 by Martinus Nijhoff Publishers.*

called the "symbolic-perceptual theory", the effectiveness of mental practice lies in the fact that it improves the cognitive component of motor activity, thus making the activity both easier to carry out and to learn (Minas, 1978 ; Wrisberg & Ragsdale, 1979 ; Ryan & Simons, 1981, 1983). Most research has been based on the second theory and has tended to prove its validity and/or invalidate the first theory (see the review by Feltz and Landers, 1983).

Nevertheless, these two theories may not be as contradictory as many studies have made them seem by presenting them as two opposing alternatives. The incompatibility between the two theories is based on the fact that processes qualified as central, cognitive, and "outflow" (not always sufficiently defined) have been too strongly opposed to peripheral, kinaesthetic and "inflow" processes (see for example Kohl and Roenker, 1983). By reformulating the two theories, they become complementary. In the "symbolic-perceptual theory", tasks should no longer be characterized by the extent to which they require cognitive and motor activity, or if not rejected altogether, this type of characterization should be refined. The "psychoneuromuscular theory" on the other hand should not be reduced to kinaesthetic feedback. Here, a more precise characterization of mental practice, defined by its relationship to actual physical practice of the action, is a critical factor.

2. COGNITIVE AND MOTOR COMPONENTS OF TASKS

Any theoretical approach that acknowledges the links between cognitive and motor processes must of course differentiate these two types of processes. But relevant differentiation should not, however, become separation. This problem, partly a result of how the "motor skill" is defined, has been the pitfall of many studies on mental practice. Two possible cases exist :

1) The task does not fit the definition of motor skill or action, since the motor component is almost insignificant. This is the case of the task defined as a "low motor" task by Ryan and Simons (1983) : "A stylus is moved through a maze pattern by the rotation of two handles, one controlling movement in the horizontal plane and the other controlling movement in the vertical plane. By coordinating both handles it is possible to move the stylus in any direction". In the "low motor" situation, "the maze consisted of only horizontal and vertical pathways... Thus, at no time was movement of both hands required at once and the motor involvement was minimal". It was indeed so minimal (at least for a normal adult) that we cannot really call it a motor action, and it would be more appropriate here to consider it as a cognitive task of maze learning. The same remark may be applied to one of the tasks used by Wrisberg and Ragsdale (1979), the McCloy blocks test of multiple response, in which the motor component appears very elementary (turn the blocks over and set them down) as compared to the cognitive component (choose the block to turn it over according to the rules). It should be emphasized here that there is no symmetry between the idea

that there are motor operations in certain mental skills (for example moving the men on a chessboard) and the idea that there are mental operations in motor skills (tennis, golf...). In the first case, the motor operations play no other role than that of exteriorizing the result of mental operations involved. In the second case, it is the mental operations that determine the motor operations.

2) The motor skill studied is in fact made up of two actions, a cognitive and a motor one (the latter naturally comprised of its own mental and motor components). This is for example the case of the skill studied by Minas (1978) : "ball throwing into a particular sequence of bins... the subject's task was to anticipate which bin was the target at any point in the sequence... Having made his guess... the subject had to aim balls at his choice of bin". This skill is very clearly composed of two quite different and independent tasks : one of sequence learning, the other of ball throwing. The first is entirely cognitive, the second is motor, but not entirely so : the cognitive component of ball throwing is far from minor. Ryan and Simons (1981) specified some of the cognitive elements in throwing tasks as "how to hold the ball or dart, how the arm is to be extended, how the ball is released...". Unfortunately, these authors are not interested in the cognitive aspects of this motor action, and in their "high motor" task (in which the maze pattern was rotated 45° and thus the constant coordination of both hands was required) they feel that the necessary bimanual coordination did not increase the cognitive requirements.

Thus, if it is important to differentiate between the cognitive and motor components of a skill, the term "motor action" (or task) should be applied only to cases in which dependence (interdependence ?) exists between them. Certain studies have shown that mental practice has a positive effect on motor actions of this type, for example rotary pursuit tracking (Rawlings, Rawlings, Chen, & Yilk, 1972 ; Kohl & Roenker, 1980, 1983), throwing tasks (Clark, 1960 ; Mendoza & Wichman, 1978), swimming skills (White, Ashton, & Lewis, 1979) and gymnastic skills (Jones, 1965 ; Phipps & Morehouse, 1969). If mental practice essentially improves the cognitive component of the motor task, two cognitive intervention modes can be identified : one related to planning and organizing the motor sequence, and a second related to the motor programming and control of program execution. For example, when studying the physical actions of children, Hauert, Mounoud and Mayer (1981) based their research on the hypothesis that "representations are involved in both logical organization of the actions (or logical action procedure) and in the development and use of spatio-temporally defined action programs". This distinction is congruent with the argument that "mental practice effects are found in early and later stages of learning" (Feltz & Landers, 1983).

In early stages of learning ("verbal-motor stage", Adams, 1971), mental practice can contribute considerably to the construction of an image of the action, that is, the definition of the operations and their execution order, the conditions to be taken into account, and the "logical" aspects of the action. The Soviet psychologist Galperine (1966) has termed this an "orienting basis" : in other words a model of the action, which he defines as "a system of representations of the action and its product, the initial properties of the material and their successive transformations, plus all the cues the subject actually uses to carry out the action". In this case, the type of mental practice used is not relevant : the fact that the subject is involved in a cognitive activity concerning the action and its conditions suffices (mental rehearsal, but also model observation, reading task descriptions, etc. ; see the various mental practice techniques identified by Singer, 1972, cited by Weinberg, 1981). In later stages of learning, when the motor action becomes generalized and automatized, when learning without knowledge of results can occur (the expression "later stage" ought to be more precisely defined), the fact that mental practice can be effective suggests that it can contribute to the development of motor programming and control. It is precisely with regards to this cognitive aspect of motor action that the "psychoneuromuscular" hypothesis may provide an explanation.

3. MOTOR CONTROL AND MENTAL PRACTICE

Using a bilateral transfer procedure in a rotary pursuit task, Kohl and Roenker (1983) showed that the amount of bilateral and unilateral transfer after skill imagery was functionally equivalent. This is convincing and apparently decisive evidence in favor of an interpretation of skill imagery (or mental practice) mechanisms in terms of "outflow" processing, rather than in terms of "inflow" processing relying on kinaesthetic feedback. These authors were thus led to conclude that the subliminal neuromuscular activity detected by EMG is nothing more than a simple effect of imagery, or even an "artefact". This "outflow" processing must be more precisely defined, and I will present a number of comments aimed at better characterizing the mental practice of an action and its relationship to the physical practice of that action.

The first issue is whether movement can be programmed in the same way in mental practice as in physical practice. In physical practice, according to Schmidt (1975), five sources of information are necessary for the subject to generate the response specifications and the expected sensory consequences of the movement : the desired outcome, the particular initial conditions, the past actual outcomes, the past response specifications and the past sensory consequences. Only the initial conditions are not directly accessible in mental practice, but their representation by the subject does not appear to be an insurmountable problem. One might ask whether it is even necessary, in mental practice, to evoke the expected sensory consequences of the movement since there is no longer any usable response feedback to compare with them. The question still seems relevant to us in that for certain authors, anticipated feedback does not simply serve as a reference but may also be "the basis on which commands are organized" (Kelso & Wallace, 1978). Motor programming may thus be considered as the same in mental practice as in physical practice.

The second issue concerns how this program is triggered. Is the process identical in both mental and physical practice? According to Mackay's theory (1981), mental practice and physical practice have the same underlying mental component, and the elements of this component are activated in the same way in both cases ; there is a triggering mechanism under voluntary control which activates the elements of the mental component in a serial order (but not those of the motor component, which are only primed during mental practice). In an another perspective, Pickhenhain (1984) states that during mental practice "the efferent impulses of the complex motor program... reach all parts of the central nervous system which serve as subprogram effectors of the whole process of realization", the real movement being inhibited. This "involvement of as many lower levels of the central nervous system as possible in mental reproduction of the leading motor program... supplies the higher centres with the necessary reinforcing feedback information", thus explaining some of the learning effects of mental practice. The triggering of the program may therefore occur during mental practice as well as during physical practice. This is an important consideration, in that program triggering can allow internal feedback loops to be used.

Now as far as program execution is concerned, let us go back to the subliminal neuromuscular activity observed in mental practice. Even if this activity is not a source of kinaesthetic feedback, it can nevertheless be considered as evidence of program triggering. As Pickhenhain (1984) noted, given the subthreshold innervation recorded by the EMG, we can see "how precisely the subject is able to reproduce his trained motor program mentally and how well he executes his ideo-motor training program". The mental execution here is an exact duplicate of the actual execution. An important question, raised by Wehner, Vogt, and Stadler (1984) remains unanswered : "It is unclear if motor commands are actively inhibited or mainly non-activated".

A final important aspect of mental practice is related to the instructions given to subjects during experiments ("internal imagery" instructions, Epstein, 1980) and by questionnaires aimed at measuring kinaesthetic imagery (Hall, Pongrac, & Buckolz, 1985). Subjects are asked to attempt to "feel" themselves making the movement. In other words, they are explicitly oriented towards evoking the kinaesthetic feedback of the movement. Thus, although the subject does not perform the movement, he can evoke a kinaesthetic image of it. This image is a dynamic one, and in the timing of afferent information represented in it we should find the timing of the efferent motor commands. This appears to us as a possible and important source of feedback, not so much resulting from the specific kinaesthetic information linked to the imagined movement, as from the spatio-temporal structure of that information. The fact that researchers agree on the abstract nature of movement representation in motor programming lends weight to this idea. Keele (1981), for example, redefines the motor program as a non-specific muscular representation. The same is true for the idea of generalized motor program (Schmidt, 1982) which only deals with the general characteristics of the movement, namely, its invariants.

In this perspective which stresses those points common to motor programming and control in both mental practice and physical practice, it makes a difference which type of mental practice is used : it should be real mental rehearsal, with "internal imagery", a "first-person perspective" (Mahoney & Avener, 1977 ; Epstein, 1980), one most likely to evoke and trigger the motor program.

REFERENCES
1. Adams, J.A. (1971). A closed-loop theory of motor learning. Journal of Motor Behavior, 3, 111-150.
2. Clark, L.V. (1960). Effect of mental practice on the development of a certain motor skill. Research Quarterly, 31, 560-569.
3. Denis, M., & Carfantan, M. (1985). People's knowledge about images. Cognition, 20, 49-60
4. Epstein, M.L. (1980). The relationship of mental imagery and mental rehearsal to performance of a motor task. Journal of Sport Psychology, 2, 211-220.
5. Feltz, D.L., & Landers, D.M. (1983). The effects of mental practice on motor skill learning and performance : A meta-analysis. Journal of Sport Psychology, 5, 25-57.
6. Galperine, P. (1966). Essai sur la formation par étapes des actions et des concepts. In Recherches psychologiques en U.R.S.S. Moscou : Editions du Progrès, 114-132.
7. Hall, C., Pongrac, J., & Buckolz, E. (1985). The measurement of imagery ability. Human Movement Science, 4, 107-118.
8. Hauert, C.A., Mounoud, P., & Mayer, E. (1981). Approche du développement cognitif des enfants de 2 à 5 ans à travers l'étude des caractéristiques physiques de leurs actions. Cahiers de Psychologie Cognitive, 1, 33-54.
9. Jacobson, E. (1932). Electrophysiology of mental activities. American Journal of Psychology, 44, 677-694.
10. Jones, J.G. (1965). Motor learning without demonstration of physical practice, under two conditions of mental practice. Research Quarterly, 36, 270-276.
11. Keele, S.W. (1981). Behavioral analysis of movement. In V.D. Brooks (Ed.), Handbook of physiology, Vol. 2, Motor control. Bethesda : American Physiology Society, 1391-1414.
12. Kelso, J.A.S., & Wallace, S.A. (1978). Conscious mechanisms in movement. In G.E. Stelmach (Ed.), Information processing in motor control and learning (pp. 79-116). New York : Academic Press.
13. Kohl, R.M., & Roenker, D.L. (1980). Bilateral transfer as a function of mental imagery. Journal of Motor Beha-

vior, 12, 197-206.
14. Kohl, R.M., & Roenker, D.L. (1983). Mechanism involvement during skill imagery. Journal of Motor Behavior, 15, 179-190.
15. Mackay, D.G. (1981). The problem of rehearsal or mental practice. Journal of Motor Behavior, 13, 274-285.
16. Mahoney, M.J., and Avener, M. (1977). Psychology of the elite athlete : An exploratory study. Cognitive Therapy and Research, 1, 135-141.
17. Mendoza, D., & Wichman, H. (1978). "Inner" darts : Effects of mental practice on performance of dart throwing. Perceptual and Motor Skills, 47, 1195-1199.
18. Minas, S.C. (1978). Mental practice of a complex perceptual-motor skill. Journal of Human Movement Studies, 4, 102-107.
19. Phipps, S.J., & Morehouse, C.A. (1969). Effects of mental practice on the acquisition of motor skills of varied difficulty. Research Quarterly, 40, 773-778.
20. Pickhenhain, L. (1984). Towards a holistic conception of movement control. In H.T.A. Whiting (Ed.), Human motor actions : Bernstein reassessed (pp. 505-528). Amsterdam: Elsevier Science Publishers B.V. (North-Holland).
21. Rawlings, E.I., Rawlings, I.L., Chen, S.S., & Yilk, M.D. (1972). The facilitating effects of mental rehearsal in the acquisition of rotary pursuit tracking. Psychonomic Science, 26, 71-73.
22. Richardson, A. (1967). Mental practice : A review and discussion. Part 2. Research Quarterly, 38, 263-273.
23. Ryan, E.D., & Simons, J. (1981). Cognitive demand, imagery, and frequency of mental rehearsal as factors influencing acquisition of motor skills. Journal of Sport Psychology, 3, 33-45.
24. Ryan, E.D., & Simons, J. (1983). What is learned in mental practice of motor skills : A test of the cognitive-motor hypothesis. Journal of Sport Psychology, 5, 419-426.
25. Sackett, R.S. (1934). The influence of symbolic rehearsal upon the retention of a maze habit. Journal of General Psychology, 10, 376-395.
26. Schmidt, R.A. (1975). A schema theory of discrete motor skill learning. Psychological Review, 82, 225-260.
27. Schmidt, R.A. (1982). Motor control and learning : A behavioral emphasis. Champaign, Illinois : Human Kinetic Publishers.
28. Singer, R.N. (1972). Readings in motor learning. Philadelphia : Lea and Febiger.
29. Wehner, T., Vogt, S., & Stadler, M. (1984). Task specific EMG characteristics during mental training. Psychological Research, 46, 389-401.
30. Weinberg, R.S. (1982). The relationship between mental preparation strategies and motor performance : A review and critique. Quest, 33, 195-213.
31. White, K.D., Ashton, R., & Lewis, S. (1979). Learning a complex skill : Effects of mental practice, physical practice and imagery ability. International Journal of

Sport Psychology, 10, 71-78.

32. Wrisberg, C.A., & Ragsdale, M.R., (1979). Cognitive demand and practice level : Factors in the mental rehearsal of motor skills. Journal of Human Movement Studies, 5, 201-208.

IMAGERY AND SKILL ACQUISITION

JOHN ANNETT

DEPARTMENT OF PSYCHOLOGY, WARWICK UNIVERSITY, COVENTRY CV4 7AL, UK

ABSTRACT

The acquisition of motor skills involves a variety of cognitive processes, including the ability to form 'motor' images. The paper discusses the relationship between motor and verbal codes and betweeen overt and imaginary actions with respect to a serial motor task, specifically, tying a bow. Two theories of mental practice are discussed in the light of observations on verbal explanations of bow tying and an experiment comparing physical and mental practice.

1. INTRODUCTION

Skills may be acquired by reference to any of three different sources of information. First, objects and events in the environment may often determine both the form and the occasion of an action, for instance reaching out to catch a ball or steering a vehicle along a route. A second major source is the actions of other humans which are observed and imitated. Third, we have the ability to follow verbal instructions, that is to accept information coded verbally and turn it into appropriate actions. This paper is concerned primarily with the second and third cases and in general with the processes by which symbolic information is translated into action and vice versa.

2. ACTION AND LANGUAGE

The mechanisms of imitation and verbal instruction which typify these two routes between input and output have been relatively neglected in the study of the acquisition of perceptual-motor skills and I have (e.g. Annett, 1982, 1985) outlined a scheme which may help to bring some of the issues into a clearer focus. This is illustrated in figure 1.

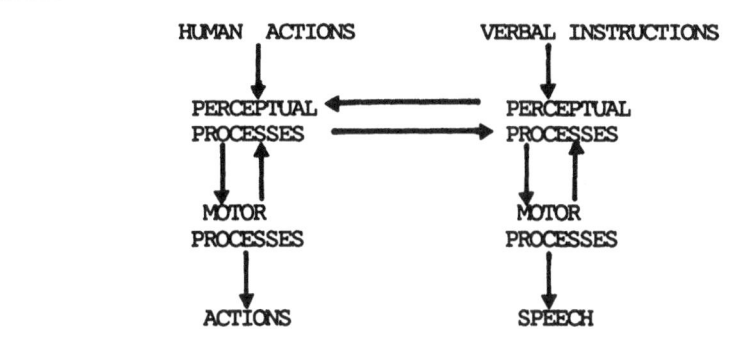

Figure 1. Relationships between action and language.

259

M. Denis et al. (eds.), Cognitive and Neuropsychological Approaches to Mental Imagery, 259–268.

The diagram shows some simple experimental paradigms and draws attention to problems which require clarification. The vertical dimension simply indicates inputs which are (normally visual) patterns of action which may lead, by imitation, to an output of analogous form. The horizontal dimension simply indicates that some of these inputs and outputs are action patterns whilst others are verbally coded. Perceptual and motor mechanisms are indicated separately on the diagram but, as I have argued elsewhere (Annett, 1982), there is good reason to regard them as very closely interconnected and probably even sharing some brain processes. The diagram symbolises this assertion with arrows in both directions between the perceptual and motor processes.

Of particular interest in the present context is the two-way arrow joining the two vertical arrays, which I call the action-language bridge. This simply represents the obvious fact that it is possible to translate in both directions, from words to actions and actions to words. We know rather little about how this is accomplished. In practical terms verbal instructions which result in actions, or the modification of actions, must cross the action-language bridge. A similar translation, but in the opposite direction, would have to occur in the case of someone asked to give a running commentary, of a boxing match, for example. The symptoms of some types of apraxia which are attributable to the disconnection of motor and verbal centres (Geschwind, 1965) indicate that the action-language bridge is more than just a theoretical abstraction.

The first part of this paper describes some exploratory studies with a simple experimental paradigm which clearly involves translation across the action-language bridge. Subjects are asked to give a verbal explanation of how they carry out a familiar task which is normally carried out without the intervention of language. What happens in this simple situation is described both qualitatively and quantitatively in an attempt to build a model of the operation of the action-language bridge.

2.1. STUDIES OF VERBAL EXPLANATIONS OF FAMILIAR SKILLS

Subjects are simply asked "tell me, in as much detail as you can how you....". Various familiar tasks have been used, such as climbing a ladder, mounting and riding a bicycle, and performing a forward roll but this paper concerns only the task "...take two ends of string and tie them together to make a bow". The subjects' verbal explanations are recorded, analysed and timed. Some experiments have involved the use of secondary tasks and these have been described elsewhere (Annett, 1985, 1986).

In the present series of experiments video recordings were made of subjects in three different conditions. The first condition simply requires the subject to explain how to tie a bow. In the second condition the subject is provided with a piece of wood approximately 30 x 15 x 1.5 cm. to which two pieces of string (approx 40 cm) are attached and is simply asked to tie them together into a bow. In the third condition the subject is presented with the board and strings and asked to demonstrate how to tie a bow, giving a verbal commentary at the same time. We now have recordings of some 50 subjects in all three of these conditions and the following discussions relate to this data set.

In these recordings the use of a mixer enabled us to dub onto the video a centisecond time base and, in a corner of the picture, an oscilloscope trace of the voice track. This latter enables the identification of the beginning and end of verbal episodes even when the video is played back at slow speeds (including frame by frame) to permit analysis of the movements.

2.2. RESULTS

Most of the interesting results are qualitative although several quantitative indices have contributed to our understanding of the processes underlying performance in this situation. First, subjects find it impossible to comply with the task instructions without resorting to imagery. On receiving the instruction to explain how to tie a bow subjects typically turn their eyes away from the face of the experimenter towards the ceiling and pause before replying. Replies normally come slowly with frequent hesitations. The one or two subjects in the hundred or more tested who have totally failed to give an explanation have given as their reason the inability to form or hold onto images.

In this task, at least, the translation between action and language is accomplished by the use of imagery. It would appear to be necessary either to directly perceive or to form a clear image of an action in order to give a verbal description and it is for this reason I have drawn the action-language bridge between the two boxes representing 'perceptual' rather than 'motor' processes.

After they have provided their explanations subjects are questioned about their imagery using the questionnaire in figure 2 .

---

1. I visualised myself performing the task clearly/vaguely/not at all.
2. I visualised someone else performing the task C/V/N.
3. I visualised myself from a point outside myself/through my own eyes.
4. I was aware of the colour of the string C/V/N.
5. I was aware of the texture of the string C/V/N.
6. I was aware of an object to which the string was attached C/V/N.
7. I was aware of the environment (indoors/outdoors) C/V/N.
8. I could feel the string C/V/N.
9. I could feel myself making the movements C/V/N.
10. My imagery was predominantly visual/non-visual/a mixture.
11. The action was continuous (like a movie)/a series of stills/a mixture.
12. It was easy/difficult/neither to form images.
13. It was easy/difficult/neither to hold images once formed.
14. It was easy/difficult/neither to describe the images in words.
15. Talking disrupted the images a lot/a little/not at all.

Figure 2. The Action-imagery questionnaire.

The responses reveal a number of features. First, the imagery is predominantly visual. Although only a minority of subjects claim they could "feel the string" many assent to the statement "I could feel myself making the movements". This sense of active involvement is subjectively separable from quasi-sensory impressions such as feeling the texture or seeing the colour of the string and would seem to correspond to the classical "sense of effort".

About half of the subjects claim to experience the imagery as a kind of movie and feel able to control its speed whilst others experience a series of "stills" corresponding to critical aspects of the task. Almost all subjects experience the imagery from an egocentric viewpoint, as if through their own eyes. In other imaginary tasks, such as gymnastic exercises, subjects not infrequently take an external viewpoint and report imaging a model, identified as themselves, performing the task.

Turning to the verbal protocols, considerable variation is found in both the quality and quantity of the explanations. A detailed account is given in Annett (1986) but, briefly, no very clear relationship has emerged between characteristics of the imagery and characteristics of the verbal explanations, and this despite the fact that having some sort of imagery appears to be necessary for any kind of verbal account. Finding the appropriate words seems to constitute a task in itself over and above that of forming the images. This point is demonstrated by a comparison of the two sets of protocol in figure 3 obtained from the same subject, once when giving an explanation from memory and once when asked to tie a bow and explain the procedure when actually performing the task. Over the sample of data so far analysed the verbal protocols from these two variations are virtually indistinguishable.

(a)   You take hold of both ends of the string...

(b)   um...you take both ends...

(a)   cross the right one over the left one...

(b)   cross the right one over the left...

(a)   and underneath to make a knot...

(b)   and underneath...

(a)   make a loop in what is now the right hand string...

(b)   make a loop with what is now the right hand one...

(a)   pass the left underneath...

(b)   cross the left hand one over...

(a)   and pull the loop through...

(b)   pull a loop through...

(a)   tighten by pulling both loops...

(b)   tighten the bow by pulling both loops.

Figure 3. Sample protocols of a subject explaining how to tie a bow, (a) from memory and (b) demonstrating with string.

A comparison of the three conditions shows that it does take rather longer to give an explanation without the physical presence of the string than when actually performing the task, in fact about 55 seconds on average as compared with 30 seconds when the string is present and physically manipulated. By comparison the mean time for the same group of subjects to physically tie a bow, but without having to explain what they were doing was only 9 seconds. Thus the additional burden of attaching words to actions requires a threefold increase in performance time. The time penalty resulting from having to create images is an additional 25 seconds or more than twice as long as executing the basic task.

A particularly significant feature of the results is that many subjects feel the need to make hand gestures either to supplement their explanations or, perhaps, to make it easier to generate appropriate images and words. Gestures are of interest in this context because they might, on a simplistic interpretation of figure 1, have a role in the generation of imagery. The psychoneuromuscular theory of mental practice asserts that motor imagery is essentially the activation of the entire motor system as if physically carrying out the imagined task except that the final output stage of muscular activation is inhibited. Small movements and EMG activity accompanying mental practice have typically been taken as evidence for this hypothesis. If the suppression of gestures made it more difficult to form images and to give explanations this would tend to support the psychoneuromuscular theory.

One group of 10 subjects was required to tap rhythmically with the preferred hand and another group of 10 subjects was required to sit on their hands whilst giving their explanations of how to tie a bow. Neither of these constraints affected the quality (or quantity) of the explanations the subjects were able to give but those who were required to sit on their hands were less likely to report kinaesthetic sensations accompanying their imagined performances. This result is not very helpful to the psychoneuromuscular theory and a closer look at the form of spontaneous gestures gives even less comfort.

(a) Fingers slightly curled and pointing down. Both strings grasped and immediately brought together.

(b) Hands bent back, fingers pointing up. Hands shake synchronously with stressed words.

(a) Strings held at fingertips and crossed with small finger movements.

(b) Hands approach each other, right forefinger pointing.

(a) Hands close together, fingers form loops, first left then right.

(b) Hands well apart, right hand makes circling movement.

(a) Hands move apart with short jerk to tighten bow.

(b) Hands move apart, synchronously with stressed word.

Figure 4. Sample of movements when tying a bow (a) and when explaining without string (b).

From the video recordings it is possible to compare the hand movements made whilst actually tying a bow with those found accompanying verbal explanations in the absence of real string. On a detailed analysis it is clear that whilst there are family resemblances the two sets of movements differ in a number of ways, some of which are illustrated in the verbal descriptions in figure 4 .

The example in figure 5a shows what the subject's hands are doing whilst saying "you make a loop...". The actual movement required to make a loop involves the fingers of both hands, one hand to hold the loose end and a finger on the other hand inserted under the string to pull it out into a loop. Typically, and as shown in the example in figure 5b the hand movements made during an explanation do not simply replicate those made during an actual bow-tying performance but might be said to symbolise them. In many cases the movement of the hand and fingers represents the spatial pattern made by the string itself rather than the movements actually made by the hand and fingers in manipulating the string. Differences of this kind between actual bow-tying and explanatory gestures are typical and this leads to the conclusion that the skill is represented centrally in an abstract or spatial form which can generate both actions and images but the representation is not just a simple motor programme activated when tying a bow either physically or in imagination.

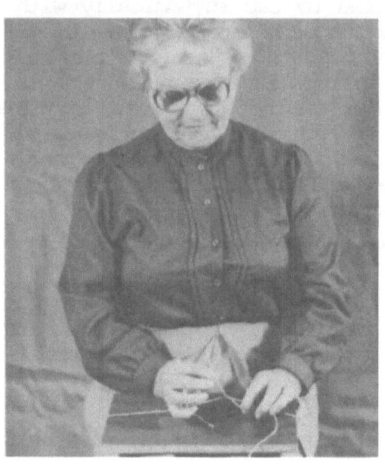 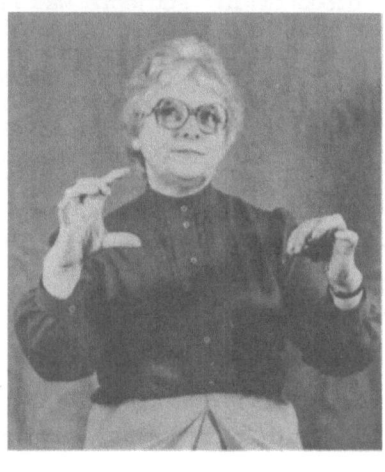

(a)   (b)

Figure 5. Position of hands in making a loop (a) and position of hands in describing how to make a loop (b).

3. A THEORY OF MENTAL PRACTICE

The principal alternative to the psychoneuromuscular theory of mental practice may be called the 'symbolic rehearsal' theory. The essence of this type of theory is that motor and symbolic aspects of performance are separable and each is capable of modification through practice. MacKay (1981, 1982) has proposed that serial skills, of which language production would be a typical example, can be understood as the activation of series of 'nodes' arranged in a hierarchical fashion. At the top of the hierarchy are mental or conceptual nodes which correspond to the core meaning of the phrase to be spoken and these are elaborated by syntactic and phonological nodes further down the hierarchy with nodes controlling actual muscle contraction at the lowest level. In silent speech or mental rehearsal only the higher level nodes are activated. In speech production the network of nodes is activated from the top down but in speech perception the same nodes are activated as it were from the bottom up. MacKay proposes that when a node is activated it 'primes' all the nodes connected to it and this, at least temporarily, lowers the activation threshold of that node. The effect in a well rehearsed sequence would be progressively faster production and MacKay (1981) demonstrated clear effects on the rate at which word sequences could be produced after mental practice. The theory is in effect a modern version of the old 'Law of Exercise' abandoned by Thorndike more than half a century ago.

MacKay (in a private communication) suggested that the bow tying task might be represented in a node structure as shown in figure 6. Several predictions could be made from the theory, including improvement with both physical and mental practice, but more rapid initial improvement with the latter. During both mental and physical practice activation spreads down the nodes shown in figure 6 thus activation of the 'knot 1' node will prime both the preparation and execution nodes of knot 1 but not the corresponding nodes of knot 2. Similarly activation of the preparation node will prime both the grasp and cross nodes but not the intertwine and pull tight nodes.

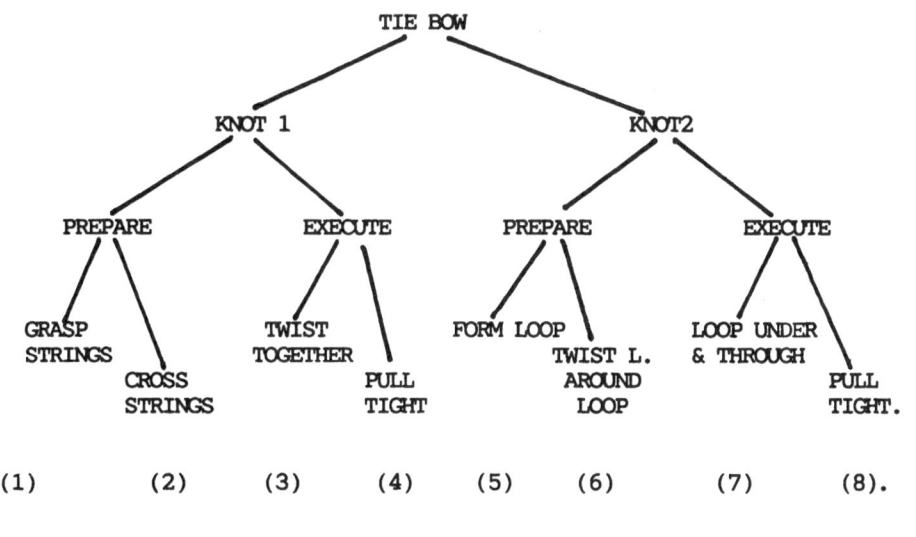

Figure 6. Hypothetical node structure underlying bow tying.

If priming does work in the way suggested by the theory then the transitions between phases of the task should be shorter where they connect to a single node than when when the connections are more remote, thus transitions 1-2, 3-4, 5-6 and 7-8 should be faster than 2-3, and 6-7 whilst the transition 4-5 should be slowest. One might expect these differences to be reflected in hesitations in the verbal explanations.

4. SOME PRELIMINARY DATA

A total of 40 subjects were given 12 trials each of both physical and mental practice in bow tying. Subjects timed themselves by pressing a switch before beginning the bow and pressing the same switch on completion of the task. Half the subjects carried out their mental practice trials first (MP1) whilst the other half began with twelve trials of physical practice (MP2). Instruction and preliminary practice using a different task ensured that they were familiar with the apparatus and procedure, including mental practice, before the experiment proper.

The principal results are shown in table 1. The average time for tying the bow of 6.7 seconds indicates that subjects were following the instruction for speed since performance with this particular apparatus when speed is not stressed gives a mean of about 9 seconds. The average mental practice trial takes much less time, 4.5 seconds, as predicted by the theory but whereas there is a significant reduction in performance time for physical practice, mental practice shows no such improvement.

Condition	Trial 1	Trial 12	Mean of 12 trials	
MP1	4.53	4.10	4.27	(Seconds)
MP2	4.94	4.72	4.77	"
PP1	8.11	6.21	6.78	"
PP2	7.89	6.46	6.55	"

Table 1. Time to complete imaginary (MP) and physical (PP) bow tying.

The data also suggest a small effect on mental practice times of task order, that is mental practice is slightly slower if physical practice has been done first, but this effect is not statistically significant. Subjects were asked to give subjective estimates of their times on the 12th. trial for both physical and mental practice, expressed as a percentage of the time for their first trial. Subjects who had experienced physical practice first attributed more improvement to this than to mental practice but the reverse was true for those who experienced mental practice first.

The prediction concerning the hesitations between stages of bow tying was tested by analysing data already recorded on video of subjects giving verbal explanations. A total of 33 were found who used the method of bow tying assumed by the node structure in figure 6 and the speech pauses between the stages of the explanation were measured. The results show that 5-6 is consistently the longest pause with a mean of 6.7 seconds with 7-8 next longest at 5.2 seconds. The pause between 4 and 5 which was predicted to be longest took 4.58 seconds on average thus overall the data do not support the predictions.

5. DISCUSSION

It is presumed that when a motor skill is acquired some kind of mental representation is laid down which can be reactivated at need to support an overt performance or a mental rehearsal or to serve as an information source for a recoded version of the skill such as a verbal specification or description. The two exploratory studies described above indicate some of the subjective and functional features of the representation of a familiar skill, tying a bow.

It would appear that it is only possible to translate from the 'action' mode to the 'verbal' mode via the use of imagery. The verbal system does not have direct access to any modality-neutral representation of the skill but can only describe what it 'sees', probably making use of learned habits of naming.

Although there may well be differences between skills, such as between 'open' and 'closed' skills or whole body and manipulative skills, images of the skill of bow tying are largely visuo-spatial in character. This finding should not surprise anyone familiar with the recent literature on motor control which emphasises the implementation of 'intentions' or the specification of outcomes rather than the production of rigid motor patterns. For many skills it would be quite unproductive to store copies of patterns of muscular contractions. The most helpful images one can have in the explanation task represent functional criteria, for example that the strings shall be crossed, rather than movements as such. This same feature is also reflected in the gestures made by subjects during the course of their explanations. Gestures rarely mimic the movements made when actually performing the task but rather symbolise the spatial characteristics which identify an intermediate or a final goal such as a loop or a bow.

It follows that the mental rehearsal of a skill is not necessarily or simply the activation of a motor command system up to, but stopping short of, some final stage which sets the musculature in motion. It is more probably a review of images representing criterial stages which must be completed if the outcome of the action is to be a properly tied bow.

The predictions from MacKay's theory, which proposes an incomplete activation of the motor command system as an account of mental practice, have not been confirmed on the preliminary experiment reported here. The mental performance of the familiar task of bow tying does not improve with practice whilst physical performance does and the stage transitions predicted as requiring longer and shorter activation times do not conform to predictions. It seems that mental bow tying is not physical bow tying infinitely attenuated but something quite different, an alternative rather than a 'cut down' version of the real thing. Future investigators should therefore be cautious in making the traditional assumptions about the relationship between physical and mental or imaginary practice.

ACKNOWLEDGEMENT
I am grateful to Don MacKay for his suggestions which led to the second experiment described in this paper.

REFERENCES

1. Annett, J. (1982). Action, language and imagination. In L. Wankel, and R. Wilberg, (Eds.), Psychology of Sport and Motor Behavior: Research and Practice. Edmonton: University of Alberta.
2. Annett, J. (1985). Motor learning: a review. In H. Heuer, et al. (Eds.), Motor Behavior: Programming, Control and Acquisition. Berlin: Springer.
3. Annett, J. (1986). On knowing how to do things. In H. Heuer, and C. Fromm (Eds.), Generation and Modulation of Action Patterns. Berlin: Springer.
4. Geschwind, N. (1965). Disconnection syndromes in animals and man. Brain, 88, 585-644.
5. MacKay, D.G. (1981). The problem of rehearsal or mental practice. Journal of Motor Behavior, 13, 274-285.
6. MacKay, D.G. (1982). The problems of flexibility, fluency and speed-accuracy trade-off in skilled behavior. Psychological Review, 89, 483-506.

MEDIATION IN LEARNING COMPLEX CYCLICAL ACTIONS

HAROLD T.A. WHITING

DEPARTMENT OF PSYCHOLOGY, INTERFACULTY OF HUMAN MOVEMENT SCIENCES,
THE FREE UNIVERSITY, AMSTERDAM, THE NETHERLANDS

ABSTRACT
    A general framework to the field of motor control/motor learning is
sketched in order to signal points of contact/dispute with the field of
Imagery. The distinction between the 'image of the act' and the 'image of
achievement' is presented and used to distinguish metric from topological
characteristics of movements. The use of these, and other parameters, as
dependent variables in 'imitation' research is discussed together with the
distinction between 'echokinetic' and 'synkinetic' paradigms for research
in this sub-field. The Chapter concludes with a brief discussion of an
initial experiment on mediation via a dynamic video model in the learning
of complex cyclical actions and the significance of the results for
research in the field of Imagery.

1. INTRODUCTION

    In writing this paper I find myself in something of a dilemma! The
dilemma is occasioned by the feeling that, not having carried out any
experimental work that might be construed to be concerned directly with
imagery, I am something of an intruder in the field. I feel impelled,
therefore, at the outset to try to justify the inclusion of my paper in a
text on imagery per se. Let me try to do this by, first, sketching a more
general framework to the field of motor control/motor learning. In so doing
I will be forced to signal a number of problems apparent within the
different theoretical positions being taken. This will lead me, in turn, to
a distinction made by myself and den Brinker (1982) between what we term
the 'image of the act' and what Pribram (1971) termed the 'image of
achievement' and hence to the sub-programme of research on imitation we
have recently initiated under the more extensive rubric of 'complex motor
actions'. It will not have escaped the reader's notice that this conceptual
distinction provides at least face validity for points of contact with the
field of imagery.

2.   MOTOR CONTROL/MOTOR LEARNING
2.1. Motor systems v. action systems

    In the current literature on motor control, and to a lesser extent
motor learning, two contrasting perspectives are to be distinguished,
perspectives that might suitably be labelled 'motor systems' and 'action
systems' approaches (Meijer & Roth, 1987). These should be seen as families
of theories rather than single theoretical approaches. In what follows,
therefore, it should be noted that comments made about action systems
approaches are restricted to those perspectives that lay emphasis on
natural/physical interpretations of motor control rather than those which
take an even stronger functional position (e.g. Reed, 1986).

269

M. Denis et al. (eds.), Cognitive and Neuropsychological Approaches to Mental Imagery, 269 277.
© 1988 by Martinus Nijhoff Publishers.

These two contrasting approaches to motor control/motor learning bring with them different sets of assumptions, and hence interpretations, of the way in which movements are controlled and coordinated. The motor systems approach, stemming as it does from artefactual machine analogies assumes the presence of devices within the CNS that, when activated, produce coordinated movements (Kugler, 1986) i.e. the emphasis is on more-or-less detailed prescriptions for control giving rise to conceptual metaphors - well recognised in this workshop - like 'frames', 'schemas', 'motor programmes' or to the identification of neural substrates such as central pattern generators. In contrast, the focus in the natural/physical perspective is on self-organising systems - on intrinsic symmetries (patterns of invariance) and how they are sustained under some scale changes and broken under others (Kugler, 1986). It is not, to my mind, that proponents of the natural/physical approach wish, necessarily, to deny mental representation, but rather wish to question its relevance to an understanding of motor control. The turning point in this whole debate would appear to centre around the question posed by Kugler (1986) as to how many ontologies one would wish to invoke. The natural/physical approach to movement organisation, following on the normal programme of physical science, is concerned 'to discover the simplest and most general self-contained description of natural events' (Kugler, 1986) - a rigorous application of Occam's razor. In such an approach mental representations, at least for the time being, would appear to be an unnecessary luxury!

In the context of motor learning these contrasting approaches are interesting in that they, presumably, give rise to differing interpretations of the phenomenon and, hence, to ideas about how training might be optimally organised although, it has to be said, that neither approach really provides a meaningful framework to this end. It might, however, be speculated that those adopting a motor systems perspective would, for example, be predisposed to discover how motor programmes or schemas come to be optimally established, i.e. the extent to which movements might come to be centrally represented. One proposal in this respect has come to be known as the 'variability of practice' hypothesis (Schmidt, 1975). It is difficult even to be speculative about the predictions that might be made by those adopting a natural/physical approach since statements about motor learning are few and far between. What does seem clear, however, is that they might well want to assert that movements per se are not learned! Following Gelfand & Tsetlin (1962), for example, they might want to maintain that biological systems discover the organisation of functional space by successively attempting to solve motor problems posed by the environment - defined in terms of a one-degree of freedom control system (did I achieve the goal I set myself or not?). The iterative provision of solutions to problems of a similar kind would - following Bernstein (Whiting, 1985) - lead to the discovery of how the instantaneous dynamics of the system might best be exploited to bring about the required functional outcome. The prediction might well be once again, albeit from a different perspective, presenting the learner with variable practice within a particular class of problem.

2.2. Motor learning

Perhaps the most striking characteristic of motor learning is the nature of the progress to be observed as the learner moves from exhibiting the variant movement forms that characterise him as a beginner to exhibiting a relatively invariant form as he becomes more expert (Tyldesley & Whiting, 1977). Given this remarkable invariance in the movement form of the expert it is, perhaps, not surprising that those who embrace a motor systems approach would want to invoke the 'default' argument of the availability of motor programmes. It is difficult, for them, to conceive of another mechanism which might lead to the same degree of replicability. Surprisingly, however, such proponents have little to say about how these invariant movement forms (general motor programmes - Shapiro & Schmidt, 1982) come to be established. In a similar way, while from the natural/physical perspective there is experimental evidence available about the effects of disturbing existing coordinative structures (movement forms) or the consequences of driving the system on a sensitive parameter, there is little to be found about how nested sets of coordinative structures have the capacity, via learning, to become autonomous structures. What this means, in effect, is that there is very little known about the early stages of learning a novel skill (a skill in which a novel movement form is required - what Fitts and Posner (1967) refer to as the 'cognitive stage' of skill learning).

These kinds of deficiency have been the factors prompting us to direct attention, specifically, to this very early stage of skill learning in a structured research programme which has been running for a number of years and which is destined to continue for some time yet.

2.3. 'Image of the act' and 'image of achievement'
In searching for the dependent variables that might be worth pursuing in the context of such early learning we (Whiting & den Brinker, 1982) have distinguished between what we term the 'image of the act' (an abstract topological representation of movement form) and what Pribram (1971) refers to as the 'image of achievement' (a momentary representation of the external forces to be overcome in solving a motor problem). The nature of the image of achievement can be operationalised on the basis of the experience of babies with the estimation of weight (Bower, 1977). When an object is handed to a baby of about 9 months of age, the arm falls down as the baby takes the object but is quickly adjusted. At about twelve months of age, the baby is able to anticipate the weight correctly on repeated presentations - anticipation cannot, however, be transferred to an object of different weight. This ability has been grasped by about 18 months of age: the baby is able to predict weight without the necessity of prior grasping. Runeson and Frykholm (1983) in a series of studies addressed to the kinematic specification of dynamics as an informational basis for person-and-action perception, operationalise this concept further. Using Johansson's (1973) patch-light technique they were able to show that the 'lead-in' movements of a person lifting a box allow perception of what weight the lifter expects (i.e. his image of achievement) and, also, that a person lifting a box cannot deceive observers about the weight of the box, only convey the deceptive intention.

In early learning situations - as has been described for babies 'lifting' weights and as is apparent for novices learning new movement forms in phylogenetic skills - inaccuracies in both images are likely to be encountered. It would seem that the best way for an 'actor' to discover the properties of one of these images would be to keep the properties of the other as stable as possible while this was being explored. Thus, in coming to a relatively invariant 'image of the act', we hypothesise that the learning situation should be so structured that the field of external forces to be overcome be kept relatively constant while the actor gives his attention to establishing a reliable and appropriate 'image of the act'.

In other words - and unlike the predictions to be made from, for example, the 'variability of practice hypothesis' of Schmidt (1975) - the introduction of variation in environmental conditions (including required movement parameters) should be postponed in the process of learning until an adequate 'image of the act' has been developed under one of the many conditions under which the act has, eventually, to be executed i.e. the 'image of the act' has first to be developed as a holistic unit, a gestalt, before it can be manipulated to serve acts under changed conditions. It should be noted that this is not a plea for a form of training that 'grooves-in' a stable 'image of the act' but is more in keeping with Bernstein's (Whiting, 1985) conception of training as being 'repetition without repetition' in the sense that the actor repeatedly attempts to solve the same motor problem by means which are adjusted from occasion to occasion. The updated 'image of the act' is distilled out of repeated attempts to solve the same class of problem.

Although we have not pursued some of the predictions from the distinction here being made, it is worthwhile in the context of the content of the present volume to draw the reader's attention to past work in the psychological literature on both 'forced-response guidance learning' (Holding, 1965) and mental practice. A greater cognisance of the distinction, here being made, between the 'image of the act' and the 'image of achievement' and the use of dependent variables that reflect this distinction, might, we maintain, lead to more meaningful research paradigms as well as interpretations of the existing literature.

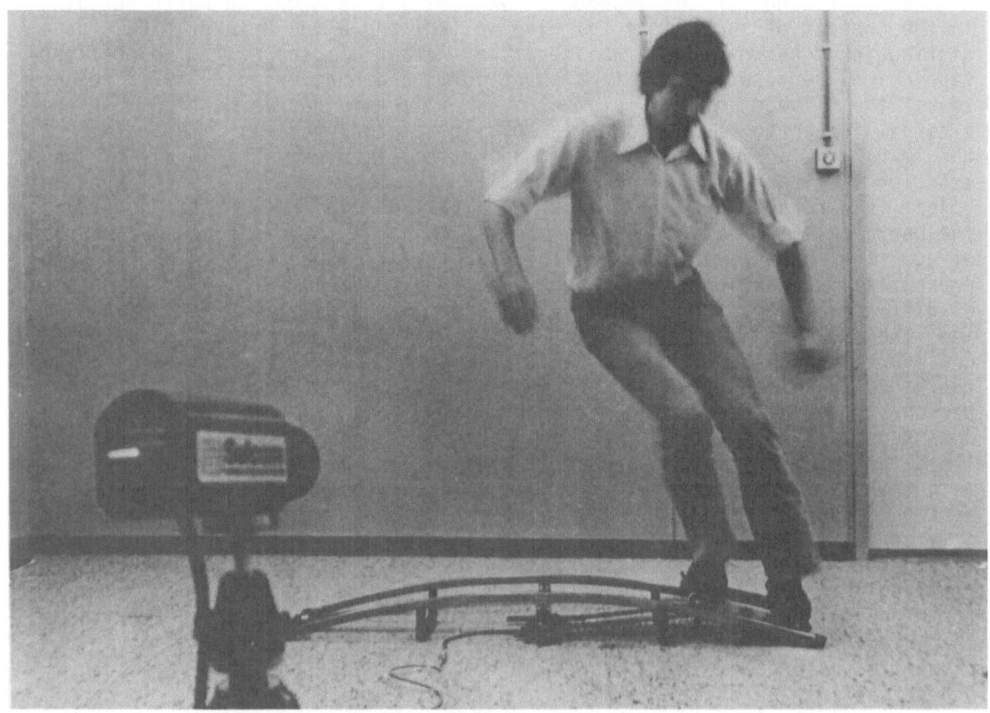

FIGURE 1. The ski-simulator apparatus. (The platform on which the subject stands can, with the aid of slalom-type ski movements, be made to move to and fro over a pair of rigid, bowed steel rails. Strong springs ensure that the platform returns to its resting position in the middle. Light emitting diodes attached to the centre of the platform allow its movement characteristics to be monitored via a SELSPOT system).

2.4. Dependent variables in motor learning research

We have not, ourselves, pursued these latter interesting research lines although in the context of 'imagery' they have much to offer. Instead, we have concentrated attention on the earliest stages of learning complex cyclical actions in the form of slalom-type ski movements on a simulator (Fig. 1) and discrete actions as exemplified by the attacking forehand drive in table-tennis. I shall restrict myself in what follows to the cyclical actions.

From the outset, it was our intention to utilise two classes of dependent variable stemming from the distinction made between the 'image of the act' and the 'image of achievement' namely, movement form and an operationalisation of the external forces to be overcome in terms of amplitude and frequency of movement. However, it quickly became apparent that there is another class of qualitative variable that might be important in both movement and movement production. This is well signalled in Hopkins and Prechtl's (1985) approach to the development of movements during early infancy. As they point out, an infant's general movements can be quantified in terms of their individual properties (i.e. their metrical or form topological dimensions) but this, in itself, would say nothing about whether the movements were smooth or jerky. This is catered for by adding an additional dimension to our list of potential dependent variables - a measure of 'fluency' (Δ acceleration).

The experimental work in which we have been involved has made use of amplitude, frequency and fluency of movement as dependent variables (Bootsma, den Brinker & Whiting, 1985; den Brinker, Stabler, Whiting & van Wieringen, 1985; den Brinker, Stabler, van Wieringen & Whiting, 1986; Whiting, Bijlard & den Brinker, 1987), earlier work (den Brinker & van Hekken, 1982) having demonstrated that these were good indices of learning. Unfortunately, in these early experiments the problem of determining movement form had not been resolved. Progress in this respect is now being made.

2.5. Imitation learning

Perhaps the most interesting of our experiments to date in the present context is that on 'imitation learning' since it is generally asssumed that imitation involves some kind of imagery mediation. Although the literature on the imitation of motor acts is relatively limited - particularly outside the baby literature - imitation per se is far from being a new concept. As Scheerer (1986), in his excellent overview, has so succinctly traced, imitation, as a phenomenon, has been repeatedly 'rediscovered'. Scheerer traces the philosophical traditions through cosmology, the theory of art, anthropology and education, ethics and religion before concentrating attention on 18th century German empirical psychology. He concludes that, in evolutionary thinking about imitation, a dichotomy is to be discerned between 'cognitivistic' and maturational/ emotional approaches to imitation that provides more insight into the history of the concept than the customary assumption that the drive or instinct theory of imitation was, eventually, superceded by a learning process.

Preyer (1882), a pioneer in the description and explanation of early infant activity, was responsible for a four-fold classification of infant behaviour, i.e. impulsive, reflective, instinctive and ideational. Under ideational were included early imitative acts which, to Preyer, were evidence of cerebral activity operationalised in the form of volition (Butterworth, 1986). The theoretical significance of such imitative movements was that, according to Preyer, they were always guided by mental representations. It is interesting to see this contention being returned to in the more recent approach of Carroll and Bandura (1982) to observational learning in the more general framework of social learning theory. Their contention being that motor learning, via observation, is mediated by conceptual representations. Central to Bandura's (1977) social learning theory of imitation is the role of symbolic representations. He proposes two such systems - closely analogous to Paivio's (1986) dual coding theory - a spatial (imaginal) and a verbal. Verbal mediation, in establishing categorical similarities, enables people to very quickly 'represent' and 'retain' model behaviour. The spatial representation system, it is suggested, plays its most important role in that developmental phase when the capacity to verbalise is not present. But, one has to agree with Williams (1985) that while it is clear that people can watch the movements of others and produce similar movements themselves, it is not particularly helpful merely to know that this is achieved by means of the 'construction of a central representation that serves as an internal model for response production' (Bandura, 1977). Nevertheless, the departure point of Williams (1985) - who, to my mind, has carried out some of the most meaningful work on the imitation of motor acts in recent years - is very much within this frame of interpretation. To Williams:

> ". . . movement imitation involves the 'pick-up' of selected spatio-temporal parameters of modelled movements which are embodied into a general motor programme which is used for, or facilitates, the production of, these movements."

All Williams' work has been carried out using an echokinetic paradigm.

Prinz (1985), in discussing ideo-motor phenomena, distinguishes between echokinesis - off-line reproduction of a movement - and synkinesis - on-line completion of a movement sequence. He proposes that echokinesis always requires spatial as well as temporal correspondence between the model and its copy, the spatial correspondence can be of two kinds, based on the topology of the body (use of corresponding body parts) and the geometry of environmental space (generation of corresponding movement trajectories).

The above discussion forms the background to the sub-programme on imitation we have recently initiated. A first experiment (Whiting, Bijlard & den Brinker, 1987) has recently been completed. From a whole range of possible experiments which might have been initiated on the basis of what has been written above, we opted for a synkinetic paradigm. There were two major reasons in this respect: in the first case, no work could be found in the literature adopting this kind of paradigm and in the second such procedure is ecologically similar to what happens in certain real-life skiing instruction situations. Basically, the design allowed comparisons to be made between subjects who were required to learn to make fluent slalom-type ski movements (of large amplitude and high frequency) on a ski-simulator (Fig. 1) under the conditions that they had the benefit or not of the availability of a dynamic video model of an expert performer on the simulator during training trials. Dependent variables were, as previously specified, amplitude, frequency and fluency of movement of the simulator platform on which subjects were required to stand. Results, after five days training, confirmed that subjects having the advantage of the availability of an expert dynamic model during training showed superior fluency in the movements of the simulator platform as well as less variable fluency of movement and less variable frequency of movement. The latter two measures are highly correlated since maintaining a relatively constant frequency leads to more fluent movements. No significant differences in amplitude or frequency were apparent. In as far as fluency is one of the criteria of skilled performance it must be concluded that the availability of a dynamic model during training has a positive, mediating effect, on the skill level of the performer. The use of the term 'mediating effect' rather than imitation per se is deliberate since subjects who had the benefit of the availability of a dynamic model during training did not copy, exactly, the movement parameters of the platform as indexed by amplitude, frequency and fluency (in the absence of the appropriate analysis it is not possible to make a similar statement with respect to movement 'form'). The effect of the availability of a dynamic model, we are claiming is more that of 'regulatory' in the manner envisaged by Ricoeur (1966):

"Whatever explanation is adopted, it has to deny the reflex character of imitation forcefully: imitation never presents the stereotyped, isolable, irrepressible characteristics of a reflex. A similar action has perhaps a primitive motor power, but it is a power of regulation and not of mechanical production."

While a number of interpretations of these results are possible (Whiting, Bijlard & den Brinker, 1987) the interesting question, in the present context, is the part played by imagery in the mediation process. At one extreme, it might be proposed - by invoking, for example, Prinz's (1985) principle of immediate similarity based matching - that it plays no part. On the other hand the results might be explainable as an artefact of subjects, who had the benefit of a model during training, adopting the movement form of the model (mediated by an 'image of the act') and this, in turn, leading to superior 'fluency' of movement. The latter interpretation would give rise to further interesting work on the nature and role of such imagery.

Prinz's principle of immediate similarity-based matching between perceived and generated event configuration is based on the assumption that two principles underlie the variables which might most lend themselves to observational learning. In the first place, event generation tends to rely more on pattern in time than pattern in space. Secondly, with respect to both spatial and temporal patterns, the parameters of the to-be-generated motor event tend to be based on some abstract, higher order representation of the perceived event. If, he proposes, ideo-motor event generation relies on the use of parameters of these higher order representations of spatial and temporal patterns, this should become apparent in closer fits between imitated and imitating movements - in the high as compared to the low-order functions.

Future work in our own sub-programme on imitation will try to tease out some of these problems further. It is expected that imagery and mental practice will, in the long-term, become central issues. In the short-term, a replication of the reported experiment utilising an echokinetic paradigm is likely to produce important differences which may require alternative explanations.

REFERENCES

1. Bandura, A. (1977). Social learning theory. Englewood Cliffs, N.J.: Prentice-Hall.
2. Bootsma, R.J., Brinker, B.P.L.M. den & Whiting, H.T.A. (1985). Complexe beweginshandelingen op sportgebied. Nederlands Tijdschrift voor de Psychologie, 41, 14-26.
3. Bower, T.G.R. (1977). A primer of infant development. San Francisco: Freeman.
4. Brinker, B.P.L.M. den & Hekken, M.F. van (1982). The analysis of slalom-ski type movements using a ski-simulator apparatus. Human Movement Science, 1, 91-108.

5. Brinker, B.P.L.M. den, Stabler, J.R.L.W., Wieringen, P.C.W. van &
    Whiting, H.T.A. (1985). A multidimensional analysis of some persistent
    problems in motor learning. In: D.G. Goodman and R.B. Wilberg (Eds.),
    Differing perspectives in motor control and motor learning. Amsterdam:
    North-Holland.
6. Brinker, B.P.L.M. den, Stabler, J.R.L.W., Whiting, H.T.A. & Wieringen,
    P.C.W. van (1986). The effect of manipulating knowledge of results on
    the learning of slalom-type ski movements. Ergonomics, 29, 31-40.
7. Butterworth, G. (1986). Some problems in explaining the origins of
    movement control. In: M.G. Wade and H.T.A. Whiting (Eds.), Motor
    development in children: aspects of coordination and control.
    Dordrecht: Martinus Nijhoff.
8. Carroll, W.R. & Bandura, A. (1982). The role of visual monitoring in
    observational learning of action patterns: making the unobservable
    observable. Journal of Motor Behavior, 14, 153-167.
9. Fitts, P.M. & Posner, M.I. (1967). Human performance. Belmont:
    Brooks/Cole.
10. Gelfand, I.M. & Tsetlin, M.L. (1962). Some methods of control for
    complex systems. Russian Mathematical Surveys, 17, 95-116.
11. Holding, D.H. (1965). Principles of training. London: Pergamon.
12. Johansson, G. (1973). The visual perception of biological motion and a
    model for its analysis. Perception and Psychophysics, 14, 201-211.
13. Kugler, P.N. (1986). A morphological perspective on the origin and
    evolution of movement patterns. In: M.G. Wade and H.T.A. Whiting
    (Eds.), Motor development in children: aspects of coordination and
    control. Dordrecht: Martinus-Nijhoff.
14. Meijer, O.G. & Roth, K. (Eds.) (1987). Complex movement behaviour:
    'the' motor-action controversy. Amsterdam: North-Holland.
15. Paivio, A. (1986). Mental representations: a dual coding approach.
    Oxford: University Press.
16. Preyer, W. (1882). Die Seele des Kindes. Leipzig: Grieben.
17. Pribram, K.H. (1971). Languages of the brain. New Jersey:
    Prentice-Hall.
18. Prinz, W. (1987). Ideo-motor action. In: H. Heuer and A.F. Sanders
    (Eds.), Perception and action. Berlin: Springer-Verlag.
19. Reed, E.S. (1986) Applying the theory of action systems to the study of
    motor skills. In: O.G. Meijer and K. Roth (Eds.), Complex movement
    behaviour: 'the' motor-action controversy. Amsterdam: North-Holland.
20. Ricoeur, P. (1966). Freedom and nature: the voluntary and the
    involuntary. Illinois: North-Western University Press.
21. Runeson, S. & Frykholm, G. (1983). Kinematic specification of dynamics
    as an informational basis for person-and-action perception:
    expectation, gender recognition and deceptive intention. Journal of
    Experimental Psychology: General, 112, 585-615.
22. Scheerer, E. (1986). Pre-evolutionary conception of imitation. In: G.
    Eckhardt, W.G. Bringmann and L. Sprung (Eds.), Contributions to the
    history of developmental psychology. Paris: Mouton.
23. Schmidt, R.A. (1975). A schema theory of discrete motor skill learning.
    Psychological Review, 82, 225-260.
24. Shapiro, D.C. & Schmidt, R.A. (1982). The schema theory: recent
    evidence and developmental implications. In: J.A.S. Kelso and J.E.
    Clark (Eds.), The development of movement control and coordination. New
    York: Wiley.
25. Tyldesley, D.A. & Whiting, H.T.A. (1977). Operational timing. Journal
    of Human Movement Studies, 1, 172-177.
26. Whiting, H.T.A. (Ed.) (1985). Human motor actions: Bernstein

reassessed. Amsterdam: North-Holland.

27. Whiting, H.T.A., Bijlard, M. & Brinker, B.P.L.M. den (1987). The effect of the availability of a dynamic model on the acquisition of a complex cyclical action. The Quarterly Journal of Experimental Psychology, 39A, 43-59.

28. Whiting, H.T.A. & Brinker, B.P.L.M. den (1982). Image of the act. In: J.P. Das, R.F. Mulcahy and A.E. Wall (Eds.), Theory and research in learning disabilities. New York: Plenum.

29. Williams, J.G. (1985). Movement imitation: some fundamental processes. Unpublished Ph.d. thesis, University of London, 1985.

University, Rotterdam, Netherlands, 1972.

21. Smith, F.A. 1981 and N.J. Brinkman, M.P.C.M. Krijn, 1982. The struc-
    ture, stability and dynamics of a macromolecular... The structure of a complex.
    ... the structure. J. ... University of ... ... Netherlands, 1981.

22. Watson, J.D. ... ...
    ... ... Vol. 73, pp 335-339.
    ... ...

23. ... ... fundamental processes.
    Proceedings ... ... 1968.

3.3. DISCUSSION OF PART 3

EMPIRICAL APPROACHES TO A FUNCTIONAL ANALYSIS OF IMAGERY AND COGNITION

MARK A. MCDANIEL

UNIVERSITY OF NOTRE DAME, NOTRE DAME, IN, U.S.A.

ABSTRACT

In investigating the role of imagery in learning, several approaches including material manipulation, instructional manipulation, presentation of interfering tasks, and individual differences have been adopted. The applicability of these approaches for investigating the functional role of imagery in other cognitive activities, in particular, problem solving and motor skill learning, are considered. It is argued that these approaches, or some variants of these approaches, can be fruitfully applied to imagery research in areas other than verbal learning. Possible pitfalls of each approach are discussed as well.

1. INTRODUCTION

My charter as a special discussant was to comment on the paper sessions held during the second day of the workshop. The preceding chapters have conveyed the excitment and fruitfulness of each participant's efforts during that second day, efforts generally concerned with the functional role of imagery in problem solving, motor learning, and skill acquisition. I would add little by revisiting those particular efforts here. Consequently, I will adopt the modest objectives of discussing several possible approaches to investigating the role of imagery in cognition, relating these approaches to some of the themes covered during the second day of the workshop, and identifying possible pitfalls associated with each approach.

In investigating the role of imagery in cognition, the underlying assumption is, of course, that people can form a mental image and/or have some specialized system for encoding and processing nonverbal information emanating from either perceptual input or from long-term memory. This assumption has received strong empirical support that need not be reviewed here (e.g., Kosslyn, 1980; Baddeley, this volume). The trick is to find ways to elicit imagery and to do so in such a way as to be able to demonstrate that effects attributed to imagery are in fact due to imagery processing per se. Because much of the work on the functional nature of imagery has focused on imagery effects in verbal learning, this area has an established set of techniques for studying the influence of imagery. Using these techniques as a foundation, I will briefly describe their use in memory research and then examine each technique's potential for more general application to investigations of imagery in problem solving, motor learning, and skill acquisition.

2. VARYING THE MATERIALS

One approach in studying the role of imagery in verbal learning has been to vary the to-be-learned stimulus material. Most typically the concreteness of the to-be-learned material is varied (see Paivio, 1986), with the expectation that concrete material will be processed imaginally and verbally, whereas abstract material will be processed only verbally. Thus, any concreteness effects in remembering might be thought to be due to imagery processing. The question for present purposes is whether the same type of approach might be extended to study the role of imagery in problem solving, acquisition of motor skills, and other tasks involving cognitive components. For motor skills, on the dimension of concreteness, the answer seems to be no, for the simple reason that motor

M. Denis et al. (eds.), Cognitive and Neuropsychological Approaches to Mental Imagery, 281–291.
© *1988 by Martinus Nijhoff Publishers.*

tasks are ordinarily concrete as evidenced by the ubiquitous use of demonstration in the teaching of motor skills (cf. Whiting, Bijlard, & den Brinker, 1987). Motor tasks vary on a number of other dimensions, however. One common distinction is between "open skills" and "closed skills" (see Newell, Quinn, Sparrow & Walter, 1983). Another dimension that seems potentially important is one that might be referred to as functional and non-functional. For example, joy-stick movement patterns (randomly determined by an experimenter; Chevalier-Girard & Wilberg, 1980) would be non-functional, whereas performing movements such as combing one's hair (Engelkamp & Zimmer, 1985) would be functional. Clearly, there are many more dimensions that could be enumerated. The point here is simply that the role of imagery may differ in the acquisition or memory of movement patterns as a function of the type of pattern being investigated (this is the case for other variables associated with motor learning, such as knowledge of results, Newell et al., 1983). Thus, while imagery is apparently useful for aiding memory of movement lists that are composed of joystick patterns (Chevalier-Girard & Wilberg, 1980), or useful for acquiring random movement patterns (Goss, Hall, Buckolz, & Fishburne, 1986), it is not clear apriori whether imagery would be equally useful in remembering other types of more functional movement patterns.

For problem solving, varying the concreteness of materials to elicit imagery is in principle possible. Kaufmann, in the course of the workshop, indicated that imagery use in problem solving would depend on the concreteness of the problem. Across problem domains it seems reasonable to assume that some problems are more concrete than others, and it also seems reasonable to link imagery use with concrete problems more so than with nonconcrete problems. To proceed further, however, and try to determine if imagery plays any functional role in problem solving would require, it seems, that similar problems be couched in more concrete or less concrete terms. Problem solving appears to be an especially interesting and tractable domain in which to do this because the very same problem can be presented in different isomorphic surface forms (Hayes & Simon, 1974). Thus, one might present a problem in a form that does not invite visuo-spatial representation and another form that invites a visuo-spatial representation and compare the efficacy of problem solving on the two forms of the problem. For instance, in Carroll, Thomas, and Malhotra's (1980) work, a design problem that required satisfying as many of 19 constraints as possible was presented in spatial terms (assign offices along a corridor to different employees) or in temporal terms (assign a production sequence to different manufacturing processes). The spatial isomorph but not the temporal isomorph prompted subjects to sketch a pictorial representation of the problem situation, and more of the constraints were satisfied for the spatial than the temporal isomorph. This implies that nonverbal processing can be important in the problem solving process. As another example, syllogism problems can be presented in very abstract, symbolic form or in terms of premises with concrete referents. Interpretation of differing patterns due to the concreteness of syllogism problems should be undertaken cautiously, however, because although concrete premises might afford more imaginal processing they may also invite solution strategies based on declarative knowledge and/or affective responses (cf. Howard, 1983).

Another way to manipulate the materials to induce a verbal versus visual approach to solving the problem is to present the problem either in pictorial or verbal form or to present supplementary information either in verbal or visual (pictures or diagrams) form. For example, in work on problem solving by analogy the analogs might be presented either in verbal or visual form (see Beveridge & Parkins, 1987). Similarly, in work on transfer of training, the training can either be perceptually based or verbally based (e.g., Katona, 1940). In addition to establishing the importance of visually represented information in problem solving, this approach can also be effectively used to determine the mechanism(s) by which this information facilitates problem solving. In Beveridge and Parkins (1987) this was done by varying the particular visual analogs presented, and in so doing, varying the properties of the visual information.

There are several potential problems with the technique of varying the nature of the problem solving materials. One is that a verbal presentation does not ensure that visuo-spatial imagery will not be employed. For instance, in Gick and Holyoak's (1980) work on analogical problem solving it seems that verbally presented analogical stories may have induced visuo-spatial representations. Another problem is that the <u>content</u> of the material presented may covary with the format of the presentation. In Katona's (1940) work with matchstick problems, the verbal training group was given the arithmetic principle: "All lines with double function must be changed to lines with single function." The visual training group was shown how to solve the problem in a step-by-step fashion, with shading used to highlight the squares to be left intact. Visual training was found to produce superior problem solving performance relative to verbal training on subsequent matchstick problems, perhaps implying that visual imagery is superior to verbally induced problem-solving strategies (Kaufmann, 1980, p. 158). An alternative conclusion based on the content or on the comprehensibility of the instruction cannot be ruled out, however. The verbal training involved presentation of a general scheme or principle, while the visual training involved presentation of specific operations or steps. As Helstrup pointed out in the workshop, these are different strategy levels. Pre-training that varies on these levels can lead to different problem solving performance, even when the format (verbal--visual) of the training is held constant (McDaniel & Schlager, 1986). Thus, more telling designs would be those that factorially vary content and format of supporting materials.

3. VARYING THE INSTRUCTIONS

An extensively used method for investigating the role of imagery in learning is to instruct subjects either to use imagery to encode the material or to use some kind of encoding task that is nominally nonimaginal in nature (e.g., Bower, 1972; McDaniel & Kearney, 1984). In some circumstances this technique has been successful in demonstrating the unique mnemonic properties of images. For example, McDaniel and Einstein (1986) demonstrated that the bizarreness of a sentence frame in which three target nouns were embedded significantly affected recall when subjects were instructed to image the sentences but not when subjects were not instructed to use imagery, implying that the bizarreness effects were unique to imaginal encoding.

For studies of problem solving and motor learning, employing an instructional approach to manipulating imagery would appear to be straightforward at first blush. In Carroll et al.'s (1980) work described above, to confirm that the visuo-spatial representation prompted by the spatial isomorph was instrumental in aiding solution attempts, subjects given the temporal isomorph were instructed to think of the problem in spatial terms and to use a pictorial representation. Given these instructions, subjects performed as well on the temporal isomorph as did subjects on the spatial isomorph. Or consider a hypothetical experiment with the monk problem (this problem involves proving that a particular monk, who begins his ascent of a mountain at sunrise on one day and begins his descent at sunrise on the next day, must cross one spot on the path at exactly the same time each day). To investigate the role of imagery, one might simply instruct some subjects to try to solve the problem by employing imagery, while not instructing other subjects to employ imagery. If imagery is an effective device for solving this particular problem, then we would expect the imagery group to outperform the nonimagery group (in fact, imagery does seem to be useful in solving this problem; cf. Howard, 1983; Mayer, 1983). One might even take stronger measures in implementing the nonimaginal group and instruct that group to verbalize aloud during problem solving, a procedure that Kaufmann assumes invokes a linguistic strategy (Kaufmann, 1980, p. 161).

In terms of investigating the role of imagery in motor skill acquisition, subjects instructed to imagine the actions can be contrasted with subjects given no such instructions. Several different types of questions might be addressed with this approach. Paralleling the verbal learning paradigms, one could ask whether instructions to use an imagery strategy to encode lists of arbitrary movement patterns increases memory for those movement patterns relative to a control given no imagery instructions (it appears that imagery instructions do facilitate recall of the movement lists, Chevalier-Girard & Wilberg, 1980). Or one could examine the differential influence of instructions to engage in imaginary practice versus instructions to engage in physical practice on the proficiency of performing a particular motor task (Savoyant, this volume). Another comparison of interest in terms of motor skill acquisition is that between subjects instructed to use imagery in mental rehearsal and subjects instructed not to use imagery in their mental practice (cf. Goss et al., 1986).

There are several important considerations, however, when using instruction to study the role of imagery in cognition. One is that the particular wording of the instructions may produce demand characteristics for subjects to simulate imagery use instead of actually using imagery to perform a cognitive process. That is, according to Pylyshyn (1984), in some problem solving tasks, for instance those based on "imagining" a map to make a judgement about locations on the map, care must be taken that the instructions do not imply to subjects that the subjects should try to simulate the actual situation depicted in the problem. The idea is that in the map judgment task, subjects instructed to image may try to respond as if they were using an actual map in producing their responses; a response based on this strategy may or may not involve imagery (e.g., it could involve knowledge that is represented amodally, Pylyshyn, 1984).

The wording of the instructions may be even more critical when trying to investigate the role of imagery in motor skills learning. This is due to the possibility that imagery relating to motor movements may involve at least two different nonverbal subsystems, a visual imagery system and a motor program system (Engelkamp, this volume; Engelkamp & Zimmer, 1985; Engelkamp & Perrig, 1986). Or put another away, there may be two distinguishable types of imagery, motor and visual imagery (cf. Kosslyn, Holtzman, Farah, & Gazzaniga, 1985; Goss et al., 1986). Ideally, then, studies in motor skills learning using instructions to image would distinguish between instructions to invoke motor imagery versus those that invoke visual imagery. That is, subjects might be instructed on any of the following: image somebody else performing the task, image yourself doing the task, or image the kinesthetic sensations involved performing the task (see Savoyant, this volume). Further, Savoyant's (this volume) identification of two distinct "cognitive intervention modes" (planning and organizing versus motor programming and control) for enhancing the cognitive component of motor skills, raises the possibility that imagery rehearsal and type of imagery rehearsal (visualizing one's self, visualizing a model, kinesthetic imagery) could have differential effects depending on the mode targeted. Savoyant hints that this could be the case. If possible, then, it would be informative to vary instructions such that they target particular modes of intervention.

For problem solving, the particular function of the image might also need to be specified in the instructions. This is clearly the case for tasks for which one strategy (but not the only strategy) is to scan an image, such as tasks requiring judgments about the presence or absence of a key location on a previously presented map. In these experiments, one issue is whether or not time to scan between two imaged locations is a function of conveyed distance. However, unless subjects are given precise instructions designed to induce scanning of an image that traverses only the shortest distance between a starting location and the target location, subjects will use imagery but not necessarily in connection with a scanning strategy (Kosslyn, 1980, Chapter 3).

More generally, information processing theories of problem solving (e.g., Newell & Simon, 1972) distinguish between representational stages of problem solving and search stages. Perhaps either or both stages may be influenced by imagery. For example, expert physicists appear to first represent a problem in a visual, physical format (by sketching the problem elements) before applying the appropriate computational formulae to arrive at the solution (Larkin, 1979). In this instance, we might characterize the process thusly: solvers represent the problem in a global, visual fashion and then proceed to compute (construct) the solution nonimaginally with mathematical expressions. But it also might be the case that in other instances like the monk problem described above, imagery extends beyond a representational function and is also intimately involved in generating or searching for a solution. Indeed, on Kaufmann's (1980; see also his paper in this volume) perspective, imagery is useful for novel or difficult problems because it facilitates construction of (or search for) solution alternatives, often in the form of visual analogies. An example given by Gorden (cited in Kaufmann, 1980) is that of the problem of inventing a jacking mechanism, not bigger than four-by-four inches, yet able to extend out and support four tons. The problem was solved by elaborating on the pictorial analogies of an Indian rope trick wherein an initially soft rope is stiffened until it can be climbed. This prompted the analogy of a penis erection that suggested a hydraulic principle and so on. Thus, the use of visual analogy for productive thinking or creation of a novel solution appears to be different from the use of imagery to sketch a picture of the problem description before applying known computational procedures or principles to arrive at a solution. Consequently, investigations of the role of imagery in problem solving that vary instructions might profit from tailoring the instructions such that more precise functions of imagery can be examined (e.g., one might instruct the subject to proceed by using visual analogy if this were of interest or one could instruct the subject to proceed by sketching the problem elements before searching for a solution, e.g., Paige & Simon, 1966).

Given that the particular problem information to be represented visually is specified, an additional concern is that the quality or nature of the visual material generated may significantly impact the degree of facilitation evidenced (e.g., Beveridge & Parkins, 1987). This occurred in Paige and Simon's (1966) study, in which subjects were asked to sketch diagrams representing the information in algebra story problems. Integrated diagrams were associated with successful performance, whereas a series of diagrams in which each represented a sentence in the story problem was not associated with successful generation of the solution. Clearly, inattention to differences in performance as a function of the type of visual information produced could lead to spurious conclusions concerning the efficacy of imagery in problem solving. Thus, if the instructions stimulating visual representation specify covert (i.e., mental images) rather than overt (i.e., sketches) use of visual information, then some sort of experimental debriefing to assess the nature of the visual information used might be warranted.

Even when the particular instructions have been carefully developed, interpretational issues can still emerge. Of primary concern is that instructions may not exclusively control subjects' cognitive processes. Processing not mentioned in the instructions may be spontaneously employed by the subject so that subjects given imagery instructions may also employ other nonimaginal strategies, and subjects given nonimaginal or control instructions may use imagery. This type of "leakage" has been found in memory studies (e.g., McDaniel & Kearney, 1984), and it seems reasonable to assume that the same could occur in studies focusing on imagery strategies in other cognitive tasks. Preventing or mitigating spontaneous use of imagery may be especially difficult in studies of motor learning because simply performing the task may invoke mental imagery (Engelkamp & Zimmer, 1985). In general, using post-experimental probes (e.g., McDaniel & Kearney, 1984) to assess the degree to which subjects complied with the instructions seems to be an indispensible adjunct to varying instructions. It provides some convergence for the assumption that subjects used the assigned strategy (for those tasks in which subjects actually can or do effectively control their processing), and in the event that subjects' strategies do not conform to instructions, subjects can either be replaced or the results can be interpreted in light of the subject feedback. Of course, in situations where the majority of the subjects have not limited their strategies to those instructed, the role of imagery may still be uncertain. Moreover, the accuracy or validity of subjects' feedback might be questioned. If so, a more sophisticated methodology will need to be considered. One such methodology is described next.

4. INTERFERING TASKS

The interfering task paradigm involves having the subject concurrently perform some secondary task along with the task of primary interest. Sometimes for learning studies, the secondary task is presented immediately upon completion of the primary encoding task (Engelkamp & Zimmer, 1985). The idea is to demonstrate that imaginal processes, and/or some limited capacity mechanism dedicated to processing and maintaining visuo-spatial information, are necessary for the primary task by selectively disrupting performance on the primary task with a visual but not a verbal secondary task. For instance, Logie (1986) has demonstrated that when subjects are instructed to use a mnemonic presumed to involve imagery (e.g., the peg-word mnemonic), recall performance is disrupted by a visual but not a verbal interference task. Also, recall is affected little, if at all, by the visual interference task if the material is learned by rote (verbal rehearsal). The papers in this volume by Baddeley and his associates describe particulars of this methodology and illustrate its effectiveness in studying the characteristics of the visuo-cognitive characteristics of working memory (see also Logie, 1986).

The interference methodology appears to be tractable for studying the use of imagery (and the use of visuo-spatial working memory) in more complex cognitive and perceptuo-motor tasks. For instance, the use of visuo-spatial memory in acquiring proficiency at a complex computer game has been implicated by applying this methodology (Logie, Baddeley, Mane, Donchin, and Sheptak, this volume). Logie et al. extended the typical methodology by analyzing the disruption in performance on the secondary task due to the concurrent computer game activity, as well as vice versa, and by showing that mutual interference was greater in general for the visual than for the verbal secondary tasks. Importantly, however, the patterns of disruption changed as subjects gained greater experience with the computer game. Thus, this methodology appears to be sensitive to a changing role played by visuo-spatial processing in the course of skill attainment.

The selective interference methodology can also be successfully used to implicate activation of visual imagery in performance of motor tasks (see Engelkamp, this volume). Further, Engelkamp's paper suggests that by selecting appropriate interference tasks, separate nonverbal subsystems can be identified (in this case separate motor and visual imagery systems). Such successes with the methodology offer the possibility of providing experimental tests regarding speculations presented at the workshop concerning the existence or nonexistence of other imagery systems, e.g., haptic (Baddeley), olfactory (Andreani; see also Lyman & McDaniel, 1986).

The tractability of the concurrent task methodology for studying the use of imagery in more complex cognitive and perceptuo-motor tasks gives it an advantage over material or instructional manipulations. Consider the computer game studied by Logie et al. It would seem very difficult to manipulate the game, i.e., the materials (so as to demonstrate differences in performance due to presumed differences in imagery use), without also fundamentally changing the nature of the task. The same would be true for studying how people learn to classify visual patterns (e.g., Posner & Keele, 1968); changing these materials would fundamentally change the task. Using instructions to vary the use of imagery in the computer game would also appear to be intractible because instructions to not use visual information in memory would presumably be difficult, if not impossible, for subjects to implement. This assumption is based on the finding that storage of visual information in the visuo-spatial sketchpad can be obligatory, occurring even with unattended visual material (Logie, 1986), and once information is stored in working memory, it is difficult not to use that information for the criterial task (Reitman, 1974). In these cases, then, the interference paradigm would seem to be most useful.

There are potential pitfalls with the selective interference paradigm. One problem is that the cognitive load of the interfering tasks may be so high that general interference occurs, interference that is in addition to the specific verbal, visual or motor component of the interfering task (see Logie et al., this volume). Such general interference may override or mask any selective disruption effects. The problem extends beyond that of adequately piloting the interfering tasks. If a selective interference effect is not found or is not as robust as it might be, does one conclude that the interfering tasks are not entirely appropriate or does one conclude that the different primary task conditions do not differentially activate imagery? Both kinds of conclusions can be found (e.g., Engelkamp & Zimmer, 1985; Logie, 1986). Perhaps one way of avoiding, or at least mitigating, the potential circularity is to use a number of secondary tasks to provide convergence (as Engelkamp and Logie et al. reported at the workshop). Also, a priori theoretical analysis of the processing requirements of the secondary task can strengthen the case. For instance, Logie (1986) assumed that a secondary task that requires a comparison of similar visual patterns will require a decision component that is amodal, thus leaving open the possibility that this kind of visual secondary task could interfere somewhat with a verbal primary task. On the other hand, a visual secondary task involving material similar to that above but not requiring any judgements or decisions would be expected to interfere only with the visual primary task. This pattern obtained as predicted.

5. INDIVIDUAL DIFFERENCES

A fourth useful experimental technique is one employing individual differences. The idea underlying this technique is that if imagery is involved in the performance of a particular task, then the performance of individuals who are proficient at generating mental images should be better than, or at least different from, that of individuals who are not as proficient with visual imagery. Individual differences can be "manipulated" either by classifying subjects as "high imagers" or "low imagers" using appropriate psychometric instruments (e.g., Denis, 1987; although see Katz, 1983, for a cautionary note) or by selecting subjects based on differential experience (e.g., Cocude; Cornoldi & de Beni, both in this volume). The advantages of an individual differences approach are similar to those of the selective interference paradigm; in particular, instructions and materials can be held constant, thereby eliminating problems that arise (see above sections) when attempting to vary some aspects of the instructions and materials while holding other aspects constant. The individual differences approach has the additional advantage over the selective interference paradigm of being usable with any task, whereas selective interference may be difficult to orchestrate with some tasks.

The individual differences approach has been used successfully to demonstrate the role of imagery in learning and memory (e.g., Cornoldi & de Beni, this volume; Denis, 1987; Ernest, 1987) and in the acquisition of movement patterns (Goss et al., 1986). Several papers in this volume illustrate the use of this technique in other contexts. Denis supports his notions regarding the role of imagery in text processing by demonstrating that high imagers display different reading time patterns than low imagers (see also Denis, 1987). Cocude demonstrates that individual differences in experience with mental control and concentration techniques produce differences in image maintenance times but not image generation times. This work has important theoretical significance, supporting modular approaches to mental imagery in general, and Kosslyn's (1980) notions regarding the existence of separate subroutines for image generation and image maintenance in particular. It offers a complementary approach to recent work that has examined image dysfunction due to physiological impairment (Kosslyn et al., 1985). Cocude's work, by demonstrating dissociative facilitation of imagery processes as a function of individual differences, suggests that performance of image processing subroutines can be improved, and raises the challenge of identifying the mechanisms by which such improvement might occur.

An individual differences approach offers great promise for application to other issues in imagery and cognition. One such issue concerns the existence of nonvisual imagery processing. By demonstrating that low-imagery subjects, subjects with no visual experience (individuals congenitally blind from birth), or subjects with visual imagery dysfunction due to neurological deficits can perform well on tasks that appear to require or afford some sort of nonverbal processing, one can begin to implicate imaginal processing that is at least partially different from visual imagery (Ernest, 1987; Kosslyn et al., 1985). Similarly, differential performance for groups of subjects that are equated on a visual imagery individual difference measure but differ on a nonvisual imagery measure (e.g., kinesthetic), implicates the influence of a nonvisual imagery component in cognition (e.g., Goss et al., 1986). Another issue has to do with the functional equivalence of visual imagery and perception. Finke and his colleagues (see Finke, 1980) have shown that individual differences in reported vividness of imagery influence the degree to which results in imagery conditions mimic results in perception conditions. Based on these types of data, Finke (1980) has argued that imagery and perception share at least some information-processing mechanisms.

An individual differences approach to studying the role of imagery in cognition could also help provide converging evidence for extant notions regarding the role of imagery in concept formation and in problem solving. For instance, regarding classification of visual patterns, one view is that some subjects may employ an imagery strategy to form a representation of a visual category and to make subsequent classification decisions, while others may employ a more verbal or rule-based strategy (cf. Mayer, 1983). If it were the case that high and low imagers differed in their concept formation patterns and strategies, then this would provide additional suppport for the idea that at least some concept formation strategies are imaginal in nature. Further, if the imagery strategy were predominantly used by high imagers and the rule-based strategy were used by low imagers, then a better understanding of who uses each kind of strategy and why would be at hand.

Straightforward distinctions in performance between high and low imagery individuals like that sketched above may be too much to expect, however. Remarking on another type of task in which both imagery and nonimaginal strategies were possible, Katz (1983) hypothesized, "it is doubtless the case that even those who employed the nonimaginal strategy would have been shown to possess imaginal abilities on standard tests" (p. 47). Katz (1983) suggests that "high" versus "low" imagery is too simplistic a conceptualization for predicting who will use imagery and when, and he advocates development of a more complex individual difference composite based on the complete personality. The point he emphasizes is that an individual's choice to use imagery may depend on a host of factors that are in addition to, or perhaps independent of, whether the individual is classified as having high or low imagery ability.

There are several other considerations and/or drawbacks to an individual differences approach. One is that it can be expensive in terms of the number of subjects that need to be tested or at least screened. As with any individual differences work, including subjects that score near the median on the individual difference measure may mask or obscure individual difference effects (e.g., Denis, 1987); therefore, the experimental groups submitted for analysis may often only include subjects that score at the extremes (e.g., in Goss et al., 1986, only 24% of the subjects completing the imagery questionnaire were acceptable candidates for the study). Another, perhaps more important, consideration involves selecting an appropriate individual difference measure. One might use vividness of generated images, one might use the tendency to habitually generate images, one might use the ease with which images are formed and manipulated, one could measure the degree of kinesthetic imagery (cf. Savoyant, this volume), and so on. This workshop has identified yet another potentially important individual difference measure relating to imagery, that of the span of the visuo-spatial sketchpad (Wilson, Scott, & Power, in press). The problem is that ambiguous results can occur because of failure to identify the best measure (cf. Goss et al., 1986). Clearly, in some cases, selection of a particular measure will be guided by the research question being addressed. For example, recent work has suggested that the functional capacity of working memory may be intimately related to the efficacious use of mnemonic imagery strategies in children (Pressley, Cariglia-Bull, Deane, & Schneider, 1987). Confirmation and refinement of this view in terms of involvement of the visuo-spatial sketchpad would obviously involve using an individual difference measure directed at visuo-spatial sketchpad span. Alternatively, in investigating the relation between imagery ability and the acquisition of movements, it appears that the ease of forming both visual and kinesthetic images is a better measure than a measure focusing on visual imagery alone (Goss et al., 1986).

Even if the choice of a particular measure is clear cut, there can still be uncertainty regarding what that measure is tapping. For instance, differences in rated vividness of imagery could be due to differences in using the rating scale, to differences in the degree to which similar imagery processing mechanisms are activated, or to differences in the particular mechanisms in the system that are activated (Finke, 1980). The general assessment has been that imagery ability tests are psychometrically primitive (Katz, 1983), and consequently issues of validity and the processes underlying the presumed skill being measured need continued attention to enhance an individual differences approach to studying imagery and cognition.

6. CONCLUSIONS

This chapter has suggested several empirical approaches for investigating imagery and cognition. Each particular approach was found wanting in one respect or another, however, with each having its own particular hurdles to surmount. Consequently, compelling evidence for the role of imagery in processes like problem solving or perceptuo-motor skill acquistion will likely necessitate the programmatic use of all the techniques discussed. Sets of studies are needed in which the techniques are varied across studies, and the different techniques also need to be used in concert within one study. For example, one can vary the materials and the instructions so that imagery effects would be expected to obtain only under particular instructional--material combinations (e.g., Engelkamp & Perrig, 1986), or one can factorially vary instructions, materials, and individual differences (Denis, 1987). This kind of factorial approach mitigates the plausibility of interpretations based on demand characteristics, spontaneous use of strategies, or other alternatives. While one might be able to argue with the results based on one technique on some grounds and argue with the results based on another technique on other grounds, it would be difficult to derive an integrated alternative account (to imagery processes) for a set of results derived from two or more converging techniques. The promise of this kind of multi-pronged attack has been convincingly demonstrated in the arena of imagery and learning of verbal materials (e.g., Engelkamp & Zimmer, 1985; Paivio, 1986). Hopefully, the next decade will see a similar multi-pronged approach systematically applied to the study of imagery in other cognitively-based processes like problem solving, motor learning, and skills acquisition.

ACKNOWLEDGMENTS

I am grateful to Brian Lyman for his comments on an earlier version of this chapter. Participation at this conference was made possible in part by a grant for partial travel expenses from the Institute for Scholarship in the Liberal Arts, University of Notre Dame. The author is now at Department of Psychological Sciences, Purdue University, West Lafayette, IN, U.S.A.

REFERENCES

1. Beveridge, M., & Parkins, E. (1987). Visual representation in analogical problem solving. Memory & Cognition, 15, 230-237.
2. Bower, G. H. (1972). Mental imagery and associative learning. In L. W. Gregg (Ed.), Cognition in learning and memory. New York: Wiley.
3. Carroll, J. M., Thomas, J. C., & Malhotra, A. (1980). Presentation and representation in design problem solving. British Journal of Psychology, 71, 143-153.
4. Chevalier-Girard, N., & Wilberg, R. B. (1980). The effects of image and label on the free recall of organized movement lists. In P. Klavora and J. Flowers (Eds.), Motor learning and biomechanical factors in sport. Toronto: Publications Division, School of Physical and Health Education, Unversity of Toronto.
5. Denis, M. (1987). Individual imagery differences and prose processing. In M. A. McDaniel and M. Pressley (Eds.), Imagery and related mnemonic processes: Theories, individual differences, and applications. New York: Springer/Verlag.
6. Engelkamp, J., & Perrig, W. (1986). Differential effects of imaginal and motor

encoding on the recall of action phrases. Archiv für Psychologie, 138, 261-272.

7. Engelkamp, J., & Zimmer, H. D. (1985). Motor programs and their relation to semantic memory. The German Journal of Psychology, 9, 239-254.

8. Ernest, C. (1987). Imagery and memory in the blind: A review. In M. A. McDaniel and M. Pressley (Eds.), Imagery and related mnemonic processes: Theories, individual differences, and applications. New York: Springer/Verlag.

9. Finke, R. A. (1980). Levels of equivalence in imagery and perception. Psychological Review, 87, 113-132.

10. Goss, S., Hall, C., Buckolz, E., & Fishburne, G. (1986). Imagery ability and the acquisition and retention of movements. Memory & Cognition, 14, 469-477.

11. Hayes, J. R., & Simon, H. A. (1974). Understanding written problem instructions. In L. W. Gregg (ed.), Knowledge and cognition. Potomac, MD: Erlbaum.

12. Howard, D. V. (1983). Cognitive psychology: Memory, language, and thought. New York: Macmillan.

13. Katona, G. (1940). Organizing and memorizing. New York: Columbia University Press.

14. Katz, A. N. (1983). What does it mean to be a high imager? In J. C. Yuille (Ed.), Imagery, memory, and cognition: Essays in honor of Allan Paivio. Hillsdale, N.J.: Erlbaum.

15. Kaufmann, G. (1980). Imagery, language, and cognition. Bergen, Norway: Universitetsforlaget.

16. Kosslyn, S. M. (1980). Image and mind. Cambridge, MA: Harvard University Press.

17. Kosslyn, S. M., Holtzman, J. D., Farah, M. J., & Gazzaniga, M. S. (1985). A computational analysis of mental image generation: Evidence from functional dissociations in split-brain patients. Journal of Experimental Psychology: General, 114, 311-341.

18. Larkin, J. H. (1979, April). Models of strategy use for solving physics problems. Paper presented at the American Educational Research Association Meeting, San Francisco.

19. Logie, R. H. (1986). Visuo-spatial processing in working memory. The Quarterly Journal of Experimental Psychology, 38A, 229-247.

20. Lyman, B. J., & McDaniel, M. A. (1986). Effects of encoding strategy on long-term memory for odours. The Quarterly Journal of Experimental Psychology, 38A, 753-765.

21. Mayer, R. E. (1983). Thinking, problem solving, and cognition. New York: Freeman.

22. McDaniel, M. A., & Einstein, G. O. (1986). Bizarre imagery as an effective memory aid: The importance of distinctiveness. Journal of Experimental Psychology: Learning, Memory, and Cognition, 12, 54-65.

23. McDaniel, M. A., & Kearney, E. M. (1984). Optimal learning strategies and their spontaneous use: The importance of task-appropriate processing. Memory & Cognition, 12, 361-373.

24. McDaniel, M. A., & Schlager, M. (1986). Discovery learning and transfer of problem solving skills: A cognitive approach. Unpublished manuscript, University of Notre Dame, Notre Dame, IN.

25. Newell, A. & Simon, H. A. (1972). Human problem solving. Englewood Cliffs, N.J.: Prentice-Hall.

26. Newell, K. M., Quinn, J. T., Jr., Sparrow, W. A., & Walter, C. B. (1983). Kinematic information feedback for learning a rapid arm movement. Human Movement Science, 2, 255-269.

27. Paige, J. M., & Simon, H. A. (1966). Cognitive processes in solving algebra work problems. In B. Kleinmutz (Ed.), Problem solving: Research, method and theory. New York: Wiley.

28. Paivio, A. (1986). Mental representations: A dual coding approach. New York: Oxford University Press.

29. Posner, M. I., & Keele, S. W. (1968). On the genesis of abstract ideas. Journal of Experimental Psychology, 77, 353-363.
30. Pressley, M., Cariglia-Bull, T., Deane, S., & Schneider, W. (1987). Short-term memory, verbal competence, and age as predictors of imagery instructional effectiveness. Journal of Experimental Child Psychology, 43, 194-211.
31. Pylyshyn, Z. W. (1984). Computation and cognition. Cambridge, MA: MIT Press.
32. Reitman, J. S. (1974). Without surreptitious rehearsal, information in short-term memory decays. Journal of Verbal Learning and Verbal Behavior, 13, 365-377.
33. Whiting, H. T. A., Bijlard, M. J., & den Brinker, B. P. L. M. (1987). The effect of the availability of a dynamic model on the acquisition of a complex cyclical action. The Quarterly Journal of Experimental Psychology, 39A, 43-59.
34. Wilson, J. T. L., Scott, J. H., & Power, K. G. (in press). Developmental differences in the span of visual memory for pattern. British Journal of Developmental Psychology.

PART 4

IMAGERY, ACTION, AND EMOTION IMAGERY AND THE BRAIN

4.1. IMAGERY, ACTION, AND EMOTION

IMAGES AND ACTIONS IN VERBAL LEARNING

JOHANNES ENGELKAMP

DEPARTMENT OF PSYCHOLOGY, UNIVERSITY OF SAARBRUECKEN,
D-6600 SAARBRUECKEN, F.R.G.

ABSTRACT

This paper presents a selective survey of our investigations concerning sensory and motor memory systems. It is shown that motor programs are part of the memory representation of action phrases such as "to comb one´s hair", that motor programs are not normally activated during the verbal processing of action phrases but only after enacting the action and that this activation has specific effects on memory performance when action phrases are learned. It is furthermore shown that motor programs form a partially independent subsystem of memory, distinguishable from a verbal as well as from a visual-sensory memory storage.

1. INTRODUCTION

The influence of images on verbal learning and on other types of tasks has been studied for a considerable time. Images of concrete nouns have thereby been in the centre of interest (e.g. Paivio & Begg, 1981; Kosslyn, 1980; Wippich, 1980). This holds true even for interactive imagery where the interaction of persons and objects has been studied (Bower, 1972; Begg, 1978). Images of verbs, particularly images of action verbs, have been far less intensively investigated. The study of actions has been almost totally neglected until recently (e.g. Cohen 1981, 1983). The influence of both - of actions and of images of actions - has been the topic of our research in Saarbruecken for the last couple of years (for reviews see e.g. Engelkamp 1986a, 1987; Engelkamp & Zimmer, 1985). What I want to do here, is to give a selective review of this work. The most important and global result of our studies can be stated in this way: Information processing of identical verbal action phrases is different in the case of standard verbal learning, forming images, and performing actions symbolically. The verbal phrases in our experiments have always been action phrases such as "smoke a cigarette" or "clench a fist". Put in a more speculative way the main result could be summarized in this way: A motor memory system has to be distinguished from a verbal and a visual-imaginal system, henceforth referred to as imaginal system.

I will now give you some brief information about four groups of data which support this conclusion: data on differential quantitative recall, data on selective interference, data on recognition and data on differential qualitative recall.

2. DIFFERENTIAL QUANTITATIVE RECALL

In our first experiments subjects had to learn identical lists of about 50 acoustically presented action phrases under different encoding conditions. One group received a standard learning instruction (= listening only). A second group learned the same list by forming images of the actions. A third

M. Denis et al. (eds.), Cognitive and Neuropsychological Approaches to Mental Imagery, 297–306.

group saw, while listening, a model performing the actions symbolically on a TV screen. A fourth group finally enacted the actions symbolically. After the presentation of all items a free recall test was given. Figure 1 shows the results of several experiments of this type.

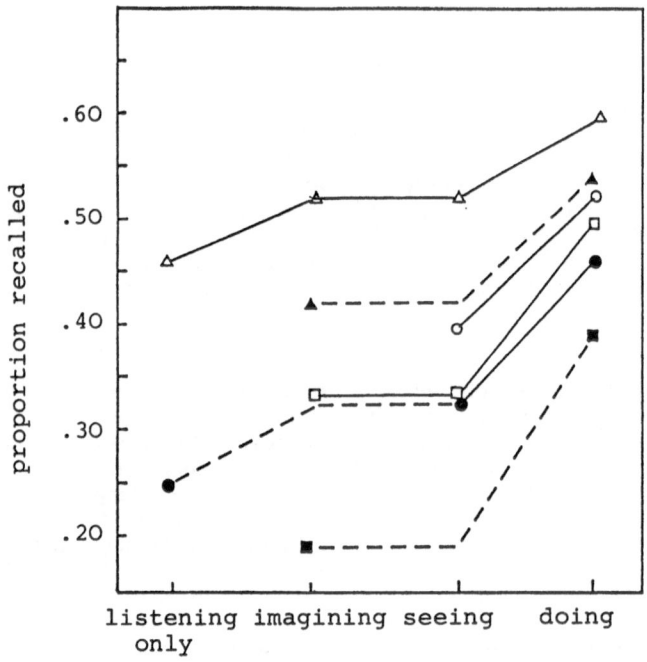

FIGURE 1. Synopsis of mean recall scores of action phrases under different encoding conditions. Data from the following experiments are included: △ Engelkamp & Krumnacker 1980, Exp. 1; ▲ Zimmer 1984, Exp. 2; ○ Engelkamp & Zimmer 1983, real object; □ Zimmer & Engelkamp 1984, Exp. 1; ● Engelkamp & Zimmer 1983, imaginal object; ■ Engelkamp & Krumnacker 1980, Exp. 2. Broken lines are intrapolations.

The results are clear-cut. Listening only leads to the worst memory performance, doing to the best. Performance with imagining and seeing lies between the above.

The different encoding conditions result in different information processing. One specific aspect which we were interested in, was whether we could locate the memory effect of motor encoding more specifically. We therefore tried to find out whether planning to perform the action alone is sufficient to produce the same memory performance as planning and executing the action. To achieve this goal we invented a situation in which all subjects participated in the following three experimental conditions: to plan, to plan and execute the action, and to watch how another person performs the action. For this purpose subjects were tested together in groups of three. They were told that we had carried out several experiments with actions and that we had noticed that it was not equally easy to perform them. Therefore we were interested in collecting ratings on how easily the different actions could be performed. The task was to rate how easily the actions could be performed. To get ratings and performances from as many subjects as possible - both aspects would be important to generalize the results - we always invited groups of three subjects. Two of them alternately had to perform the actions and the third assessed the actions. Which one of the two actually had to perform the action was indicated by the experimenter immediately after presentation of the action phrase. Further, the roles were changed in the course of the experiment so that each of them would function in each role equally often.

After the presentation of all 48 items there was an unexpected free recall. The result was clear-cut again. Planning and executing the action led to better recall performance than planning only or watching, both of which led to almost identical performances (Zimmer & Engelkamp, 1984).

What can we conclude from this result? Firstly, to plan an action does not result in the same information processing as planning and executing it does. Secondly, to plan has as good an effect on recall as watching someone else performing the act. Therefore, there is some effect of planning on memory. And finally the effect of doing can probably not be explained by motivational factors which were comparable under the three conditions of this experiment.

We assume that information processing with doing is different from information processing with verbal or imaginal encoding because of the activation of motor programs. According to Summers (1981) a motor program presents a set of muscle commands that enables the execution of an action. Thus a motor program is not only a description of a movement but the information that allows the movement to be made. This information is activated to its full extent in the context of doing and to a minor extent in the context of planning an action. It is normally not activated when listening to an action phrase and trying to understand its meaning or to form an image of its action.

We further assume that these motor programs form a partially-independent information-processing system analogous to the system formed by images. Are there arguments to support this latter assumption?

3. SELECTIVE INTERFERENCE

It is widely accepted that processing a list of items within one system leads to a decline of memory performance compared with processing the same items via two systems (e.g. Bosshardt, 1975; Janssen, 1981). The reason for this can be seen in the reduced distinctiveness of the memorial representation of each item if only one system is involved.

Following this logic we provided our subjects with 48 action phrases. Half of them had to learn the items by alternately forming an image or an action. These subjects started either with forming an image or with enacting an action. The other half of the subjects had to encode all the items in one manner. A quarter encoded all items imaginally and a quarter in a motor way. After one presentation of all items a free recall test was given. Figure 2 shows the result (Zimmer, Engelkamp & Sieloff, 1984).

Relative recall performance is shown on the ordinate. The diagram indicates that imaginal learning is impaired more by imaginal than by motor interference and that motor learning is disturbed more by a motor than by an imaginal distracting task. Similar results have been observed by Zimmer and Engelkamp (1985) and by Hulme (1978) and Saltz and Donnenwerth-Nolan (1981).

From these findings it can be concluded that processing a list of items by imagining or enacting them makes them more similar to each other than processing them by partly imagining and by partly enacting them. We think what makes the items more similar is the activation of images in one case and the activation of motor programs in the other. Thus there seems to be good reason to claim different memory sub-systems, one for imaginal and one for motor processing.

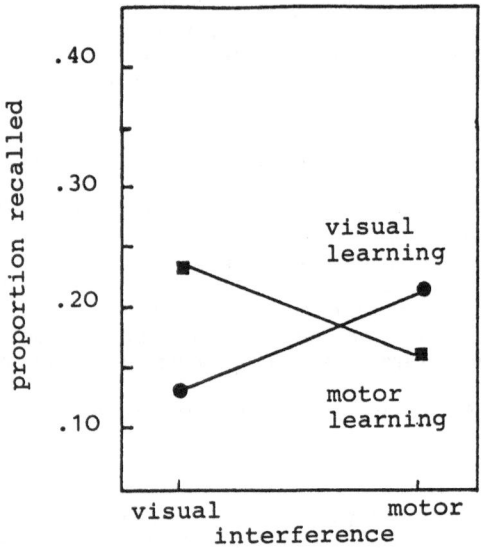

FIGURE 2. Selective modality-specific interference effects between a visual or a motor learning and interference task.

4. RECOGNITION

It is of course not enough to state that performing an action activates motor programs and that activating motor programs has a better effect on memory than activating an image or conceptual information. We have to think of what makes activation of motor programs as efficient for a memory task as free recall.

One widely accepted assumption is that recall performance is based on retrieval processes on the one hand and recognition processes on the other (e.g. Brown, 1976; Wessels, 1984, pp.194-197). While a good retrieval schema has a positive effect on item generation, good distinctiveness of a memory unit improves recognition, that is, it allows the identification of the generated items as members of a to-be-learned list. It is our assumption that activation of the motor program makes an item more distinct as compared with activating its image or only the conceptual information. According to this assumption the good performance in free recall under the experimental condition of doing is at least in part the result of the good distinctiveness of the memory traces under this encoding condition.

Can we prove this? One way is to study recognition because it is supposed to be based mainly on the distinctiveness of items. Engelkamp and Krumnacker (1980) have reported better recognition performances for identical action phrases if they were motor encoded than if they were learned under a standard verbal learning instruction or encoded imaginally (cf. also Zimmer, 1984). Although this result is compatible with the distinctiveness hypothesis, it is not very convincing because items which are better freely recalled are usually also better recognized.

To make a better argument for this hypothesis we have used a more complex design. Before I comment on the logic of the experiment, I will briefly describe it. Subjects learned three lists of action phrases in a two-trial learning task. The first list, the i(dentical) list, was composed of common action phrases such as "das Papier schneiden" (to cut the paper), which were presented in the first and again in the second trial. In the second list the action phrases in the second trial were not identically repeated but with a similar surface structure. The verb was identical but the object was changed, so that the motor programs of the two phrases were different. "Den Apfel pflücken" (to pick an apple) was for example changed to "die Blume pflücken" (to pick the flower). This was the d(ifferent) list. The third list, the s(imilar) list, contained action phrases which were changed in the second trial too, but in this case the motor programs of the two phrases were similar. An example is "das Brett annageln" (to nail down the board) and "die Leiste annageln" (to nail down the skirting board). With respect to the surface structure, the second and the third groups of items were similarly constructed: the verbs were identical and the nouns differed. They differed with respect to their motor components. The two paired items of the d-group had different motor programs, while the items of the s-group had similar motor programs. Table 1 illustrates the three types of learning material.

TABLE 1. Examples of the learning material used

item group	examples of items in the first trial	second trial	item relation with respect to surface structure	motor program
i-items	to cut the paper	to cut the paper	identical	identical
d-items	to pick the flower	to pick the apple	similar	different
s-items	to nail down the board	to nail down the skirting board	similar	similar

At the end of the second trial a common recognition test was given for the items of both trials. Old items were mixed with new ones. Recognition times were measured.

What is the logic behind the experiment? We assume that motor encoding makes items more distinctive and therefore, identical items should of course be recognized faster under motor than under verbal encoding. If this effect is due to the activation of motor programs it should be even more pronounced with d-items, because here motor program information is different whereas verbal information is similar. S-items however should be equally difficult to recognize under motor and under verbal encoding because their verbal information as well as their motor program information is similar. We therefore expect comparable recognition time with s-items. Figure 3 shows the results.

Identical and different items are recognized faster after motor than after verbal encoding and this difference is larger for d-items than for i-items. S-items, however, are recognized equally fast after verbal and motor encoding (Zimmer, 1984, Exp. 6, and 1986).

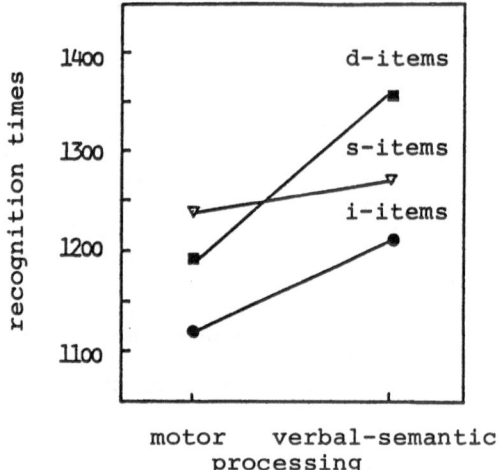

FIGURE 3. An illustration of the mean recognition times for the item groups with d(ifferent), s(imilar) or i(dentical) movement, dependent on the encoding condition.

This experiment provides further support for the idea that specific motor information is activated in the context of doing and not under a standard verbal learning instruction and that it is the motor information that makes memory traces particularly distinctive.

5. DIFFERENTIAL QUALITATIVE RECALL

In my opinion the most convincing arguments for the claim of different modality-specific memory systems in the context of verbal learning are those based on qualitatively different memory effects. With qualitatively different effects I mean effects that are observed depending on which memory sub-systems are involved. It is not sufficient to show that performance is better if one system is involved than it is if the other is involved. It has to be demonstrated that the same variable brings about an effect in one system and none in the other or, even better, that it produces opposite effects in both systems.

To demonstrate such qualitative effects one has to reflect upon the functional characteristics of the systems that one wants to distinguish. To do so, the functional properties of the contrasted systems have to be characterized in more detail. That is, one has to specify the organizational structure of each system and to elaborate on differences of the processes that work on these structures. What follows is a report on one such effort.

As to the imaginal system it is generally assumed that several pieces of information can be processed in it simultaneously, at least in the sense that the result of the process is available for a couple of seconds as a whole. The system may be considered to consist of a buffer into which a certain amount of visual information can be placed to form a visual unit. In the case of verbal information this means that several pieces of verbal information can be made to form larger units by transforming them into the imaginal system.

One way to show this is to use interactive imagery in paired associate learning (PAL). In interactive imagery subjects are asked to form a single image out of a pair of verbal items. If one does so, this is the recall pattern that one can observe: Cued recall (CR) is better than free recall (FR). In brief, this is the explanation for this pattern. Interactive imagery forms an integrated unit of each word-pair that can easily and with great probability be retrieved if one element of a pair is given as a cue (cf. Begg 1978). With FR each pair has to be retrieved. That means that not all units are found. Therefore CR is better than FR.

Let us now compare what happens if word-pairs are encoded in a motor mode. I assume that the units of the motor system are motor programs (MP). If one performs actions the MPs are activated. Since performing actions relies on motor skills their integration should follow the rules of skill acquisition. This means that in order to put two items that describe verbal actions into one larger MP, more than one presentation and the corresponding motor processing is necessary. To integrate two MPs into one larger one, practice is required. Thus to motor encode two verbal action phrases does not integrate the two items immediately. Therefore there is little use in giving the subjects a CR. On the other hand, as I have shown above, doing the item makes it episodically more distinctive than imagining it does. FR should therefore benefit from this condition. This is one reason why action phrases are freely recalled better if encoded in a motor mode than imaginally as has been demonstrated repeatedly (e.g. Engelkamp & Zimmer, 1983; Zimmer, 1984).

Summing up these considerations lead to the expectation that in a PAL experiment with pairs of action verbs that are encoded in a motor mode, there should be no advantage of CR over FR. On the contrary, CR should be worse than FR. If on the other hand the same verb-pairs have to be learned by forming images, there should be the usual advantage of CR over FR.

To test this hypothesis the same pairs of verbs had to be learned by one group of subjects under an imaginal encoding instruction and by an other group under a motor encoding instruction. Both groups were first given a FR and then a CR. The result is shown in Figure 4.

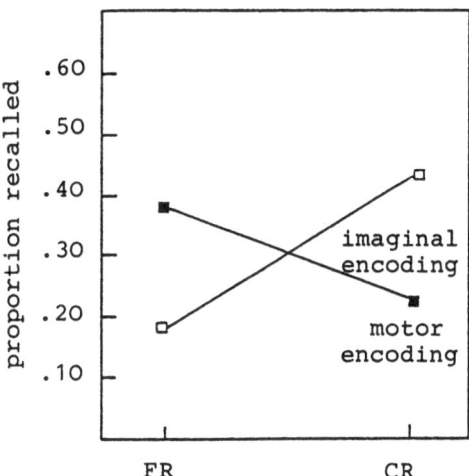

FIGURE 4. Mean proportion of verbs recalled in free recall (FR) and cued recall (CR) under imaginal and motor encoding.

As expected, CR is better than FR under imaginal encoding while under motor encoding the reverse holds true (Engelkamp, 1986b).

The main conclusion from this and similar experiments that I have conducted (Engelkamp, 1986b, c) is as follows: The imaginal and the motor system obey different rules. It is obvious that while information can easily be combined into new units in the imaginal system, such an integration needs practice in the motor system. The imaginal and the motor systems should be characterized by different functional properties.

As a whole I consider it heuristically useful to claim a motor memory system besides an imaginal one. The units of the motor memory system are considered to be motor programs whose activation makes the actions which they are part of episodically particularly distinctive but which do not integrate several actions without practice. Thus the activation of images and motor programs influence verbal recall of action phrases in a different way.

6. FUTURE PERSPECTIVES

Having reached this stage, we have begun to work in three fields to make further progress.

a) Since we consider the demonstration of qualitative differences as particularly important for the assumption of different modality-specific subsystems we have looked further for such differences. One important question in this context is, for instance, whether the role of elaboration in encoding is the same within the different sub-systems. Our results indicate that there is no elaboration effect in the motor system (Zimmer, 1984; cf. also Cohen, 1983).

Another question is which kind of information is made available by the motor as compared with other sub-systems. Results of some experiments show that information of movement pattern is made available by activating motor programs, which means that it is accessible faster under motor encoding than under verbal or imaginal encoding (Engelkamp & Zimmer, 1984; Engelkamp, 1985).

b) A second field is the comparison of the subjective lexicon of nouns and verbs. As the motor system is tightly connected with action and these again with the linguistic form of verbs and as the imaginal system is strongly associated with objects and scenes which again are usually represented by nouns, a systematic comparison of the mental representation of concrete nouns and action verbs seems desirable.

Three aspects of this comparison form our main focus of interest:
- the organizational structure of nouns and verbs in memory;
- the modality-specific aspects of the representation of nouns and verbs;
- the activation processes with nouns and verbs.

c) Finally we are working on a multimodal memory model that is based on the assumption that there are partly independent modality-specific sub-systems with their proper functional characteristics. In this context we are studying the literature to find evidence for different effects of these sub-systems on categorizational, predicative and memorial processes.

ACKNOWLEDGEMENTS

This work was supported by grant En 124/7 from the Deutsche Forschungsgemeinschaft.

REFERENCES

1. Begg, I. (1978). Imagery and organization in memory: Instructional effects. Memory & Cognition , 6, 174-183.
2. Bosshard, H.G. (1975). The influence of visual and auditory images on the recall of visual and auditory presentation mode. Psychological Research,

$\underline{37}$, 211-227.

3. Bower, G.H. (1972). Mental imagery and associative learning. In L.W. Gregg (Ed.), Cognition in learning and memory. New York: Wiley.

4. Brown, J. (1981). An analysis of recognition and recall and of problems in their comparison. In J. Brown (Ed.), Recall and recognition. New York: Wiley.

5. Cohen, R.L. (1981). On the generality of some memory laws. Scandinavian Journal of Psychology, $\underline{22}$, 267-281.

6. Cohen, R.L. (1983). The effect of encoding variables on the free recall of words and action events. Memory & Cognition, $\underline{11}$, 575-582.

7. Engelkamp, J. (1985). Aktivationsprozesse im motorischen Gedächtnis. In D. Albert (Ed.), Bericht über den 34. Kongreß der Deutschen Gesellschaft für Psychologie in Wien 1984. Göttingen: Hogrefe.

8. Engelkamp, J. (1986a). Motor programs as part of the meaning of verbal items. In I. Kurcz, E. Shugar & J.H. Danks (Eds.), Knowledge and language. Amsterdam: North-Holland.

9. Engelkamp, J. (1986b). Nouns and verbs in paired associate learning: Instructional effects. Psychological Research, $\underline{48}$, 153-159.

10. Engelkamp, J. (1986c). Differences between imaginal and motor encoding. In F. Klix & H. Hagendorf (Eds.), Human memory and cognitive capabilities. Amsterdam: North-Holland.

11. Engelkamp, J. (1987). Modalitätsspezifische Gedächtnissysteme im Kontext sprachlicher Informationsverarbeitung. Zeitschrift für Psychologie (in press).

12. Engelkamp, J. & Krumnacker, H. (1980). Imaginale und motorische Prozesse beim Behalten verbalen Materials. Zeitschrift für experimentelle und angewandte Psychologie, $\underline{27}$, 511-533.

13. Engelkamp, J. & Zimmer, H.D. (1983). Zum Einfluß von Wahrnehmen und Tun auf das Behalten von Verb-Objekt-Phrasen. Sprache & Kognition, 2, 117-127.

14. Engelkamp, J. & Zimmer, H.D. (1984). Motor program information as a separable memory unit. Psychological Research, $\underline{46}$, 283-299.

15. Engelkamp, J. & Zimmer, H.D. (1985). Motor programs and their relation to semantic memory. German Journal of Psychology, 9, 239-254.

16. Hulme, C. (1979). The interaction of visual and motor memory for graphic forms following tracing. Quarterly Journal of Experimental Psychology, $\underline{31}$, 249-261.

17. Janssen, W.H. (1981). Vorstellung und Wahrnehmung: Eine Prüfung ihrer Beziehungen mit Hilfe des selektiven Interferenzparadigmas. Zeitschrift für Semiotik, 3, 339-352.

18. Kosslyn, S.M. (1981). Image and mind. Cambridge: Harvard University Press.

19. Paivio, A. & Begg, I. (1981). Psychology of language. Englewood Cliffs, N.J.: Prentice Hall.

20. Saltz, E. & Donnenwerth-Nolan, S. (1981). Does motoric imagery facilitate memory for sentences? A selective interference test. Journal of Verbal Learning and Verbal Behavior, $\underline{20}$, 322-332.

21. Summers, J.J. (1981). Motor programs. In D. Holding (Ed.), Human skills. New York: Wiley.

22. Wessells, M.G. (1984). Kognitive Psychologie. New York: Harper & Row.

23. Wippich, W. (1980). Bildhaftigkeit und Organisation. Darmstadt: Steinkopff.

24. Zimmer, H.D. (1984). Enkodierung, Rekodierung, Retrieval und die Aktivation motorischer Programme. Arbeiten der Fachrichtung Psychologie der Universität des Saarlandes Nr.91, Saarbrücken.

25. Zimmer, H.D. (1986). The memory trace of semantic or motor processing. In F. Klix & H. Hagendorf (Eds.), Human memory and cognitive capabilities. Amsterdam: North-Holland.

26. Zimmer, H.D. & Engelkamp, J. (1984). Planungs- und Ausführungsanteile motorischer Gedächtniskomponenten und ihre Wirkung auf das Behalten ihrer verbalen Bezeichnungen. Zeitschrift für Psychologie, 192, 379-402.

27. Zimmer, H.D. & Engelkamp, J. (1985). An attempt to distinguish between kinematic and motor memory components. Acta Psychologica, 58, 81-106.

28. Zimmer, H.D., Engelkamp, J. & Sieloff, U. (1984). Motorische Gedächtnis-Gedächtniskomponenten als partiell unabhängige Komponenten des Engramms verbaler Handlungsbeschreibungen. Sprache & Kognition, 3, 70-85.

ON THE DISTINCTION OF MEMORY CODES: IMAGE VERSUS MOTOR ENCODING

WALTER J. PERRIG

INSTITUT FUER PSYCHOLOGIE, UNIVERSITY OF BASEL, SWITZERLAND

ABSTRACT

Memory literature distinguishes a whole variety of memory codes or systems, even within high level cognition. It can be shown that these distinctions are justified mainly on introspective or operational levels. There is usually only weak empirical support for the theoretical distinction between different memory systems. As a consequence arguments are presented for an unitary conception of mind, and unification in the use of theoretical terms in memory research. In an experimental demonstration it is shown how this conception of memory can be used to interpret behavioral data, which otherwise is explained in terms of verbal, visual and motor systems.

1. INTRODUCTION

In dealing with our environment we receive and process information from different input channels. It seems plausible to assume that when we receive information through different sensory systems or sensory modalities, we also somehow store modality-specific traces of these inputs in some kind of memory. Because of the obvious differences between the sensory systems we are easily ready to assume that in a theory of memory the modality-specific traces have to be represented as different types of memory or memory codes. Theoretical notions like verbal, visual, auditory, motor, semantic, propositional, conceptual and other codes or memories seem to respond to this assumption. In this paper I will focus on the question of what the justifications for these theoretical distinctions in memory are. I will discuss this question on three levels of description: the introspective, the operational and the theoretical level.

On the introspective level we rely on the subjectively experienced phenomena of different sensory inputs as mentioned above. Theoretical classifications of memory types at this level serve heuristic purposes, at best, and there is no way of measuring objectivity, reliability and validity of a memory typology.

On the operational level we define what is meant by a certain type of memory by specifying the performances preceding the measurement of characteristic forms of memory. We can speak of visual, auditory or motor memory and simply mean that the stored information was processed by a specific modality. In the simplest case this means that the information was presented to the visual or auditory system. Similarly, memory types can refer to tasks where the input is not necessarily restricted to a specific channel; rather it is the way an information is processed. In this sense the same verbal information - an auditory or visual input - can be visualized, rehearsed, verbalized or enacted. Sometimes a part of a

M. Denis et al. (eds.), Cognitive and Neuropsychological Approaches to Mental Imagery, 307–316.
© 1988 by Martinus Nijhoff Publishers.

complex information process will be dominated by some modality-specific action and we are ready to label the resulting memory trace accordingly, e.g., as motor code. In all these cases we relate output performances directly to the preceding task. At this operational level - strictly speaking - we simply do a task analysis. We observe by means of behavioral measures characteristics of memory, following well-standardized test situations. Operationally, memory is subject to experimental manipulations, and thus we have a way to establish internally valid reliable facts. But in cognitive psychology we are not satisfied by stating behavioral contiguities. More importantly we want to find out what mediates test performance. The central question focuses on the processes which underly the observed behavior. When we discuss memory from this perspective, we switch to the third, the theoretical level.

On the theoretical level the label "memory" refers to a hypothetical construct. At this level we want to know how the encoding, storage, and retrieval of information works, and here we come to the representational reference of the label memory code.

2. MULTI-SYSTEM VERSUS UNITARY THEORIES OF HIGH-LEVEL COGNITION

We can roughly distinguish two theoretical positions in the conceptualization of high level processes: Multi-system theories versus unitary conceptions of mind. Proponents of multi-system theories postulate the existence of different representational formats (codes), based on different principles, which can account for the experimentally produced differences in memory performances. So we are taught to distinguish between a verbal system and several nonverbal processing systems. Focusing on a verbal and a visual system, we consequently have to separate these two systems, starting from peripheral sensoric stimulation to high level cognition. Here, different codes mean different cognitive systems. A representational structure represents system-specific information, bound to one specific cognitive faculty: In the verbal system words are represented, and in the visual system sensory images are stored. Complex interactions between the two systems and among all other systems to be defined must be specified.

In an alternative view, a unitary conception of high level cognition is proposed. In this model special-purpose "peripheral" systems for processing perceptual information and coordinating motor performance are distinguished. However, behind these systems lies a common or unitary cognitive system. Within this high level cognitive system different representational codes can be distinguished. But the essential assumption is that all these different codes are governed by principles which are common to the cognitive high level information processing system. The same processing architecture is able to deal with different data structures which vary in content and organization.

To which position do we have to give more weight? We will take a concrete example to show in what way the two theoretical positions might differ. Let's focus on concreteness and encoding effects in memory for sentences. Concrete sentences are remembered better than abstract sentences, and a sentence like "The man is feeding the dog" is recalled better if subjects are previously instructed to use visual mental images in processing the sentences than if they are not.

In order to explain these facts the multi-system theory will argue that concrete sentences have access to information stored in a nonverbal processing system while processing abstract sentences is restricted to the verbal system. The unitary conception will argue that content and form of the conceptual data structure will differ, depending on the material processed, and on the way this material was processed. How this could be described is shown in the following example, distinguishing a propositional from an image (or model) representation. The propositional code represents facts in abstract form. In the example "The man is feeding the dog" we have a minimum of defining features for the feeding action, the man and the dog. If we store such a sentence propositionally, we do not know (the information is not in the data structure) what kind of man is feeding what kind of dog, what kind of food, but nonetheless we understand the proposition pretty well and later we are able to reproduce this sentence. Let's think about what happens if we image or visualize this sentence. At this moment the abstract propositional representation becomes specific through elaboration. The man becomes a specific man, the dog a specific dog (e.g. poodle), the food is now a sausage, which is given to the dog in a specific feeding action. This data structure now contains all the information to model the stated fact in a two or three-dimensional reference frame. From this example it seems obvious that behavioral data will differ when we observe encoding and retrieval processes.

Thus at this level of description we have an explanation for the behavioral data from both theoretical positions readily at hand. This is not surprising because first, these explanations are formulated on a very general level, and second, there is virtually no behavioral fact which could not be explained by different notational conventions. But there are differences in the theoretical implications, when we try to specify theoretical assumptions of both frameworks. In separating nonverbal from a verbal processing system the multi-system theory has to say what these alternative systems look like. We can speak of visual, auditory or motor memory, and associate a representational code with a sensory system e.g. the visual code with the visual information processing system.

One of the first problems is then to decide how many of these systems in a human being have to be distinguished. To stay with the example of vision, it would be easy to distinguish more specific subsystems in perception which serve highly unique or specific functions in the flow of processing a stimulus input. Cognitive psychology so far has not tried to elaborate on the representational basis of such subsystems. We simply do not have any empirical data to distinguish further between specifications. In the current discussion on memory codes people usually restrict themselves to the distinction between two or three different codes which are more or less explicitly related to the different sensory systems, ignoring the problem of how specific this taxonomy should be. From what we know at the present time about sensory, modality-specific representations, descriptions of these nonverbal memory systems remain vague and relatively abstract.

Another important question is: What are the criteria to distinguish between the characteristics of the information stored in the different memory systems. The verbal system is usually characterized as linear and sequential in nature while more analogous and concrete encodings are attributed to the nonverbal systems. Analogous certainly means that the stored information preserves functionally the structural relationships of physical events in the real world. But often it is said that analogous representations or image representation may even contain sensoric components, which are qualitatively completely different from the word representation of the verbal system. This is most evident in formulations like the following: "The perceptual 'literal' memory of the appearance of an object or scene is not interpreted semantically;..." (Kosslyn et al. 1979, p. 541). This represents the view that some kind of sensory representation can be reactivated, depicted in working memory, searched and semantically interpreted. According to this view, we should be able to "see" things in stored information we have overlooked when we perceived the physical event.

If we base our memory theoretic assumptions on this kind of system specific processing and representations, we finally have to ask what the biological basis of the verbal system is. When we speak of visual, auditory and other images we immediately relate them to the corresponding biological sensory system. What can we do with represented words? Do we have a similar clear cut sensory system for verbal processing? Certainly not, but of course we could also speak of word images which are auditory or visual in nature. But words are symbolic representations and refer to objects and events in the real world; more specifically they refer to the knowledge we have about them, which means that words have meaning. But what about stored visual and auditory images, don't they fulfill this function? Do they not have meaning in the sense of words? The answer to this question depends on the nature of these images. If these images are raw sensory copies of the real world, their function is primarily not a symbolic one. That is, because these images can be inspected and meaning can be extracted directly in the way we would observe events of the real world. But if these images contain the meaningful interpretation of a perceptual process, images refer to events in representing the meaning, or part of it, itself. Of course there might be a hierarchy in reference in that an abstract word may refer to many possible images, while a specific image represents one situation. Here the question remains open: What is the word, its image, its meaning, what is the image, its meaning, and consequently what are the systems processing these different components?

From what was said above about the unitary conception of mind, we have not to worry about different computational systems in high level cognition. While for the low level processing highly specific sensory systems are accepted, for the cognitive system a unitary set of principles control the processing of different data structures. One of the basic assumptions is that the quality of the information units (nodes and relations) in the data structure of the unitary cognitive system is the same. Thus the representation of "dog" in the propositional code and the representation of "poodle" in the modal code are based on the same representational conditions. Henceforth we will label this representation in the cognitive system as conceptual memory. It is this memory we have access to, when we willingly and consciously do some kind of reasoning or retrieve information. The basic feature of all the information stored in this memory is that it is semantically meaningful interpreted information. Thus this memory has no possibility of storing some kind of copy of a sensory perceptual input. What is stored in this memory therefore is always the meaningful interpreted result of a perceptual process and never a copy of a perceptual input. There is no storage of surface structures in terms of words or pictures, but rather deep structures containing the meaning. The meaning (information) stored in conceptual memory is 1) constructed during encoding (think of the interpretation of ambiguous figures), 2) subject to modifications during storage (think of the findings of Loftus' (1975) eyewitness studies) and 3) reconstructed during recall (think of Bartlett's (1932) findings).

I am not denying that the human organism is able to store some kind of sensory-perceptual copies on lower levels. On the contrary, I think from a developmental point of view, that there is even a necessity to postulate such kind of representations. How else should an organism be able to recognize identity in his/her environment, an absolute prerequisite for learning. There are findings in perceptual recognition tasks (Jacoby & Dallas, 1981) which lend support for the notion of some sensory-perceptual representations.

3. FREE RECALL HAS ONLY ACCESS TO THE CONCEPTUAL MEMORY: A HYPOTHESIS

Here I am argueing for the assumption that conscious and willingly controlled retrieval is restricted to the conceptual memory. This implies that all free recall performances can be described in the same basic terminology. When we think in terms of Fodor's theory of modularity of mind (1983), there must be some cognitive systems that are not domain-specific. When we think of the conceptual memory as a central system which delivers the interface of modular encapsulate input systems, we can follow Fodor's view that this central system has restricted access to the vertical input systems which are modular, modality-specific, but encapsulated. It is plausible to assume that representations in these encapsulated systems are of sensory nature, but that the central system has no access to these representations. This view is compatible with phenomena observed in amnesia, described in Baddeley (1982), where patients do not remember having done a specific task, but demonstrate learning when they do it again.

If we conceptualize imagery theories on this basis, we share a terminology which is also used in other memory theoretic approaches like text processing and related areas where relational and item specific processing, context availability, and levels of representations are crucial theoretical concepts (Denis, 1984; Marschark, 1985; McDaniel, 1984; Perrig & Kintsch, 1985; Perrig, 1986). Thus, instead of speaking of different, only vaguely described, processing systems, we would have a unitary pool of theoretical terms to describe high-level cognition (Anderson, 1983), making communication easier. The implications of a theoretical notion would be more strictly analyzed and tested before a new theoretical concept is introduced.

I will try to demonstrate now what kind of questions could be asked from a perspective of a unitary conception of mind if we find memory differences which intuitively depend on different sensory representations. For this I will rely on empirical findings presented by Engelkamp & Zimmer (1985). These authors found that subjects who are presented action phrases of the form "smoking a pipe" are better in recall if they image these actions than if they only listen to them, and if the subjects enact the actions symbolically, their recall is even better than that of the imagery group. How can these effects be explained in a theory of conceptual memory as described above?

First, I agree with the assumption that there must be some differences in the representation of listening, motor, and image encoding. We can distinguish an image code from a propositional code as described above, assuming that the imagery group has more representations of the former and the listening group more of the latter kind. These are different data structures in that the image representation preserves spatial relational information while the propositional representation does not (Anderson, 1983). I would also agree to distinguish a motor code from an image code as soon as enough stable distinctive characteristics for the two codes could be found. From the theoretical background sketched above, we would expect to be able to describe the recall differences in terms of familiarity, distinctiveness, meaningfulness of represented information, encoding specificity, retrieval cues, retrieval strategies, etc.

In any case, I would exclude an interpretation which assumes that during free recall we have access to a qualitatively different data structure which is sensory in nature in the sense that we have some raw sensory non-interpreted information which can be activated, inspected, and from which something can be retrieved, which had not already been noticed before.

Here we try to describe what happen if subjects are confronted with action phrases, which they have to image or to enact (to simulate symbolically), and later to recall, by using Baddeley's (1982) conception of "domains of recollection". This concept advocates the distinction of processing domains, in which certain types of information are closely related and interact strongly, whereas other types are relatively separate. In this view, recollection implies that retrieval implements a strong active problem solving aspect, where a subject can not only build up a retrieval system at time of encoding, but can actively set new retrieval cues which are effective during recall. This assumption goes together with the view that retrieval is a two-stage process in which first, potential candidates of a certain knowledge-search domain or a certain context are generated and secondly in an evaluative process are selected. What is the difference in encoding and retrieval of action phrases between a motor and an image task? Our hypothesis is that there could be differences in the retrieval cues leading to different search domains. First let's think about what happens, when subjects listen to action phrases like "to smoke a pipe", and they are asked to enact these actions. What these people experience and know at the latest at time of recall, is that all the actions they are asked to recall were actions they performed with their own body, defining a very restricted search domain. In the task where subjects have to image these actions, and if they are informed to imagine themselves doing it, the domain restriction is less evident. "To smoke a pipe" can be imaged without any visible movement of hands or face, moreover, a broad context may be integrated into the picture: room, flowers, friends, etc. A possible search domain is thus much larger than in the motor group. From this assumption and the fact that we have higher recall scores when the set of alternatives is smaller (Davis, Sutherland & Judd, 1961), we could conclude that this is one reason why the motor group has higher recall scores than the image group.

There is another quite obvious and impressive difference between the image and the motor group. While the subjects using imagery perform completely unobserved, and in a more or less familiar activity, the performance of the motor group is plainly exposed, unusual and subject to the experimenter's observation. It is plausible to assume that because of the feedback a subject has of his/her own performance or because he/she is embarrassed by the presence of an experimenter, there may be notable extraprocessing. This kind of extraprocessing would create additional retrieval cues, which could become activated later when the subject is asked to retrieve the experiment episode, thus leading to increased performance.

4. AN EXPERIMENT ON IMAGE AND MOTOR ENCODING

We conducted an experiment to see whether there is some empirical basis for our hypothesis, that the motor group in this specific task (recall of previously heard action phrases) is better than the image group, because of restriction of the search domain and probably emotional extra processing.

Method

Subjects. Twenty-six psychology students of an introductory class at the University of Basel participated in the experiment.

Materials. Twenty-five action phrases (e.g. "smoking a pipe", "washing the dishes") were used in the experiment. The whole set of phrases was taken from the experimental material used by Engelkamp and Zimmer (1985) in their studies.

Procedure and Design. The subjects were randomly assigned either to the imagery group or to the motor group. Written instructions were given to both groups. The imagery group was instructed to listen carefully to the phrases, and to form a visual image of the described action. The motor group was instructed to listen carefully to the phrases, and to imitate the described action in a simple movement. The phrases were presented by a tape recorder in intervals of 6 seconds.

Both groups received the additional remark: "It is important that you realize that only actions which you can imitate in a simple movement are described. Thus only actions are presented, which you can perform yourself". This instruction was introduced to equalize the search domain in both groups. After the 25 phrases were presented, the subjects were asked to recall in writing everything they could remember.

After the free recall task the subjects were presented again with all the action phrases they had heard before. The phrases were typed on a sheet of paper, and the subjects were instructed to read

every action phrase and to note whether they remembered having had
some kind of emotional reactions related to the action at the time
when they visualized or enacted this action. The subjects could
choose from among five categories, and were asked to indicate
whether they thought an action was somehow stupid, annoying,
strange, funny or whether they experienced nothing special.

Results

In the free recall we scored for correctly recalled verbs and
objects of the action phrases. Synonyms were accepted as correct
responses. Recall of the verbs was 55% and 61% for the imagery
group and the motor group, respectively. Percentage for correctly
recalled objects was 54% and 59%. The ANOVA revealed no statistical
significance for these differences $(F(1,24) = 2.35$ and $F(1,24) =$
1.41 for verbs and objects, respectively).

In analyzing the emotional reactions to the action phrases, we
also did not find any differences between the image group and the
motor group. The subjects of both groups said in about 60% of the
action simulations (imaging and enacting) that they experienced no
special emotional reactions. About 20% of the action simulations
were experienced as funny. In about 10% of the simulations subjects
felt somehow strange, and in 5% of the cases they felt either
annoyed or stupid. But in none of these qualitatively different
judgments we found differences between the motor and the imagery
group.

In correlating the degree to which an item was judged to have
elicited a specific emotional reaction and its probability of being
recalled, we found positive correlations in the imagery group, $r(25)$
=.44, p<.05, and $r = .31$, for the qualities "stupid" and "strange",
respectively, and negative correlations for the motor group in the
same categories $(r = -.14$, and $r = -.42$, p<.05). It seems that
bizzareness of the action improves memory in the imagery group,
while conventional items improve memory in the motor group.

After a six-month period 5 subjects of the imagery group and 10
subjects of the motor group performed in delayed memory tests. A
free recall was followed by a recognition test. The motor group was
divided into two groups. While one of the motor groups was simply
instructed, like the imagery group, to remember in writing the
action phrases heard in the experiment, the second group was again
given the information (cue) that there were only actions they could
perform themselves. In neither test we found significant
differences between the three groups.

Discussion

In this experiment we did not find differences in memory
between subjects who imaged action phrases, and subjects who enacted
them. We expected that the superior recall of the motor group,
which is usually found in experiments, comparing subjects who enact
the movement of a verbal action description with subjects who image
an action description, would be reduced if both groups, the motor
group, and the imagery group refer to the same search domain when
they retrieve the actions.

We assumed that the set of alternatives from which the correct
response must be drawn would be much more restricted in the motor
group than in the image group. While the task of a motor group

implies the restriction of actions which the subjects can perform by parts of the body, the task of the imagery group is open to a broad diversity of context situations in which the actions can be imaged. Compared to the motor group, which in retrieving the auditory information can rely on the class of performed body reactions, the imagery group possibly has to retrieve the items from a set which in its multi-dimensionality offers many more candidates or alternatives for retrieval. Considering the fact that increasing the number of possible incorrect alternatives automatically reduces the likelihood of a correct response (Davis, Sutherland, & Judd, 1961) provides an explanation for why in the kind of experiments mentioned above recall performance of the motor group is better than performance of the imagery group. As our experiment shows, this superiority is reduced if both groups during instruction are informed explicitly about the set of items from which the correct items later on should be retrieved.

We replicated this finding in another experiment. There remains the problem of a null finding. But there will be other ways to test the predictive power of our theoretical framework. In congruence with the rationale presented here, subjects instructed to image themselves doing the actions should be better in recalling the actions than subjects instructed to image someone else performing the actions. Experimental data supporting this expectation has already been collected by Engelkamp and Zimmer (personal communication). In a study done by Engelkamp and Perrig (1986) a motor group and an imagery group were presented action phrases with local attributes (e.g. smoke the pipe in the lounge), and with local prepositional objects (e.g. pick up the coin from the floor). In free recall the motor group was better than the imagery group, thus fitting with what was said above. In cued recall with the location as cue the imagery subjects remembered both phrase types equally well. The motor group remembered the phrases with prepositional locations significantly better, and the phrases with attributive locations significantly worse than the imagery group. This differential effect can easily be described in terms of attentional focus and organization at time of encoding, showing that the motor group obviously integrates locations very strongly into the stored information, if these are prepositional and integrated into the movement, but they do not if location is not an integrated part of the action. Thus considering motor and image encoding as different strategies leading to differences in the organization of the retrieval system in conceptual memory, which can be made transparent by using different kinds of memory tests, is the way to proceed in this theoretical approach.

5. CONCLUSION

In this study we presented a rationale to explain behavioral differences in memory tests between motor and image encoding groups of verbally presented action phrases without the need to refer to some kind of sensory-motor or sensory-image memory traces. It is possible to explain the superior recall of motor groups compared to imagery groups in terms of encoding and recollection (Baddeley, 1982) processes in conceptual memory. In this theoretical framework a specific task (imaging, enacting) establishes a distinctive retrieval system. This retrieval system can be described as an

organizational structure of the data stored in conceptual memory
which can be accessed and/or modified by conditions in the retrieval
situation. Here we demonstrated in one example how from this
theoretical framework operational experimental questions can be
deduced and tested. And we are optimistic that many of the
so-called distinctive features of motor and image codes, beyond the
phenomena in free recall, to stay with our example, can be explained
in the theoretical terms mentioned above.

REFERENCES

1. Anderson, J.R. (1983). The architecture of cognition.
    Cambridge: Harvard University Press.
2. Baddeley, A.D. (1982). Domains of recollection. Psychological
    Review, 89, 708-729.
3. Bartlett, F.C. (1932). Remembering. Cambridge: Cambridge
    University
4. Davis, R., Sutherland, N.S., & Judd, B.R. 1961. Information
    content in recognition and recall. Journal of Experimental
    Psychology, 61, 422-429.
5. Denis, M. (1984). Imagery and prose: A critical review of
    research on adults and children. Text, 4, 381-401.
6. Engelkamp, J., & Zimmer, H.D. (1985). Motor programs and their
    relation to semantic memory. The German Journal of
    Psychology, 9, 239-254.
7. Engelkamp, J., & Perrig, W.J. (1986). Differential effects of
    imaginal and motor encoding on the recall of action phrases.
    Archiv für Psychologie, 4, 261-271.
8. Fodor, J.A. (1983). The modularity of mind. Cambridge:
    MIT Press.
9. Jacoby, L.L. & Dallas, M. (1981). On the relationship between
    autobiographical memory and perceptual learning. Journal of
    Experimental Psychology: General, 3, 306-340.
10. Kosslyn, S.M., Pinker, S., Smith, G.E. & Shwartz, S.P. (1979).
    On the demystification of mental imagery. The Behavioral
    and Brain Sciences. 2, 535-581.
11. Loftus, E.G. (1975). Leading questions and the eye-witness
    report. Cognitive Psychology, 7, 560-572.
12. Marschark, M. (1985). Imagery and organization in the recall
    of prose. Journal of Memory and Language, 24, 734-745.
13. McDaniel, M.A. (1984). The role of elaborative and schema
    processes in story memory. Memory and Cognition. 12,
    46-51.
14. Perrig, W.J. (1986). Imagery and the thematic storage of
    prose. In D. G. Russell & D. F. Marks (Eds).
    Imagery 2. Dunedin: Human Performance Ass. in press.
15. Perrig, W.J. & Kintsch, W. (1985). Propositional and
    situational representation of text. Journal of Memory and
    Language, 24, 503-519.

SUSAN AYLWIN

DEPARTMENT OF APPLIED PSYCHOLOGY, UNIVERSITY COLLEGE, CORK, IRELAND

ABSTRACT

A modified association technique is used to show that verbal, visual and enactive (imagined action) representations employ different cognitive structures. Verbal representation uses superordinate and oppositional structures; visual imagery uses whole-part, object-attribute, and locative structures; enactive imagery is temporally and affectively organised, using transitive action and emotive structures. The Modes of Thought Questionnaire (MOTQ) assesses biases in representational style by looking at the extent to which individuals use the cognitive structures characteristic of each mode of thought. Studies on personality correlates show that verbalisers are interested in power and order, visualisers in affiliation and sensitivity to others, and enactive imagers in what Bandura called 'self-efficacy'. Current work is exploring health and illness correlates.

1. COGNITIVE STRUCTURES IN VERBAL, VISUAL AND ENACTIVE REPRESENTATIONS

Twenty years ago Jerome Bruner (1966) suggested that we each have available to us three different forms of mental representation. Each of these derives from the internalisation of one of our major ways of interacting with the world. Thus from the internalisation of language we have inner speech; from the internalisation of visual perception we have visual imagery; and from the internalisation of action we have a form of imagined action that can be called enactive imagery.

For some tasks any of these three forms of internal representation can be used. For example, in reading a novel, we can concentrate on the words and repeat them over under our breath, using inner speech or verbal representation. Or we can conjure up pictures in our mind's eye of the events referred to in the novel and follow the plot in the form of the mental movie offered by visual imagery. Or we can imagine ourselves identified with hero, heroine or villain, and follow the plot through imagined identification and action.

However, since speech, perception and action have very different functions in the real world, it seems likely that their internalised counterparts will also have different functions, and will constitute in effect different kinds of meaning systems.

This turns out to be the case. Figure 1 shows the three domains of meaning for a single word: dog. This semantic 'map' is based on the results of several association studies (Aylwin, 1977, 1981, 1985) in which people were given a stimulus word or sentence, asked to represent it verbally, visually or enactively, and to associate to their representation. Thus people were asked to say the word 'dog', or to see a mental picture of a dog, or to imagine being a dog, and to associate to their representation. (Adults are close enough to their childhood to find this no problem!)

317

M. Denis et al. (eds.), Cognitive and Neuropsychological Approaches to Mental Imagery, 317–325.
© 1988 by Martinus Nijhoff Publishers.

318

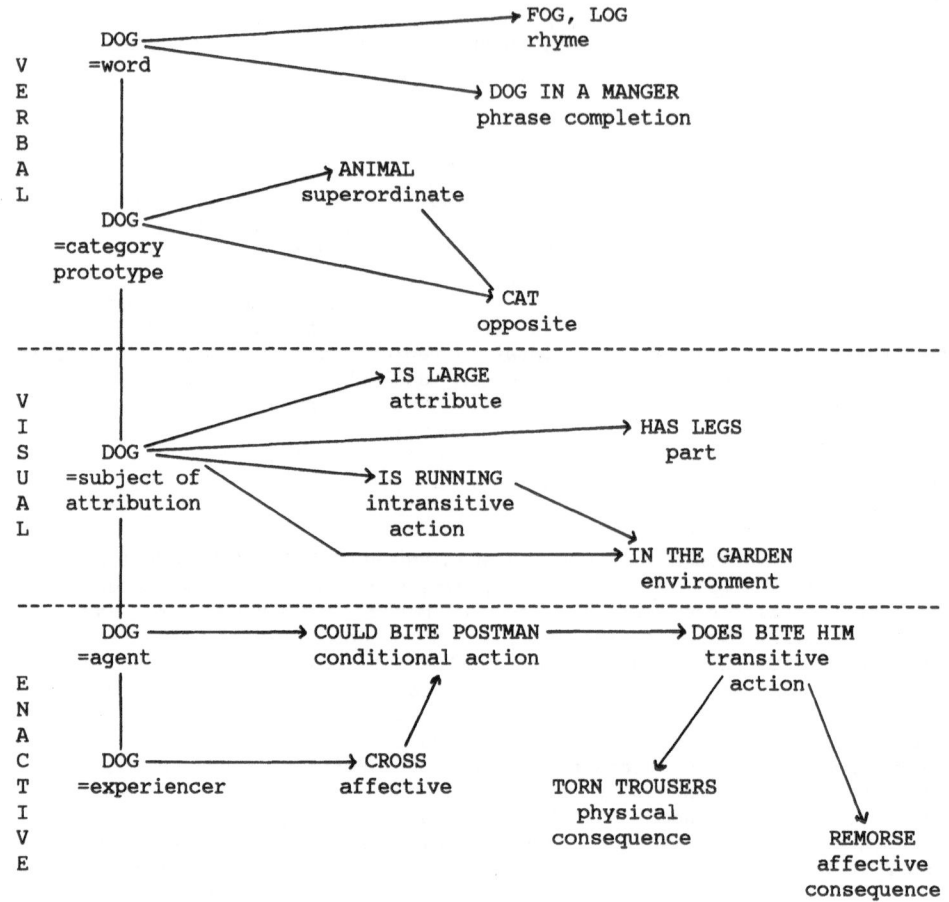

FIGURE 1. Semantic map for verbal, visual and enactive representations.

Content analyses of the associations show that each form of representation
emphasizes very different aspects of the stimulus.

For verbal representation the acoustic properties of the stimulus are
important. Rhyming associations such as 'dog--fog' are characteristic, as
are phrase completions such as 'dog--in the manger'. Verbal representation
also taps into that part of the semantic network concerned with taxonomic
or hierarchical organisation. Hence superordinate associations such as
'dog--animal', and contrast or oppositional responses such as 'dog--cat',
are characteristic.

Visual imagery is in general concerned with the static, spatial, picture-
like properties of the stimulus. When associating to a visual image of a
dog people respond with attributes and parts - 'it is large', 'it has
legs'; and there are also frequent references to the environment and to the
intransitive actions that may occur in it - 'the dog is in the garden', or
'the dog is running in the garden'.

Enactive imagery is organised temporally and affectively. In it the dog
is an agent of actions and an experiencer of feelings. The actions may be

expressed in hypothetical mode, as in the conditional - 'the dog could bite
the postman', and the actions may be carried out if they are affectively
justified - 'the dog is cross so he does bite the postman'. There is an
awareness of the possible consequences of action, both physical - 'the torn
trousers'; and affective - the 'remorse' that may follow this piece of
impulsive behaviour.

Clearly the different forms of representation are employing different
cognitive structures in making sense of the stimulus. The propositional
account of cognitive structures in imagery (Pylyshyn, 1973) asserts the
reality of the underlying propositions at a level inaccessible to
consciousness. An alternative account (Aylwin, 1985) sees the cognitive
structures characteristic of each mode of representation not as entities
themselves but as descriptions of mental transformations. In the
association studies the cognitive structure, object--superordinate,
describes the transformation of the idea of an object to the idea of its
superordinate class, for example the idea of a dog to the idea of an
animal. This view sees structures as describing transformations, and not
as generating representations. Attention is oriented by different
representational instructions to move down different cognitive or
transformational pathways. Figure 1 then becomes not a static semantic
network but a map of the possible cognitive pathways that attention may
take in the three representational modes.

2. THE MODES OF THOUGHT QUESTIONNAIRE

It seems likely that a person who attends to objects and who makes sense
of them by labelling and categorizing will be a different kind of person
from the one who focuses on appearance and location; and that both these
will differ from someone who concentrates on action and feeling. Different
representational styles can be hypothesised to be associated with different
personalities and lifestyles.

The study of the personality correlates of verbal, visual and enactive
thinking requires first a way of assessing the extent to which people use
each of the modes of thought. The Modes of Thought Questionnaire (MOTQ) was
developed for this purpose (Aylwin, 1985).

In the MOTQ people are presented with a series of stimulus-association
item pairs, each of which exemplifies a particular cognitive structure.
They are asked to represent the first item using the appropriate form of
representation, and then to rate the likelihood of the second item coming
to mind in association with it using a five-point scale. There are 13
structural subscales in the MOTQ, and from these, verbal, visual and
enactive mode scores are derived by summing across the appropriate
subscales. Sample items are given below:

Verbal subscales
say WIDE----narrow...............( ) (opposite)
say SCARLET-----fever............( ) (phrase completion)
say REGAL-----legal..............( ) (rhyme)
say ALUMINIUM-----metal..........( ) (superordinate)
  Visual subscales
see BOAT-----harbour.............( ) (environment)
see HANDKERCHIEF-----square......( ) (attribute)
see PENSIONER-----strolling......( ) (intransitive action)
see KETTLE-----spout.............( ) (part)
  Enactive subscales
be OBLITERATING-----gone.........( ) (consequence)

```
be GREEDY-----tummy ache.........(  )  (affective consequence)
be TELEPHONIST-----curious.......(  )  (affective)
be LEOPARD-----catches gazelle...(  )  (transitive action)
be SECRETARY-----could kick boss.(  )  (conditional action)
```

There is also a fourteenth subscale, called the 'cross-modal scale', because here the representational instruction is inappropriate to the structure exemplified, as in the item:

```
see WEASEL-----easel............(  )
```

where the rhyming structure is preceded by a visual instruction instead of its proper verbal one. This cross-modal scale functions as a general response bias scale.

The structural subscales of the MOTQ have generally adequate or good reliability (Aylwin, 1985), and allow an assessment of the extent to which people use particular cognitive structures.

3. PERSONALITY CORRELATES OF THE THREE MODES OF THOUGHT

We have used the MOTQ in four kinds of studies (for full details see Aylwin, 1985): (a) using an adjective rating scale to give a general impression of personality; (b) using personality tests - the Wilson and Patterson Attitude Inventory (Wilson, 1975), Rotter's Internal-External Locus of Control Scale (Rotter, 1966), and the Marlowe-Crowne test of Social Desirability (Crowne & Marlowe, 1964); (c) using tests of cognitive abilities - the General Aptitudes Test Battery (United States Employment Service, 1970), the space relations section of the Differential Aptitudes Tests (Bennett, Seashore & Wesman, 1974), and Sheehan's version of the Betts' Questionnaire upon Mental Imagery (Sheehan, 1967); and (d) looking at differences in MOTQ scores in students in different faculties - arts and social sciences, commerce, and engineering.

This work can be summarised in the form of three personality portraits which show how particular personality traits relate to the particular cognitive structures which are characteristic of each of the three modes of representation.

3.1 Verbalisers

The personality of people biased towards verbal representation can be summarised by saying that verbalisers are bureaucrats, generally oriented towards traditional values, and with a liking for power.

Verbalisers describe themselves as religious, and tend to score highly on the religion-puritanism scale of the Wilson and Patterson Attitude Inventory. This religiousness is specifically related to the rhyme subscale of the MOTQ. A possible interpretation of this is that rhymes represent the kind of soothing sonority characteristic of much religious language, where the music of the words is at least as important as their reference.

The phrase completion subscale of the MOTQ correlates with the possession of a broad vocabulary on the General Aptitudes Test Battery, and this probably relates to the use of language as a persuasive social tool, useful for gaining power and popularity, both of which appear to be ambitions for people with a strong verbal bias.

The superordinate and opposition subscales together tap the extent to which people make sense of things by slotting them into an hierarchical structure. In terms of their personalities, verbalisers seem to construe themselves according to how they fit into a socially or bureaucratically organised hierarchy. Thus verbalisers are ambitious for moving up the hierarchy, but fear the failure marked by slipping down it. They have a preference for order, and are suspicious of those violating that order: the opposites subscale correlates with militarism-punitiveness on the Wilson and Patterson Attitude Inventory.

In terms of career choice the verbal style predominates among students in the commerce faculty, many of whom will go into jobs in business or the civil service. Both these career routes appear to offer the kind of hierarchical organisation in which verbalisers will feel at home.

3.2 Visualisers

The personality of people with a strong visual bias can be summarised by saying that visualisers are Romantics, strongly oriented towards others, and concerned with affiliation and sensitivity to others.

The environment subscale of the MOTQ correlates with a number of traits indicating sensitivity both to the natural and to the social environment. Visualisers describe themselves as artistic and as capable of a sense of wonder. They also describe themselves as self-aware; and the evidence suggests that this self-awareness is an externalised version, the kind that derives from seeing oneself through the eyes of others. This accords with the fact that visualisers have an external locus of control on Rotter's Internal-External Locus of Control scale, and show a concern with social desirability on the Marlowe-Crowne scale.

The objective self-awareness of visualisers is useful for affiliative purposes, as it allows them to monitor their behaviour for its social desirability. But the disadvantage of this external perspective on the self is that it tends not to penetrate the skin, and the person using it is in danger of seeing the self as an appearance with nothing inside. This is suggested by the fact that the parts and attributes subscales of the MOTQ relate to self-descriptions of dependency, emptiness, apathy and indecision.

Generally the visual mode of thought is one that is stronger in women then in men; and in terms of career path it is found in those in the arts and social sciences, including psychology.

As a cognitive tailpiece to this visualiser portrait it is of note that imagery vividness (Sheehan 1967) correlates with all the MOTQ visual subscales, and most strongly with the attributes subscale. This makes sense, as vividness is itself a kind of attribute.

3.3 Enactive imagers

The personality of people with a strong enactive bias can be summarised by saying that enactive imagers are innovators, or perhaps more often, frustrated innovators. These people are inner-directed, concerned with what Bandura (1977) called 'self-efficacy'.

Enactive imagers describe themselves as being both intense and inhibited, and these correlate specifically with their capacity to represent internalised action (the MOTQ transitive action subscale). The intensity seems to find expression in stubbornness and aggression, and when inhibited it seems to turn inwards in depression and suicidal thoughts.

The consequences subscale of the MOTQ shows enactive imagers at their best, as patient, serious, and inventive. This is a rather different type of creativity from the dreamier artistic creativity of the visualiser. Enactive imagers are also solitary people, by their own account, which probably fits with their particular creative style. It probably also fits with the fact that their intensity isn't everybody's social cup of tea.

The affective aspects of the enactive cognitive style (MOTQ affective and affective consequences subscales) are expressed in personality in a sense of vulnerability and a liking for risks. The general association of enactive representation with strong feelings is interesting in the light of Peter Lang's (1979) work on imagery and emotion, which shows an association of emotion with participatory imagery rather than purely visual representations.

The enactive style is generally one that seems to suit men better than women. In terms of career choice an enactive bias is evident in engineering students. In support of this there is also an association of the MOTQ transitive and conditional action subscales with spatial flexibility on the space relations section of the Differential Aptitudes Tests, and on the space manipulation and form matching sections of the General Aptitudes Test Battery.

4. HEALTH AND ILLNESS CORRELATES OF DIFFERENT MODES OF THOUGHT

Our current work is extending the idea of representational styles to look at whether different cognitive styles are also related to different styles of health and illness.

This research was stimulated in part by work on a syndrome called 'alexithymia', a term which means literally 'without words for feelings'. Alexithymics are people who find it difficult to label their feelings, who have a rather deficient fantasy life, and who show an unexpectedly high level of psychosomatic complaints (Sifneos, 1973).

There are two reasons for hypothesising that verbalisers might have a tendency toward alexithymia. Firstly, verbal representation tends to avoid references to feelings. In the semantic triptych of Figure 1, verbal structures are most distant from affective structures, which are characteristic of enactive imagery. In the association studies which were the basis for Figure 1, verbal and enactive structures rarely co-occurred, though both showed some overlap with visual structures. This suggests that the representational style of the verbaliser may simply not be one which gives easy access to affect. Secondly, verbal representation does not indulge in fantasy. One of the association studies used sentence stimuli with free flowing speech as response (Aylwin, 1981). Subjects instructed to use verbal representation more often gave as their association a judgement about truth value (especially that the sentence was false or meaningless) than other subjects, and justified their assertion by reference to conventional factual knowledge. In contrast, visual and enactive representations allow their users to engage in fantasy elaborations of the sentences regardless of truth value. These two features, the alienation from affect and the alienation from fantasy, suggest an association between a verbal bias and alexithymia. And if this association holds, a further hypothesis becomes possible; that verbalisers may also be more prone to psychosomatic symptoms than people with other cognitive styles.

One of my postgraduate students, Mary Alison Durand, and I have tested out these hypotheses in a pilot study. The subjects were 152 students (115 female and 37 male), who completed the MOTQ, the Schalling-Sifneos alexithymia scale (Apfel & Sifneos, 1979), and a symptoms rating scale which asked them to rate, on a five-point scale, the frequency of occurrence of 12 minor symptoms which could be considered as open to psychological influence: backache, pains in the neck muscles, sore throat, headache, mouth ulcers, heart burn, dizzy spells, upset tummy, laryngitis, boils, warts, and insomnia.

There was partial support for the hypothesis relating a verbal bias with alexithymia. The alexithymia scale (which is scored negatively) showed only one significant negative correlation: for women (though not for men) there was an association between use of superordinate structures (one of the MOTQ verbal subscales) and tendency toward alexithymia ($\underline{r}$(110) = -.23, $\underline{p}$<.016, controlling for the cross-modal score).

There was also partial support for the hypothesis relating a verbal bias to psychosomatic symptoms. The results of correlating MOTQ mode scores with physical symptoms are shown in table 1. There is only one positive correlation: between verbalising and suffering from mouth ulcers.

mode	symptom	$\underline{r}$	$\underline{p}$
verbal	mouth ulcers	+.19	<.024
visual	boils	-.20	<.018
	upset tummy	-.26	<.002
	heartburn	-.17	<.042
	pains in neck muscles	-.19	<.022
	dizzy spells	-.18	<.032
enactive	backache	-.18	<.032

TABLE 1. Correlations of symptoms with modes of thought (controlling for cross-modal scores).

The results also show a number of negative correlations with visual and enactive ways of thinking. From the admittedly sparse data it looks as though these forms of imagery may be health-promoting ways of thinking, and that they may (though this is very tentative) confer health protection of two kinds. Firstly visual imagery may provide benefits in terms of resistance to infection, since visual imagers do not get boils (typically caused by Staphylococcal bacteria), and do not get upset tummies (some of which will be caused by infections, typically of Salmonella bacteria or viruses). Secondly, both enactive and visual thinking seem to bestow the benefits of relaxation: enactive imagers do not get backaches; and visual imagers do not get such tension and anxiety symptoms as pains in the neck muscles, heartburn, dizzy spells, or upset tummies (some of which are caused by anxiety rather than infection).

If nonverbal forms of imagery are particularly healthy ways of thinking, it ought to be possible to use them as an intervention to help people return to full health more quickly than they otherwise would.

We have tested this hypothesis out in a small way by looking at the efficacy of imagery as a treatment for the common cold. This was a study by Wilson and Aylwin, which used an imagery treatment for colds based on the Simontons' controversial treatment for cancer (Simonton, Matthews-Simonton & Creighton, 1978). The study used 40 subjects (29 women and 11 men) with heavy colds. Subjects were divided into a control group who simply rated the severity of 12 cold symptoms each day for the duration of the cold; and an imagery group who were asked to listen to a tape twice a day for four days in which they were asked first to relax, and then to imagine their immune system in a symbolic form winning a battle against the infection, also in a symbolic form. Such imagery involves both visual and enactive components.

There was no effect of the imagery treatment on the intensity of cold symptoms, but there was an effect on the <u>duration</u> of the cold. For the control group the mean duration of colds was 9.6 days, and for the imagery group it was two and a half days shorter, at 7.1 days, a difference significant at the p<.01 level. It may be that the relaxation component of the imagery treatment package is having some effect, but there also seems to be an effect of the imagery itself. Duration of colds in the imagery group correlated with imagery vividness on Marks' (1973) Vividness of Visual Imagery Questionnaire (r (18) = .50, p<.05; since the VVIQ is scored negatively this result means that more vivid imagery is associated with shorter colds). Duration of colds also correlated negatively with spatial ability on the Differential Aptitudes Tests (Bennett, Seashore & Wesman, 1974) (r (18) = -.46, p<.05).

Although the results of this study on colds do not allow any partitioning of effects between visual and enactive components of the imagery treatment, they do generally back up the findings of the symptoms study which suggested that nonverbal ways of thinking may be health-promoting.

Clearly these two studies are only a very small beginning. Our current work is attempting to replicate and extend these findings in the hope of mapping out more fully specific symptom and disease correlates of verbal, visual and enactive thinking.

In search of a theoretical framework that can encompass these findings it seems necessary to abandon or supplement an information processing model of thought, and to assume that as well as being a kind of computer the brain is also a brain, a complex biochemical mechanism capable of affecting immune processes in the rest of the body. At some level of analysis each mode of thought must have a biochemical manifestation, perhaps involving the use of different neuronal pathways and different neurotransmitter systems.

Inasfar as each mode of thought is a different way of attending to and assimilating information, each can be seen also as a different way of coping with the environment. Extending this idea only a short way suggests that each mode of thought may then also be a different way of coping with the stresses that may be part of the environment.

Recent work in the expanding field of psychoneuroimmunology is beginning to elaborate the pathways whereby stress affects the immune system, thus expanding on the early work of Selye (1983). Psychological stresses such as bereavement (Schleifer, Keller, Camerino, Thornton & Stein, 1983), exams (Kiecolt-Glaser, Gardner, Speicher, Penn, Holliday & Glaser, 1984), and frustration (McClelland, Alexander & Marks, 1982), have all been associated with lowered indices of immune functioning. Future work may show how different modes of thought may feed into the pathways described by psychoneuroimmunology, and thus act as modulators of disease processes.

REFERENCES

1. Apfel, R. J. & Sifneos, P. E. (1979). Alexithymia: Concept and measurement. <u>Psychotherapy</u> <u>and</u> <u>Psychosomatics</u>, <u>32</u>, 180-190.
2. Aylwin, S. (1977). The structure of visual and kinaesthetic imagery: a free association study. <u>British</u> <u>Journal</u> <u>of</u> <u>Psychology</u>, <u>68</u>, 353-360.
3. Aylwin, S. (1981). Types of relationship instantiated in verbal, visual and enactive imagery. <u>Journal</u> <u>of</u> <u>Mental</u> <u>Imagery</u>, <u>5</u>(1), 67-84.
4. Aylwin, S. (1985). <u>Structure</u> <u>in</u> <u>thought</u> <u>and</u> <u>feeling</u>. London: Methuen.
5. Bandura, A. (1977). Self-efficacy: Toward a unifying theory of behavioral change. <u>Psychological</u> <u>Review</u>, <u>84</u>, 191-215.

6. Bennett, G. K., Seashore, H. G., & Wesman, A. G. (1974). Manual for the Differential Aptitude Tests: Forms S and T (5th ed.). New York: The Psychological Corporation.
7. Bruner, J. S. (1966). On cognitive growth. In J. S. Bruner, R. R. Olver, & P. P. Greenfield, Studies in cognitive growth (pp. 1-29). New York: Wiley.
8. Crowne, D. P., & Marlowe, D. (1964). The approval motive: Studies in evaluative dependence. New York: Wiley.
9. Kiecolt-Glaser, J. N., Gardner, W., Speicher, C., Penn, G. M., Holliday, B. S., & Glaser, R. (1984). Psychosocial modifiers of immunocompetence in medical students. Psychosomatic Medicine, 46, 7-14.
10. Lang, P. J. (1979). Language, image and emotion. In P. Pliner, K. R. Blankstein, & I. M. Spigel (Eds.), Perception of emotion in self and others (pp. 107-117). New York: Plenum Press.
11. Marks, D. F. (1973) Visual imagery differences in the recall of pictures. British Journal of Psychology, 64, 17-24.
12. McClelland, D. C., Alexander, C., & Marks, E. (1982). The need for power, stress, immune function, and illness among male prisoners. Journal of Abnormal Psychology, 91, 61-70.
13. Pylyshyn, Z. W. (1973). What the mind's eye tells the mind's brain: A critique of mental imagery. Psychological Bulletin, 80, 1-24.
14. Rotter, J. B. (1966). Generalised expectancies for internal versus external locus of reinforcement. Psychological Monographs, 80, 1-28.
15. Schleifer, S. J., Keller, S. E., Camerino, M., Thornton, J. C., & Stein, M. (1983). Suppression of lymphocyte stimulation following bereavement. Journal of the American Medical Association, 250, 374-377.
16. Selye, H. (1983). The stress concept: Past, present and future. In C. L. Cooper (Ed.), Stress research: Issues for the eighties (pp. 1-20). Chichester: Wiley.
17. Sheehan, P. W. (1967). A shortened form of Betts' questionnaire upon mental imagery. Journal of Clinical Psychology, 23, 386-389.
18. Sifneos, P. E. (1973). The prevalence of 'alexithymic' characteristics in psychosomatic patients. Psychotherapy and Psychosomatics, 22, 255-262.
19. Simonton, O. C., Matthews-Simonton, S., & Creighton, J. L. (1978). Getting well again . Los Angeles: Tarcher.
20. United States Employment Service (1970). Manual for the General Aptitude Test Battery. Washington: US Department of Labour and Manpower Administration.
21. Wilson, G. D. (1975). Manual for the Wilson-Patterson Attitude Inventory. Windsor: NFER.

SELECTIVE ENHANCEMENT OF IMAGERY IN ANXIETY

MARYANNE MARTIN

UNIVERSITY OF OXFORD, ENGLAND

ABSTRACT
 Clinical observation has suggested that patients who suffer from disabling levels of anxiety may also experience enhanced levels of imagery. If this proposition is correct, it could arise in a number of ways. First, anxiety-related experiences in general may be accompanied by more imagery than are other types of experiences. Second, anxious people in general may experience more imagery than do other types of people. Third, specifically anxiety-related experiences of anxious people may be accompanied by a selective enhancement of imagery, relative to other types of experience. Experimental results yield evidence that anxiety and imagery are indeed related, and in particular provide support for the selective enhancement hypothesis.

1. INTRODUCTION

 Few people now doubt that there is a close link between cognition and emotion, although there is considerable debate about the exact nature of the causal relation between them. The work to be reviewed here focuses on the link between two specific elements of these general areas, namely on the link between imagery and anxiety. One need look no further for the powerful effects of imagery on emotion in general than the various forms of mood induction procedure which directly or indirectly employ visual images in order to manipulate temporarily an individual's mood (for a review see Martin, 1985a, 1986). The link between imagery and anxiety is of particular importance because clinical experience suggests that a number of emotional disorders involving enhanced levels of anxiety (e.g., generalized anxiety disorder, simple phobias, agoraphobia, and panic disorder) are associated with high levels of visual imagery. Many anxious patients experience images before and during their periods of anxiety. On questioning, they report visual images concerned with the anticipation of physical or psychosocial trauma. It is interesting to note, nevertheless, that few patients spontaneously disclose frightening visual images except in post-traumatic stress disorder without explicit, and sometimes repeated, questioning by the therapist (Beck, Emery & Greenberg, 1985; Clark & Beck, in press).
 Imagery has been used in a number of different forms of clinical therapy. For example, Freud used imagery in analysis to evoke past memories, as illustrated in the following passage about the treatment of a patient with hysteria:
 "Throughout this whole analysis I made use of the method of evoking pictures and ideas by pressing her head, a method, therefore, which would be inapplicable without the full cooperation and voluntary attention of a patient. At times her behavior left nothing to be desired, and at such periods it was really surprising how promptly and how infallibly the individual scenes belonging to one theme succeeded each other in chronological order. It was as if she read from a large picture book, the pages of which passed in review before her eyes" (Breuer & Freud, 1895/1936, p.109).

M. Denis et al. (eds.), Cognitive and Neuropsychological Approaches to Mental Imagery, 327–336.
© 1988 by Martinus Nijhoff Publishers.

Later, Wolpe (1969) developed the use of imagery in systematic desensitization, and Lazarus (1971) employed visual imagery to clarify patients' problems. In cognitive therapy (Beck et al., 1985), imagery-related interventions are frequent, constituting a major medium of treatment. On the one hand, ascertaining the content of spontaneous visual images is useful in probing an ill-defined problem, and in detecting distortions of reality that may give rise to excessive or inappropriate reactions. On the other hand, once these feared aspects of a situation are recognized, imagery can again be used in attempting to modify the distortions, and hence lead to the patient's recovery. Beck and his colleagues suggest a number of techniques for modifying images, including the turn-off technique, repetition, time projection, symbolic images, and decatastrophizing the image.

In contrast to the emphasis in anxiety upon imagery, clinical experiences of depression have characteristically stressed the role of verbal processes. Depressed patients typically ruminate about negative topics. This often takes the form of a (silent) self-commentary, embracing negative assertions about oneself or one's actions (e.g., "I am worthless", or "Everything I do goes wrong"). A number of forms of treatment for depression, such as cognitive therapy (Beck, 1976; Beck, Rush, Shaw, & Emery, 1979), attempt to modify such ruminating. This form of treatment for depression has been found to be as effective as (or more effective than) tricyclic antidepressants in the short term, and there is some evidence that it may be associated with a lower relapse rate than drug treatment (see Clark & Beck, in press).

The study of emotion by means of cognitive experimentation has led to a rather different characterisation of differences between anxiety and depression. In place of a clinically-based distinction between imagery and verbal processes, it appears that the effects of anxiety are of primary importance for perceptual processes (e.g., Mathews & MacLeod, 1985, 1986), whereas those of depression primarily affect memory processes (e.g., Clark, Teasdale, Broadbent, & Martin, 1983; Martin, 1985b; Martin & Clark, 1986). Why should perceptual and memory processes differ in this way? An explanation may be offered in terms of the differing cognitive processes that are appropriate for propagating differing emotions.

2. PROPAGATION OF EMOTION

Propagational theory proposes that the likelihood of a particular domain of cognitive processing being affected by an emotion is a positive function of the likelihood that the resulting change in that domain will itself serve to propagate the emotion in question. That is, it is hypothesised that the cognitive changes that accompany emotional change are generally of a nature that leads to either the perseveration or the intensification (or both) of the original emotional change. In the case of anxiety, it can be argued that centrally involved in its propagation is the discovery of threatening aspects of the environment. Thus on a propagational account one expects, conversely, that a major effect of anxiety will be to itself bias perception in the direction of selectively attending to negative material. In the case of depression, on the other hand, centrally involved in its propagation appears to be the continued working over mentally of unhappy memories. Thus here a propagational account leads one to expect that a major effect of depression will be to bias memory in the direction of selectively retrieving negative material.

Why should anxiety and depression exert self-propagating effects upon cognitive processing? This may occur because their cognitive effects can be highly adaptive in certain situations, and thus confer an evolutionary advantage. If one has reason to be anxious about a physical threat in the immediate environment, it is advantageous to be perceptually biased in favour of detecting such a threat. If, however, one has reason to be depressed about a previous event, then it is advantageous to be biased towards the retrieval from memory of relevant information that may assist one in working out how to deal with a similar event in the future. It may also be noted that the degree to which any individual is subject to these biases seems likely to vary considerably (e.g., to be normally distributed) over the population. Thus it may be that excessive susceptibility to these biases results in certain individuals being particularly prone to becoming anxious or depressed patients.

As noted earlier, an alternative characterisation of the cognitive effects of anxiety and depression may be cast in terms of imagery and verbal biases in place of perceptual and mnemonic biases. These two characterisations are perhaps more closely related than might at first sight appear. Imagery and perception are related at least in terms of subjective experience, and possibly in terms of functional representation. Similarly, the verbal and mnemonic categorisations are both germane to the same ruminative type of behaviour, in which information is both retrieved and articulated in a repeated manner. A series of recent experiments has concentrated in particular on investigating the hypothesised relation between anxiety and imagery processes.

3.   THREE HYPOTHESES ON IMAGERY AND ANXIETY
In principle, there are at least three plausible reasons why anxiety might appear to be linked clinically to imagery. The first is that anxious experiences might in general be more imageable than other types of experience (and patients with anxiety will of course have an unusually high proportion of such experiences). The second is that anxiety might lead to higher levels of imagery for experiences in general. The third hypothesis is obtained by juxtaposing the other two. It asserts neither that all anxious experiences are associated with enhanced imagery nor that all experiences of a person with anxiety are associated with enhanced imagery. Rather, it asserts that it is specifically the anxious experiences (relative to nonanxious experiences) of people with anxiety that are associated with higher levels of imagery.

At present, there is little evidence available enabling us to choose between the three hypotheses outlined in the preceding paragraph. However, one relevant study has recently been reported (Martin, in press); as with the two further experiments to be described it tested members of the normal population, none of whom was receiving treatment for any mental disorder. This first study provides evidence concerning the first of the three hypotheses.

3.1.   Testing the first hypothesis
Each subject was asked to bring to mind the memory of an occasion on which he or she had felt in a specified emotional state (either anxious, depressed, angry, or happy). Following this, subjects responded to a number of questions concerning the relevant memory (the same set of questions was used for each of the four types of memory). The response consisted in each case of placing a cross at what the subject judged to be the appropriate location on a horizontal scale marked at 10-point intervals from 0 ("Not at all") to 100 ("Extremely"). For example, for assessing visual imagery, the question was "How strong is your specifically visual image of the experience?", and the response scale was labelled "Not at all strong" and "Extremely strong" at 0 and 100, respectively. The questions that are of interest in the present context are shown in Table 1, with the results summarized in Table 2 (in Table 2, significant pairwise differences are those yielded by Newman-Keuls analyses).

The most striking result is that the greatest differences for all the variables were observed between negative and positive emotion. Episodes selected for their

TABLE 1. Topics and their questions (response scales in parentheses).

Topic	Question
Overall imagery	How strong is your overall mental image (i.e., mental picture, sound, etc.) of the experience? ("strong")
Visual imagery	How strong is your specifically visual image of the experience? ("strong")
Auditory imagery	How strong is your image specifically of the sound sensations? ("strong")
Olfactory imagery	How strong is your image specifically of the smell sensations? ("strong")
Gustatory imagery	How strong is your image specifically of the taste sensations? ("strong")
Tactile imagery	How strong is your image specifically of the touch sensations? ("strong")
Proprioceptive imagery	How strong is your image specifically of bodily sensations (e.g., warmth, cold, aching)? ("strong")
Colour extent	How much colour is there in the image? ("coloured")
Colour intensity	How bright are the colours in the image? ("bright")
Movement	How much movement is there in the image? ("mobile")
Stability	How stable (as opposed to fleeting) is your image of the experience? ("stable")
Self-comment	At the time, how strongly did you comment to yourself (probably silently, of course) about yourself or your actions? ("strongly")
Self-instruction	At the time, how strongly did you comment to yourself (probably silently, of course) how you ought to be behaving? ("strongly")

TABLE 2. Mean responses for four types of episode.

Topic	a Anxious	b Depressed	c Angry	d Happy	Significant differences
Overall imagery	63.1	66.7	67.4	77.0	ad
Visual imagery	61.3	59.9	65.0	78.8	ad,bd,cd
Auditory imagery	40.9	39.4	49.8	51.5	bd
Olfactory imagery	14.8	23.3	16.0	28.7	ab,ad,cd
Gustatory imagery	14.0	12.7	9.5	29.7	ad,bd,cd
Tactile imagery	29.2	34.4	27.4	52.2	ad,bd,cd
Proprioceptive imagery	42.9	41.9	40.2	59.0	ad,bd,cd
Colour extent	40.6	45.0	46.2	68.6	ad,bd,cd
Colour intensity	40.6	36.6	36.6	61.7	ad,bd,cd
Movement	40.8	33.8	49.5	53.6	ad,bc,bd
Stability	59.2	59.9	61.0	69.3	
Self-comment	63.5	68.1	67.9	49.3	ad,bd,cd
Self-instruction	61.3	59.7	56.7	37.5	ad,bd,cd

association with a positive emotion (happy) produced a response value that was numerically greater than each of those for negative emotions (anxious, depressed, and angry) for every single type of imagery question in Table 2. In the case of the questions concerning visual, gustatory, tactile, and proprioceptive imagery, and also those concerning the extent and intensity of coloured imagery, the responses for positive episodes were significantly greater in each case than each of the corresponding responses for negative episodes. Conversely, for the verbal components (self-comment and self-instruction) the responses for positive episodes were significantly lower than each of the corresponding responses for negative episodes. Figures 1 and 2 illustrate the findings for visual imagery and self-comment, respectively.

Of particular interest in the present context is that it can be seen from Table 2 that in not a single instance did the mean level of imagery for an anxious episode exceed the mean level for some other type of episode. This experiment therefore does not provide any evidence for the first of the three hypotheses outlined earlier, namely that anxious experiences are in general associated with relatively high levels of imagery. What, then, of the second hypothesis, that people with anxiety might experience in general higher levels of imagery?

3.2. Testing the second hypothesis

Three groups of twelve women each were selected from the normal population on the basis of their trait anxiety scores (Spielberger, 1966). The scores of all members of the high-anxiety and the low-anxiety groups were more extreme than the mean scores of the anxiety patients (51) and the control group (38), respectively, tested by Mathews and MacLeod (1985), while the medium-anxiety group had an intermediate score; the total range was 20 to 70.

Each subject in the study completed the Vividness of Visual Imagery Questionnaire (VVIQ) of Marks (1973). This widely used questionnaire asks respondents to think of four specific scenes, and in each case to judge (on a scale from 1 to 5) how vivid is their mental picture of each of four different aspects of the scene. For example, the first scene concerns a relative or friend of the subject, and the first aspect to be probed concerns the vividness of the exact contour of face, head, shoulders, and body.

The observed VVIQ scores ranged widely, from 32 to (the maximum) 80. The mean scores for the low, medium, and high anxiety groups were 56.1, 56.0, and 55.0, and did not differ significantly. The experiment did not, therefore, provide any evidence for the second hypothesis, that anxiety is associated with generally higher levels of imagery. We turn thus to the third hypothesis, that imagery is differentially associated with anxious and nonanxious experiences of people with anxiety.

3.3. Testing the third hypothesis

The same three groups of subjects as were described in the preceding section participated in this study. Each subject judged the imageability of each member of two groups of words. These words were the same as those used in a Stroop task by Mathews and MacLeod (1985), and consisted of 24 negative, potentially anxiety-provoking words (e.g., "disease", "foolish") together with 24 nonthreatening words (e.g., "confident", "holiday"). Imageability was assessed using the imagery procedure of Paivio, Yuille, & Madigan (1968), in which the ease of forming an image is assessed on a scale from 1 to 7. Only a small proportion of the words that were investigated are included in the extensive norms of Paivio ("Imagery and familiarity ratings for 2448 words", undated) or Toglia and Battig (1978).

Table 3 shows the mean imageability score for each word, both for each of the three groups of subject separately and also for the three groups combined.

332

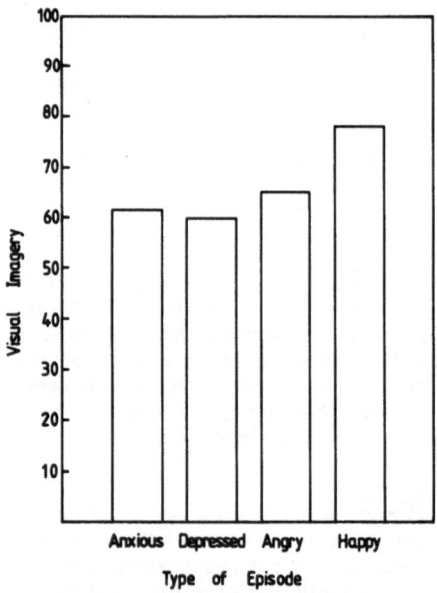

FIGURE 1. Mean judgements of visual imagery for four types of episode.

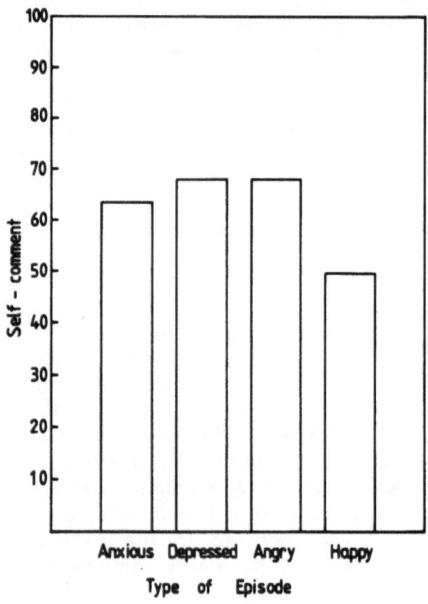

FIGURE 2. Mean judgements of self-comment for four types of episode.

TABLE 3. Mean imagery values for three anxiety groups.

Word	Low	Medium	High	Overall	Paivio
			Threat words		
Ambulance	6.67	6.75	6.58	6.67	6.67
Cancer	5.08	5.00	4.75	4.94	-
Coffin	6.33	6.67	6.50	6.50	-
Coronary	5.25	4.42	4.08	4.58	-
Criticised	3.17	3.83	2.67	3.22	-
Deathbed	5.50	5.67	5.58	5.58	-
Disease	4.58	4.50	4.08	4.39	4.87
Embarrassed	4.58	4.83	4.08	4.50	-
Emergency	5.92	5.08	5.00	5.33	5.03
Failure	3.33	3.00	3.17	3.17	-
Fatal	5.25	5.08	4.25	4.86	-
Foolish	3.50	3.00	2.50	3.00	-
Hated	2.67	4.00	3.33	3.33	-
Hazard	5.17	3.92	3.17	4.08	-
Inadequate	3.00	4.08	2.08	3.06	-
Indecisive	2.92	3.33	2.42	2.89	2.81
Inept	2.83	3.08	1.92	2.61	-
Inferior	2.92	2.92	2.17	2.67	-
Injury	6.17	5.92	5.25	5.78	5.70
Lonely	4.25	4.58	4.75	4.53	4.31
Mutilated	6.08	5.00	5.50	5.53	-
Paralysed	5.58	5.83	5.33	5.58	-
Pathetic	3.08	3.92	2.83	3.28	-
Stupid	3.42	4.00	2.83	3.42	-
			Nonthreat words		
Aloof	4.33	3.50	2.50	3.44	-
Assured	3.42	4.08	2.50	3.33	-
Bold	3.38	3.42	2.50	3.25	-
Capable	3.92	4.33	2.92	3.72	2.66
Carefree	4.42	4.58	2.92	3.97	4.34
Cocky	4.58	5.00	4.17	4.58	-
Confident	4.58	5.25	3.50	4.44	3.63
Contented	4.92	5.17	4.17	4.75	-
Entertainment	6.08	5.58	4.58	5.50	-
Genial	2.83	2.83	2.17	2.61	-
Hobby	5.83	5.42	3.58	4.94	-
Holiday	6.25	6.00	6.25	6.17	
Leisure	5.50	5.58	3.08	4.72	-
Melody	4.25	4.92	4.42	4.53	-
Merriment	5.83	4.75	3.58	4.72	-
Optimistic	4.00	4.42	3.17	3.86	3.47

TABLE 3 (cont.)

	Nonthreat words				
Word	Low	Medium	High	Overall	Paivio
Overjoyed	5.08	5.50	3.50	4.69	4.16
Playful	5.75	5.33	4.00	5.03	4.56
Reassured	2.83	3.08	2.50	2.81	–
Relaxed	4.08	4.75	3.58	4.14	
Satisfaction	3.50	3.17	2.75	3.14	–
Secure	4.08	3.50	2.33	3.31	3.41
Welcome	4.58	5.42	3.58	4.53	–
Windfall	5.42	3.67	3.83	4.31	–

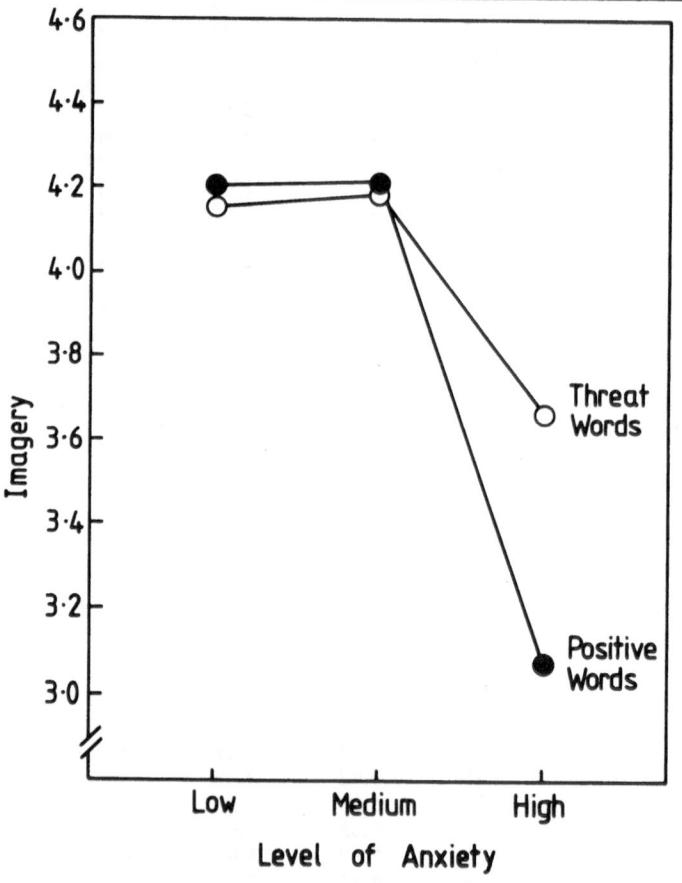

FIGURE 3. Mean judgements of imagery value for three levels of anxiety.

Also shown, where available, are the corresponding scores reported by Paivio. The agreement between the present scores and those of Paivio for the 13 words in common, $r(11) = 0.92$, was high.

Figure 3 displays the most important aspect of these results, which was that highly anxious individuals have very low levels of imagery for nonthreatening words or, alternatively expressed, yield much higher values for the ratio of imagery associated with threatening words to that associated with nonthreatening words. That is, it appears to be the balance of imagery between anxious and nonanxious experiences which is changed by high levels of anxiety.

4. DISCUSSION

The finding that high levels of anxiety are associated with a shift towards more pronounced imagery for threatening material (relative to nonthreatening material) provides support for the last of the three hypotheses outlined earlier. It appears thus that the effects of anxiety conform to the propagational theory for the cognitive effects of emotion outlined earlier, insofar as the relative enhancement of imagery for threatening material may be expected itself to lead to intensification of the anxiety state. Further, it may be noted that the fact that such enhancement appears to be only relative, and not absolute, could account for the observation that severe imagery among anxiety patients may become apparent only with detailed probing (Beck et al., 1985; Clark & Beck, in press). It is possible that overall such patients experience less imagery than do other people, but that what imagery they do experience is unusually threatening. In principle, this possibility may be examined directly by similar further research sampling among appropriate clinical populations.

5. ACKNOWLEDGEMENTS

The author thanks Tim Beck and David Clark for discussion, Kathy Clayden for experimental assistance, and the Medical Research Council for financial support.

REFERENCES

1. Beck, A.T. (1986). Cognitive approaches to anxiety disorders. In B.F. Shaw, Z.V. Segal, T.M. Vallis, & F.E. Cashman (Eds.), Anxiety disorders: Psychological and biological perspectives. New York: Plenum.
2. Beck, A.T., Emery, G., & Greenberg, R.L. (1985). Anxiety disorders and phobias: A cognitive perspective. New York: Basic Books.
3. Beck, A.T., Rush, A.J., Shaw, B.F., & Emery, G. (1979). Cognitive therapy of depression. New York: Guilford Press.
4. Breuer, J., & Freud, S. (1936). Studies in hysteria. (A.A. Brill, Trans.). New York: Avon Books. (original work published 1895).
5. Clark, D.M., & Beck, A.T. (in press). Cognitive approaches. In C. Last & M. Hersen (Eds.), Handbook of anxiety disorders. New York: Pergamon.
6. Clark, D.M., Teasdale, J.D., Broadbent, D., & Martin, M. (1983). Effect of mood on lexical decision. Bulletin of the Psychonomic Society, 21, 175-178.
7. Lazarus, R.S. (1966). Psychological stress and the coping process. New York: McGraw-Hill.
8. Marks, D.F. (1973). Visual imagery differences in the recall of pictures. British Journal of Psychology, 64, 17-24.
9. Martin, M. (1985a). Induction of depressed mood in the laboratory. American Journal of Psychology, 98, 635-639.
10. Martin, M. (1985b). Neuroticism as predisposition towards depression: A cognitive mechanism. Personality and Individual Differences, 6, 353-365.

11. Martin, M. (1986). On the induction of mood. Manuscript submitted for publication.
12. Martin, M. (in press). Imagery and emotion in episodic memory. In D.G. Russell & D.F. Marks (Eds.), Imagery 2. Dunedin, New Zealand: Human Performance Associates.
13. Martin, M., & Clark, D.M. (1986). Recall as a function of self reference in depressed mood. Manuscript in preparation.
14. Mathews, A., & MacLeod, C. (1985). Selective processing of threat cues in anxiety states. Behaviour Research and Therapy, 23, 563-569.
15. Mathews, A., & MacLeod, C. (1986). Discrimination of threat cues without awareness in anxiety states. Journal of Abnormal Psychology, 95, 131-138.
16. Paivio, A., Yuille, J.C., & Madigan, S.A. (1968). Concreteness, imagery, and meaningfulness values for 925 nouns. Journal of Experimental Psychology Monographs, 76, (1, Pt. 2).
17. Toglia, M.P., & Battig, W.F. (1978). Handbook of semantic word norms. Hillsdale, NJ: Lawrence Erlbaum Associates.
18. Spielberger, C.D. (1966). The effects of anxiety on complex learning and academic achievement. In C.D. Spielberger (Ed.), Anxiety and behaviour. New York: Academic Press.
19. Wolpe, J. (1958). Psychotherapy by reciprocal inhibition. Stanford: Stanford University Press.

IMAGES IN AUTOBIOGRAPHICAL MEMORY

MARTIN A. CONWAY

MRC, APPLIED PSYCHOLOGY UNIT, CAMBRIDGE, ENGLAND

ABSTRACT
Current models of imagery emphasise the process of imaging and give little consideration to the function images might serve. Thus, many imagery effects, such as the beneficial effects of imaging upon remembering, are not addressed by these models. This paper proposes a functional approach to imagery in which images facilitate the retrieval of information from memories of complex events. Implications of this approach for current models of imagery are considered.

1. INTRODUCTION
Recent research and theory into imagery has focussed on how imaging may occur and current models postulate mechanisms or algorithms which subserve imaging (Kosslyn & Schwartz, 1977; Pinker, this volume; Slack, this volume). As a consequence of this bias towards postulating imagery 'mechanisms', questions relating to why images occur in human cognition have been neglected. However, as Marr (1982) pointed out, models which posit mechanisms but do not consider the function of those mechanisms fail to specify the information-processing problem which a mechanism is intended to solve. Hence, perhaps, the limited explanatory range of current models.

In this paper, findings which suggest a central role for imagery in memory for complex events, and for which current 'process' models of imagery do not provide an account, will be outlined. On this basis a functional role for imagery in autobiographical memory will be considered. Finally, ways in which current models of imagery may be expanded to accommodate a broader range of imagery effects will be discussed.

2. THE 'PROCESS' APPROACH TO IMAGERY
One way in which imagery has been modelled is in terms of a 'process' in which images are 'generated' from underlying memory representations. By this approach, image generation is assumed to comprise a number of processing stages and these stages indicate the functioning of modular mechanisms or algorithms. This process of image generation is explicitly stated in a model proposed by Kosslyn & Shwartz (1977), and it is this which is considered first.

2.1. A process model
Kosslyn & Shwartz (1977; see also Kosslyn, 1980) postulated that the imaging process comprises a number of separate computational 'modules'. Three key modules considered by Kosslyn & Shwartz are the PICTURE, PUT, and FIND modules. The PICTURE module is hypothesised to locate a long-term memory description of the to-be-imaged item and to generate the corresponding image, the PUT module locates parts of the image relative to each other, and the FIND module acts as an inspection routine which

337

M. Denis et al. (eds.), Cognitive and Neuropsychological Approaches to Mental Imagery, 337–345.
© *1988 by Martinus Nijhoff Publishers.*

identifies spatial patterns in the image and passes this information to the PUT module.

Kosslyn (1980) provides an overview of findings from a range of studies which support these putative modules. For example, image generation times have been found to increase as more detail is added to an image, time to scan between parts in an image is a function of the 'distance' between the parts, and imaging smaller images takes less time than imaging larger images. More recently Kosslyn, Holtzman, Farah & Gazzaniga (1986) found functional dissociations between different types of imagery tasks performed in the right and left hemispheres of 'split-brain' patients.

However, the tasks employed by Kosslyn and his colleagues are somewhat unusual and entail the construction of types of images that are, perhaps, atypical of the types of images recurrent in everyday cognition (e.g. imaging a frying pan floating 6ft (1.8m) above a bicycle; imaging objects at subjectively small or large sizes). Furthermore, the content of images studied by Kosslyn and others has been restricted to imaging single or small sets of otherwise unrelated objects. Given this reified approach, it is important to consider what imagery function is taken as being supported by findings from such studies.

2.2. Imagery functions in the process approach

Kosslyn and his colleagues (1980) appear to regard the main function of imagery as being the vicarious manipulation of objects. For example, Kosslyn et al. (1986; p.311) comment that "Images...for many people only come to mind when they try to answer questions such as, What shape are a beagle's ears? Which is larger, a goat or a hog? Or, how would your sofa look against the opposite wall in your living room?" However, imaging isolated objects in everyday cognition or making comparisons between pairs of imaged objects may constitute relatively infrequent uses of imagery. In contrast, a frequent use of imagery may be in the recollection of past events and this is considered in further detail below.

A more developed version of this function of imagery has been proposed by Neisser (1976) and Shepard (1978). Their argument is that imagery confers a survival advantage by allowing an animal to anticipate in some analog form possible future events. So 'what to do when attacked by a lion' can be prepared for by imaging potential encounters as can 'how to behave when attending an important interview'. Thus, the process view assumes that the main function of imagery is to provide a way in which information about possible and future states of the world may be vicariously manipulated.

Perhaps the first point to note is that the imagery function assumed by the process view requires images and image manipulations which have not been investigated or considered by proponents of this view. To be adaptive, images would have to represent fairly complex scenes featuring extended action sequences. It seems unlikely that the types of mechanisms postulated by current imagery models could deliver a solution to the information-processing problems posed by such evolutionary demands. Findings within the process approach have shown that imaging is a relatively effortful and unstable process (Kosslyn & Shwartz, 1977; Kosslyn, Reiser, Farah & Fliegel, 1983). Furthermore, imagery appears to be unsuitable for certain types of manipulations (Hinton, 1979) and is inadequate for representing ambiguous states of the world (Mani & Johnson-Laird, 1982). Hence, it is unclear whether images, as currently conceived, could be used to represent complex extended actions and it has yet to be demonstrated that people can in fact use imagery in this way.

Of course imagery used in conjunction with other cognitive abilities such as the ability to build a mental model of a problem (Johnson-Laird, 1983) may form part of a very effective ability to anticipate states of the world. Yet the principle function of imagery when used in such a way may be quite different from the function of imagery assumed by the process approach and may entail imagery processes which have not been previously considered.

3. IMAGERY & REMEMBERING

It has been argued that the functional role assigned to imagery in the process approach is at least questionable. This section considers a number of findings relating to imagery which are problematic for the process approach and suggest a rather different functional role for imagery.

3.1. Remembering words

One of the most well established findings from the laboratory is that imagery gives rise to comparatively good memory performance for a variety of episodically learned verbal materials (cf. Paivio, 1972, 1986; Richardson, 1980, for reviews). The types of explanations provided for these effects typically postulate some form of privileged encoding induced by the act of imaging (Bower, 1973; Paivio, 1972). Such explanations converge on the view that imaging leads to a form of encoding which facilitates remembering.

Clearly, this is an important aspect of imagery for which any model of imagery must be able to provide some sort of account. Yet the process approach, with its emphasis on image generation and manipulation, makes no obvious predictions concerning imaging and remembering. Indeed Kosslyn & Alper (1977) found that imagery manipulations of subjective sizes of imaged objects had only small and inconsistent effects upon memory. Nevertheless, if the process approach is to (eventually) lead to a general account of imagery it should be able to at least tentatively suggest why, for example, instructions to image two items gives rise to better recall than instructions to generate a sentence containing the same two items (Bower & Winzenz, 1970).

3.2. Remembering experiences

A number of recent findings from the area of autobiographical memory demonstrate a further set of imagery effects which will have to be incorporated in any comprehensive account of imagery.

Conway & Bekerian (1987) conducted a series of primed autobiographical memory retrieval experiments. In these experiments subjects read a 'lifetime period' prime, e.g. 'Schooldays', and semantic primes, e.g. 'Furniture'. Subjects then retrieved a specific autobiographical memory to subsequently presented 'personal history' cues such as 'Holiday in Italy' or semantic cues such as 'Chair'. In one experiment (Experiment 3) the memories were rated for detail and specificity. Memories retrieved to personal history cues were rated as being reliably more specific and detailed than memories retrieved to semantic cues. However, memories retrieved to personal history cues were retrieved reliably faster than memories retrieved to semantic cues. Clearly this finding does not fit well with the claim that more detailed images take longer to retrieve than less detailed images (Kosslyn et al, 1983).

A related finding was obtained by Conway & Bekerian (1987). In this study subjects imaged typical emotional scenes and image generation times were taken. No instructions concerning the type of image were given and subjects were simply instructed to generate a specific image as quickly as possible. It was found that on over 70% of occasions subjects spontaneously retrieved detailed memories of events in which they themselves had experienced the emotion. The remaining images were comprised of scenes from television and cinema in which others experienced the emotion. In a further study Conway (in preparation) found that spontaneously retrieved autobiographical memories of emotional experiences were reliably rated as being more detailed and specific than images drawn from television. There were, however, no differences in retrieval times between the two types of memories in either experiment. Thus the claim that amount of detail determines image generation time does not appear to necessarily hold for images in the form of recalled autobiographical experiences.

A further intriguing finding in these two experiments was that subjects reliably reported marked temporary mood-shifts when imaging events they themselves had participated in. Images based on television and cinema did not, however, give rise to marked temporary mood-shifts. Thus, different types of images appear to be differentially associated with mood reinstatement.

Another area of imagery research, that of image vividness, presents a further set of problems for the process approach. Brown & Kulik (1977) found that certain types of events may give rise to highly vivid autobiographical memories. For example, in the Brown & Kulik study, subjects reported being able to bring to mind detailed and vivid images of where they were, who they were with, and what happened, when they heard about the assassination of John F. Kennedy. Similar images were reported for events of high personal importance such as the death of a close relative. Rubin & Kozin (1984) found that personal importance of an event was the best predictor of vividness of memories. Conway & Bekerian (1986) and Conway (in preparation), however, found that consequentiality, change in on-going activity, and change in emotional experience at the time the event occurred were the best predictors of vividness.

For present purposes the main point to be drawn from these studies is that the vividness of images of experienced events varies in systematic ways, and that more vivid images are associated with events of high personal importance and which represent sharp changes in experience.

3.3 Why images?

Research into imagery and memory poses two types of problems for the process approach. Firstly, findings in this area do not unequivocally support specific aspects of the process model. Secondly, many of the findings appear to lie outside the scope of the model. These findings, however, raise a number of questions concerning the function of imagery.

Perhaps the most obvious question concerns why we have images of experienced events. There are a number of reasons for regarding imagery as a poor representational form for experienced events. For instance, experienced events are typically extended in time, may involve a number of actors, different action sequences, and in some cases multiple locations (e.g. holiday in Italy; wedding day; this morning's breakfast). Clearly, an image can only represent a fraction of the information about any event and more complex memory structures must be employed for more detailed representations (Schank, 1982; Brewer, 1986). Yet it is not clear how detailed representations of complex events may be searched for specific information. The focus of recent studies (Reiser, Black & Abelson, 1985; Conway & Bekerian, 1987; Conway, 1987) has been on how autobiographical memories might be located in memory rather than on how such memories might be searched once located.

Thus, a specific information-processing problem which arises from the study of autobiographical memory is that of how to search complex memories once a memory has been accessed. One way in which this problem might be solved would be to provide some form of summary information which could be used to direct search of a memory. Possibly, images serve to represent summary information which retrieval processes may use to search a trace.

It might be objected that such summary information could be represented in a number of ways, for example as a list of features rather than in an image. Indeed there are a number of ways in which a memory might be searched and certainly not all the information associated with a memory nor all autobiographical information will be imaginal in form (Brewer, 1986; Conway, 1987). Nevertheless, images may constitute both a more economical and qualitatively different way of representing information which could not be achieved with, say, a list. For instance, information in an image may be comprised of features of an event and relations between those features. Featural relations might be implicit in the image so that various relations would only be apparent when the image was scanned in a particular way. In contrast, list scanning would be heavily dependent upon linear searches and so a list form of representation would lack the inherent informativeness of an analog representation. Furthermore, an image may represent configurations of features in which conjunctions of features were easily accessible and, possibly, these configurations and conjunctions may further assist retrieval processes. Other types of representation would not provide this economy of representation.

Images, then, may contain information which is maximally informative about a represented event – in the sense that information in the image facilitates access to other less directly accessible information in the trace – but the image itself may be accessed with minimal cognitive effort. Possibly, images are automatically generated once a complex memory trace is accessed. The information contained in an image may be employed by retrieval processes as powerful cues with which to 'probe' the trace.

Consider the following protocol (Conway, in progress) provided by a thirty-five year old subject when asked to recall her wedding-day:
"Well the first thing which comes to mind is the registry office. I can clearly see (closes her eyes) Paul who was wearing a green velvet suit, my parents and my in-laws, also Susan and Dee who were my bridesmaids and Paul's friend Ian – he was bestman – standing in a semi-circle around a big mahogany desk upon which the registrar was organising some papers. This was just before the ceremony started."

Note that the image (the subject indicated that she had been describing an image) contains information about the principle actors, actions, location, and some temporal information relating to the event. Clearly, this information could be employed to search for further specific details of the event. In fact in this protocol, the subject subsequently employed some of the above information to search for further information (and surprised herself by the recall of 'forgotten' events). Other images were generated during the course of the recall and these varied in their vividness and in whether the information they contained was employed in further attempts at recall. In general the protocols provided by a number of subjects indicated that information in images could be elaborated upon in order to access further information related to an event (see also Whitten & Leonard, 1981).

This evidence at least suggests that images may be employed to search complex memories. Images, then, may be part of a solution to the problem of how to access information within a complex memory trace. Such a view imposes constraints on any eventual model of imagery and in particular only certain types of information would be expected to be represented in images. For instance, fine-grained details, because of their lack of generality to the memory as a whole, would not facilitate retrieval and therefore would be unlikely to be preserved in an image.

4. A REPRESENTATIONAL APPROACH TO IMAGERY

The view being developed here is that a major function of imagery is to facilitate memory retrieval. In contrast to the 'process' approach, the current approach emphasises both the representational qualities of images (the type of information which images contain) and how this information may be processed (how retrieval processes can operate upon information in an image). Accordingly images should have certain fairly specific characteristics.

If images do represent information which can be exploited by retrieval processes to search a trace then, typically, the information in an image will not be unique relative to other information in the trace. For the information represented in an image to facilitate further retrieval, it must correspond to similar information stored in other parts of the memory (Tulving & Thompson, 1973). Images, to be effective retrieval aids, should represent information which maps onto many parts of a memory trace. By this argument, the information in an image should represent general information about a memory and not specific details. Images of experienced events appear to have just this property (Conway & Bekerian, 1987; Conway, in preparation).

One implication of the above line of reasoning is that images will not be veridical representations of past events. Rather, images will typically represent some aspects of an experienced event if those aspects are common to the memory representation of the whole event. Thus, it is quite possible that an image of some past event represents features of that event but the conjunction of those features in the image constitutes an experience which did not in fact occur. Images of past experiences need not then correspond to an actual experience, but only to the representation of that experience. Of course in practice, it may be that images usually correspond both to an experience and to the representation of the event of which that experience was a part. In this way then people may experience difficulties in deciding on the basis of a retrieved image whether the scene depicted by the image did in fact occur.

A further property of images which would be essential if they were to facilitate memory retrieval would be the ability to attend to various parts of an image and possibly to be able to manipulate these parts. However, as it is assumed that images do not contain details of an experience (because these serve no useful purpose in retrieval), then it seems implausible that there should be a way in which to gain a fine degree of resolution of an image. Rather, focussing on part of an image for retrieval purposes only requires a relatively crude resolving power. Similarly, the ability to manipulate information in images may relate to the function of an image for retrieval purposes and this may require only relatively simple manipulations (Hinton, 1979).

Information represented in a memory of a complex event (e.g. a holiday in Italy) may be accessed by a number of images, some of which contain fewer details than others. Furthermore, some of these images may contain information which maps onto many aspects of the event whereas other images may contain information which maps onto few aspects of the event. It does not, of course, follow that amount of information in an image correlates with the amount of event-related information that image can, potentially, be used to access. Thus, it seems reasonable to conclude that the amount of information an image contains is unlikely to be reflected in any simple way in reaction times or ratings of an image.

In terms of the retrieval function of images postulated here, it would make sense for images which access more of the trace information to be more available once the trace has been accessed. Perhaps, one way in which this is achieved is by making some images more 'vivid' than others. How this is achieved and what determines vividness are empirical questions beyond the scope of the present discussion. Nevertheless if vividness does reflect the retrieval strength of an image then it should be the case that highly vivid images are retrieved before less vivid images and give rise to the subsequent retrieval of a comparatively larger amount of event-related information than less vivid images.

One final aspect of images as retrieval aids is that they should facilitate the operation of more general retrieval processes and so help to raise the availability of related memories which they themselves cannot be used to directly access. As reported earlier, images of experienced events have been found to induce mild temporary mood-shifts. This mood-induction property of images may initiate some form of mood-congruency effect in memory (Bower & Cohen, 1982; Teasdale, 1983) and make mood-related memories more available for subsequent retrieval.

5. CONCLUSIONS

It has been argued that the explanatory power of current 'process' models of imagery does not extend to a broad range of imagery findings. This may be because of the assumption of the process approach that images are primarily employed to make vicarious manipulations of states of the world. In contrast, the representational approach to imagery emphasises the role of imagery in memory and focuses on the content of images rather than the processes by which images are instantiated cognitively. Images are considered to provide information which retrieval processes can exploit in searching for information about complex events. As Johnson-Laird (1983; p.157) has proposed "images correspond to views of models", and in this case the models are representations of experienced events.

Although the focus of the representational view is upon the nature of images and not the process of imaging, it is unlikely that these two aspects of imagery can be so simply separated. Retrieved images must be temporally maintained while retrieval processes operate upon them and this may involve representation in some form of quasi-perceptual imagery 'medium' (Kosslyn, 1980) or other temporary storage device such as a visuo-spatial sketchpad (Baddeley, 1986). Thus, characteristics of images will in part be determined by the use an image is to be put to and in part by the nature of the representational medium itself.

An approach which focusses upon properties of the representational medium, rather than the function of the representation, may not accurately distinguish between processes which are supported by the medium but are incidental to the main function of the medium. For example, the processes which mediate imaging items at different subjective sizes may be a product of the quasi-perceptual nature of the imagery medium and may serve no particular purpose in using images to search memory traces. Similarly, findings such as an increase in image generation time with increasing imagery detail may relate to properties of the imagery medium rather than images per se. In the process of creating a novel image composed of clearly separate and (in some cases) unrelated parts then processing time may be lengthened as parts are 'read' into the image as Kosslyn (1980) proposes. The operation of PUT and FIND modules may further lengthen generation time. However, for the generation of an image relating to a previously experienced event perhaps only a PICTURE module is involved and the image is read as a whole into the representational medium. In this case PUT and FIND modules may only be employed after image generation and serve to isolate features of the image upon which retrieval processes can operate. These are, however, empirical questions and it has yet to be demonstrated that people either can or do generate and manipulate images of experienced events in this way.

The main conclusion to be drawn from the above arguments is that the eventual development of a comprehensive model of imagery will have to feature, as a central part, an account of the function of imagery in human cognition. Such an approach, at the very least, compels us to consider not only what people can do with images but also the use of such images. Moreover, a model which contains an account of the sorts of information-processing problems which imagery solves may help distinguish incidental from central properties of images.

REFERENCES

Baddeley, A. (1986). Working memory. Oxford: Oxford University Press.
Bower, G.H. (1972). Mental imagery and associative learning. In L. Gregg (ed). Cognition in Learning and Memory, New York: Wiley.
Bower, G.H., & Cohen, P.R. (1982). Emotional influences in memory and thinking: data and theory. In M.S. Clark & S.T. Fiske (eds) Affect and Cognition, Hillsdale, N.J.: LEA.
Bower, G.H. & Winzenz, D. (1970). Comparison of associative learning strategies. Psychonomic Science, 20, 119-20.
Brewer, W.F. (1986). What is autobiographical memory. In D.C. Rubin (ed) Autobiographical Memory, Cambridge: Cambridge University Press.
Brown, R. & Kulik, J. (1977). Flashbulb memories. Cognition, 5, 73-99.
Conway, M.A. (1987). Verifying autobiographical facts. Cognition, 25, (in press).
Conway, M.A. Imaging emotional scenes. In preparation.
Conway, M.A. Recalling memories of emotional experiences. In preparation.
Conway, M.A. Searching autobiographical memory. In progress.
Conway, M.A. & Bekerian, D.A. (1987). Organization in autobiographical memory. Memory and Cognition, 15, 2, 119-132.
Conway, M.A., & Bekerian, D.A. (1987). Schematic representations of emotional situations. Cognition and Emotion, 2, in press.
Conway, M.A., & Bekerian, D.A. (1986). Vivid memories: encoding or recoding? Manuscript submitted for publication.
Hinton, G. (1979). Some demonstrations of the effects of structural descriptions in mental imagery. Cognitive Science, 3, 231-250.
Johnson-Laird, P.N. (1983). Mental models. Cambridge: Cambridge University Press.
Kosslyn, S.M. (1980). Image and mind. Cambridge, M.A.: Harvard University Press.
Kosslyn, S.M., & Alper, S.N. (1977). On the pictorial properties of visual images: effects of image size on memory for words. Canadian Journal of Psychology, 31, 32-40.

Kosslyn, S.M., Holtzman, J.D., Farah, M.J., & Gazzaniga, M.S. (1986). A computational analysis of mental image generation: evidence from functional dissociations in split-brain patients. Journal of Experimental Psychology: General, 114, 311-341.

Kosslyn, S.M., Reiser, B.J., Farah, M.J., & Fliegel, S.J. (1983). Generating visual images: units and relations. Journal of Experimental Psychology: General, 112, 278-303.

Kosslyn, S.M., & Shwartz, S.P. (1977). A simulation of visual imagery. Cognitive Science, 1, 265-295.

Mani, K., & Johnson-Laird, P.N. (1982). The mental representation of spatial descriptions. Memory & Cognition, 10, 181-7.

Marr, D. (1982). Vision. San Francisco: Freeman.

Neisser, U. (1976). Cognition and reality: principles and implications of cognitive psychology. San Francisco: Freeman.

Paivio, A. (1972). Imagery and verbal processes. New York: Holt, Rinehart and Winston.

Paivio, A. (1986). Mental representations: a dual coding approach. Oxford: Oxford University Press.

Reiser, B.J., Black, J.B., & Abelson, R.P. (1985). Knowledge structures in the organization and retrieval of autobiographical memories. Cognitive Psychology, 17, 89-137.

Richardson, J.T.E. (1980). Mental imagery and human memory. London: Macmillan.

Rubin, D.C., & Kozin, M. (1984). Vivid memories. Cognition, 16, 81-96.

Schank, R.C. (1982). Dynamic memory: a theory of reminding and learning in computers and people. New York: Cambridge University Press.

Shepard, R.N. (1978). The mental image. American Psychologist, 33, 125-137.

Teasdale, J.D. (1983). Affect and accessibility. Philosophical Transactions of the Royal Society, B, 302, 403-412.

Tulving, E., & Thompson, D.M. (1973). Encoding specificity and retrieval processes in episodic memory. Psychology Review, 80, 352-373.

Whitten, W.B. & Leonard, J.M. (1981). Directed search through autobiographical memory. Memory and Cognition, 9, 566-579.

EMOTIONAL IMAGERY AND COGNITIVE REPRESENTATION OF EMOTION: AN ATTEMPT TO VALIDATE LANG'S BIO-INFORMATIONAL MODEL

ALBERTO ACOSTA, JAIME VILA and ALFONSO PALMA

UNIVERSITY OF GRANADA, SPAIN

ABSTRACT
    In two experiments female students exhibiting fear of rats were differentially trained in stimulus versus response imagination. Subsequently they were presented with fear provoking and non-fear provoking scene descriptions including only stimulus propositions or including stimulus and response propositions (manipulated within subjects in Exp. I and between groups in Exp. II). Greater changes in heart rate were observed in both experiments during the description and imagination of the fear provoking scenes in the groups trained to imagine response information as compared with the groups trained to imagine stimulus information. The results are consistent with Lang's model concerning the cognitive representation of emotional imagery.

1. INTRODUCTION

    Many therapy techniques such as systematic desensitization, flooding and cover conditioning, make use of emotional images in order to modify patients' behavior. Some of these techniques can be applied "in vivo", but therapists usually prefer to apply them via the imagination, probably because real events are more difficult to control and adapt to the therapeutic context than imagined ones. However, in spite of the prevalent use of emotional images in a clinical context, theoretical models dealing with mental emotional imagery are scarce. Lang (1977, 1978, 1979) has developed one of the few models based on images as they are used and generated in behavior therapy techniques and has published some experimental data in support of it (Lang et al., 1980; Miller et al., 1981). Subsequently, Lang (1984, 1985) has generalized the model in order to deal with the cognitive events that determine the central representation and expression of emotional responses.
    Lang's model is based on Pylyshyn's (1973) and Kieras's (1978) notions on images as well as on Sperry's (1952) concept of the brain. According to Pylyshyn and Kieras, the image is an elaborated description and an integration of specific statements about the world. It is something that is functionally organized, a finite group of propositions which mediates the coding, storage and retrieval of any information, independently of its modality. On the other hand, in accordance with Sperry, Lang considers that the basic function of the brain is not to generate perceptual

M. Denis et al. (eds.), Cognitive and Neuropsychological Approaches to Mental Imagery, 347–354.

experience, but to organize and facilitate action. Lang et al. (1980, p. 180) state:

"The emotional image is seen here as a logical program of information, like those which provide a meaningful integration of stimulus input, but also organizing efferent information (somatic and visceral), and thus having the functional properties of a perceptual-motor set. Our view of the image is both propositional and constructional (Kieras, 1978; Pylyshyn, 1973). That is, the emotional image is not understood to be an internal apprehension, a picture scanned by the mind's eye, but a finite information structure in the brain which can be reduced to specific propositional units. Consonant with the concept of the image as an integration of perceptual and motor elements, the propositions which form the image structure designate both stimulus and response events."

Lang et al. (1980) and Miller et al. (1981) have published some experimental data in support of the model. In these studies control over the informational structure of the image was achieved in two ways: firstly, through differential training of the subjects in stimulus versus response imagination; and secondly, through differential manipulation of the propositional structure of the scripts presented to the subjects (including only stimulus propositions or including both stimulus and response propositions).

The results by Lang and his associates indicate higher physiological activation when the subjects are trained in response imagination and when the scripts presented to them include response propositions. Other researchers have also reported data which seem to support the model. In this context we have carried out two experiments with the purpose of improving on some methodological weaknesses encountered in the literature -such as the screening of the subjects- and to obtain an independent validation of the model.

2. EXPERIMENT I

Subjects were 24 female students evidencing fear of rats. They were assigned to three groups following a blocking procedure according to their subjective and behavioral fear scores: non-training group, stimulus-training group, and response-training group.

Subjects in the training groups had two training sessions in which they had to imagine scenes either including only stimulus propositions or including stimulus and response propositions. Subjects in the stimulus-training group were differentially reinforced for reporting stimulus information during the imagination such as colours, shapes, sizes,etc. Subjects in the response-training group were differentially reinforced for reporting response information during the imagination such as cardiac activation, muscular tension, sweating, etc.

In the laboratory session all subjects had to imagine two non-fear provoking and two fear provoking scenes. One of the two scenes of each type was presented including only stimulus propositions, the other including stimulus and response propositions. The content of the scene and type of script were balanced within each group. All the scenes were presented through earphones. Subjects were instructed to imagine the scenes as vividly as possible. In addition, trained subjects were instructed to imagine the scenes according to the training previously received. Each scene presentation had the following sequence: a) one minute relaxation period; b) description period; c) imagination period; d) quiet period.

Heart rate and electrodermal activity were recorded during the laboratory session. The dependent variables were changes in physiological activity from the relaxation period to the other periods.

Two analyses of the data were carried out: one including the non-training group and other excluding it. When the three groups were included, the results showed significant differences as a function of content of the scene and period, both in heart rate, $F (2,42)= 23.33$, $p < .00001$, and in skin conductance level, $F (2,15)= 3.84$, $p < .03$. (Due to recording difficulties two subjects in each group were excluded from the electrodermal activity analysis). Fear provoking scenes produced greater changes in heart rate during the description (mean = 7.46 bpm) and imagination (mean = 6.72 bpm) periods than non-fear provoking scenes (description mean = 2.75 bpm; imagination mean = 1.69 bpm), but not during the quiet period. In a similar way, fear provoking scenes produced greater changes in skin conductance level during the imagination period (mean = 0.0149 micromhos) than the non-fear provoking scenes (mean = -0.1272 micromhos).

When the non-training group was not included in the analysis, the results showed a significant effect of the interaction Group X Content X Period in heart rate, $F (2,28)= 3.40$, $p < .04$. In skin conductance level an effect close to significance was observed for the interaction Group X Period, $F (2,20)= 2.77$, $p < .08$, and the interaction Script X Period, $F (2,20)= 2.96$, $p < .07$. As can be seen in Figure 1, the response-training group had higher cardiac activation during the description and imagination of the fear provoking scenes than the stimulus-training group. The differences disappeared during the quiet period. Regarding skin conductance level, the stimulus-training group tended to have greater decreases throughout the periods; on the other hand, the response scripts tended to produce lesser decreases throughout the periods.

3. EXPERIMENT II

In experiment II a number of methodological variations were introduced. Type of script was manipulated between groups; three kinds of scene were used: neutral, action, and fear; in the laboratory session three scenes of each type were presented; only one training session was given; and groups were matched, in addition to subjective fear andbehavioral avoidance, in physiological reactivity to auditory stimulation.

Subjects were 72 female students evidencing fear of rats. Following a similar procedure to the one used in experiment I, they were assigned to three groups: non-training group,

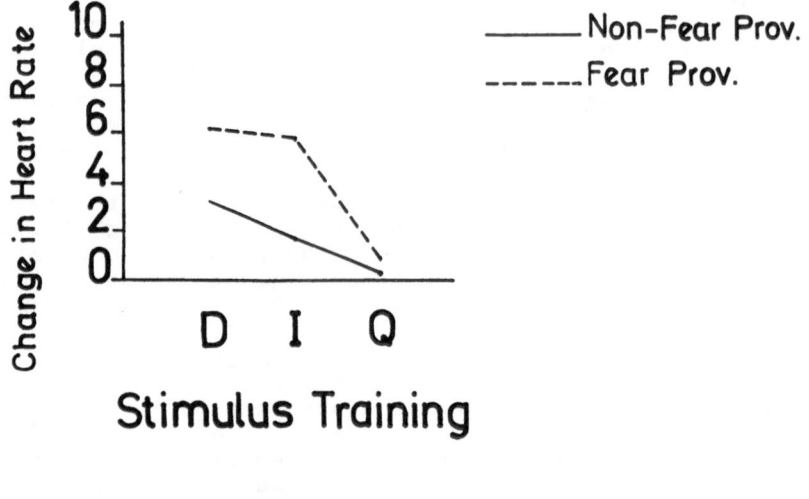

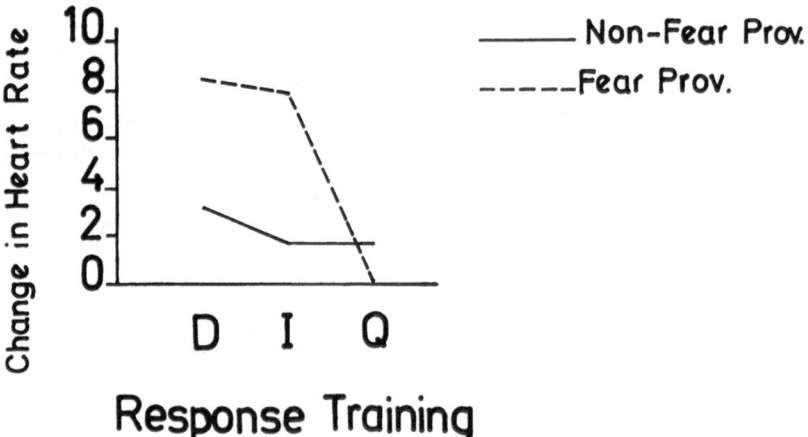

Figure 1. Change in heart rate in the training groups according
to period (D: description ; I: imagination ; Q: quiet)
and content of the scenes (Exp. I).

stimulus-training group and response-training group. Half of the subjects in each group received scripts including only stimulus propositions, the other half including stimulus and response propositions. The neutral scenes were always presented containing only stimulus propositions.

As in experiment I, two analyses of the data were carried out: including the non-training group and excluding it. In the first analysis, significant effects were obtained for the interaction Content X Period, both in heart rate, $F_{(4,264)}=$ 17.96, $p < .00001$, and in skin conductance level, $F_{(4,264)}=$ 4.38, $p < .001$. Fear scenes produced greater increases in heart rate during the description (mean = 5.21 bpm) and imagination (mean = 5.17 bpm) periods than neutral scenes (description mean = 1.89 bpm; imagination mean = 2.06 bpm) and action scenes (description mean = 1.99 bpm; imagination mean = 2.45 bpm), but not during the quiet period. Similarly, fear scenes produced greater changes in skin conductance level than neutral or action scenes (fear description mean = 0.1549 micromhos, fear imagination mean = 0.1953 micromhos, fear quiet mean = 0.1098 micromhos; neutral description mean = -0.1222 micromhos, neutral imagination mean = -0.2995 micromhos, neutral quiet mean = -0.3142 micromhos; action description mean = -0.1192 micromhos, action imagination mean = -0.1960 micromhos, action quiet mean = -0.1929 micromhos).

In the second analysis, which excluded the non-training group, in addition to the previous findings, a significant effect of the interaction Training X Content X Period in heart rate was found, $F_{(4,176)}= 2.33$, $p < .05$. As can be seen in Figure 2, the response-training group had greater increases in heart rate during the description and imagination periods of the fear scenes than the stimulus-training group.

4. DISCUSSION

In this discussion, we wish to comment on two general questions. Firstly, what is the most consistent pattern of results in our experiments? Secondly, do our results support Lang's theoretical model?

With regard to the first question, our most important finding is clearly the significant effect of training on certain physiological indices of activation when only the two training groups are included in the analysis. Greater changes in heart rate were observed in both experiments in the response-training group during the description and imagination of fear provoking scenes, as compared with the stimulus-training group. Therefore, training seems to be the most consistent independent variable to produce differences in physiological activation.

With regard to the second question, in general our results do not strictly coincide with those obtained by Lang and his associates (Lang, 1979; Lang et al., 1980), but we believe they are not contrary to his model. Lang found that subjects trained in response imagination when presented with scripts including response propositions, are the most physiologically aroused during the imagination of fear scenes. Accordingly,

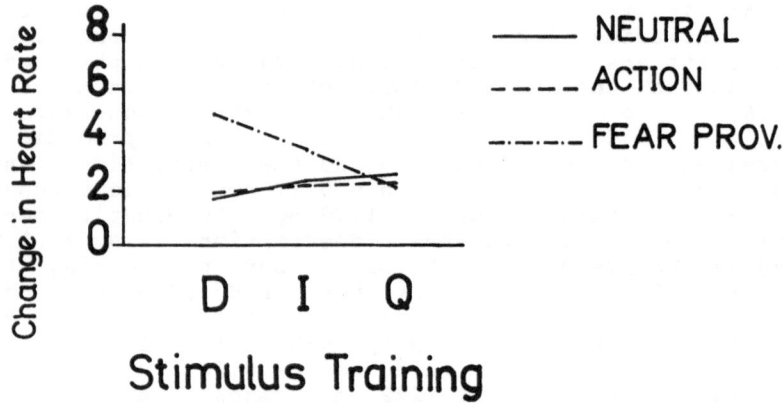

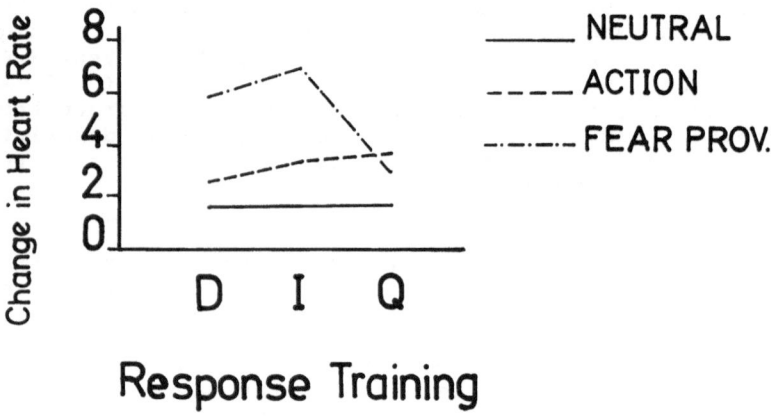

Figure 2. Change in heart rate in the training groups according to period (D: description ; I: imagination ; Q: quiet) and content of the scenes (Exp. II).

response training plus scripts with response propositions seem to be the main factors in Lang's experiments. Our data, however, indicate that training on its own seems to be sufficient. This discrepancy can be explained by the difference in instructions given to the subjects. Lang instructed his subjects to ignore those aspects of the scripts which were not congruent with the training they had previouly received. In our experiments no such instructions were given. Therefore we believe it is likely that subjects learned through the training sessions a general processing strategy that they applied in situations similar to the training one. Thus the change in the type of script, without specific instructions to pay attention to it, may not be an important factor in making the subjects change the training strategy they had already learned. We believe the relevant aspect of Lang's model is the differentiation between the processing of response information and that of stimulus information. This differentiation can indeed be achieved by manipulating different variables: training, scripts or instructions, or any combination of the three. Whether simple main effects or interaction effects are found seems to be irrelevant. The specific effect would depend on the particular procedure used.

Finally, we would like to conclude with two further comments. First, which aspects of Lang's theoretical model are really supported by our data? We believe that within Lang's model there are implicitly at least two different aspects: one related to the nature of mental representation --which he assumes to be propositional-- and the other related to the relevance of considering response information within the representation of emotion. Our data are probably irrelevant to the problem of the nature of representation but we think they support the second aspect of the model, that is the importance of including visceral response information within the structure of emotional imagery. The last comment is concerned with the feasability of linking different research approaches in the study of emotion as Lang's bio-informational model does: the clinical, the psychophysiological and the cognitive psychology approach. We are sure clinical psychology has benefitted from this closer relationship with experimental cognitive psychology and psychophysiology. We hope the reverse will also be true for cognitive psychology and psychophysiology.

REFERENCES

1. Kieras, D. (1978). Beyond pictures and words: Alternative information-processing models for imagery effects in verbal memory. Psychological Bulletin, 85, 532-554.
2. Lang, P.J. (1977). Fear imagery: An information processing analysis. Behavior Therapy, 8, 862-886.
3. Lang, P.J. (1978). Anxiety: Toward a psychophysiological definition. In H.S. Akiskal & W.L. Webb (Eds.), Psychiatric diagnosis: Explorations of biological predictors. New York: Spectrum.

4. Lang, P.J. (1979). A bio-informational theory of emotional imagery. <u>Psychophysiology</u>, 16, 495-512.
5. Lang, P.J. (1984). Cognition in emotion: Concept and action. In C.E. Izard, J. Kagan & R.B. Zajonc (Eds.), <u>Emotions, cognition and behavior</u>. New York: Cambridge University Press.
6. Lang, P.J. (1985). The cognitive psychophysiology of emotion: Fear and anxiety. In A.H. Tuma & J.D. Maser (Eds.), <u>Anxiety and the anxiety disorders</u>. Hillsdale, N.J.: Erlbaum.
7. Lang, P.J., Kozack, M.J., Miller, G.A., Levin, D.N. & McLean, A.,Jr. (1980). Emotional imagery: Conceptual structure and pattern of somato-visceral response. <u>Psychophysiology</u>, 17, 179-192.
8. Miller, G.A., Levin, D.N., Kozack, M.J., Cook, E.W., McLean, A.,Jr. & Lang, P.J. (1981). Emotional imagery: Individual differences in imagery ability and physiological responses. <u>Psychophysiology</u>, 18, 196.
9. Pylyshyn, Z.W. (1973). What the mind's eye tells the mind's brain: A critique of mental imagery. <u>Psychological Bulletin</u>, 80, 1-22.
10. Sperry, R.W. (1952). Neurology and the mind-brain problem. <u>American Scientist</u>, 40, 291-312.

4.2. IMAGERY AND THE BRAIN

EVIDENCE FOR SHARED STRUCTURES BETWEEN IMAGERY AND PERCEPTION

FRANCK PERONNET
INSERM, U280, LYON, FRANCE

MARTHA J. FARAH
PSYCHOLOGY DEPARTMENT, CARNEGIE-MELLON UNIVERSITY,
PITTSBURGH, PA, U.S.A.

and MARIE-ANNE GONON
INSERM, U280, LYON, FRANCE

ABSTRACT
    The evoked activity mapping during a task in which a mental image interacts with the detection of a stimulus was recorded. We found a systematic effect of imagery on the evoked potentials showing a greater early negativity when the image and the stimulus were the same than when they were different shapes. Further we found that this effect was maximal over the occipital regions of the scalp. These two results converge to indicate that imagery engages perceptual representations in the visual system proper.

1. INTRODUCTION

    The idea that mental imagery is self generated activation in perceptual representational structures is the subject of intense debate in cognitive psychology. One research strategy used to support the claim that mental imagery engages perceptual representations is to observe the ways in which concurrent imagination and perception affect one another. Segal and Fusella (1970) found that imagery exerts a systematic effect on perception in tasks in which a subject forms images while detecting faint signals. This implies that there is some common locus of processing for imagery and perception at which they interact. Recently it has been shown that the interaction between imagery and perception is content-specific. For example, imaging an "H" facilitates detection of "H's" more than detection of "T's" and vice versa (Farah, 1985). A content-specific interaction implies that the shared locus of the imagery and perceptual systems, at which they interact, represents information about the content of the image and stimulus sufficient to distinguish between, for example, "H's" and "T's".
    This work was undertaken in order to study this content-specific effect of image on perception while recording topographically mapped evoked potentials (EPs) : by recording the EP to a stimulus at 16 different scalp positions, we can roughly localize the electrical activity that accompanies stimulus processing. In this way we could expect to localize

357

M. Denis et al. (eds.), Cognitive and Neuropsychological Approaches to Mental Imagery, 357–362.

not only in space but also in time the content-specific interaction between imagery and perception, and thereby put constraints on the locus of the representations accessed by both imagery and perception.

This would tell us two things. First, it would tell us the location on the brain of the shared representations for imagery and perception. For example, whether or not the shared representations occur in modality-specific visual cortex. Second, it would tell us the time course of the interaction between imagery and perception, for example, whether the shared representations are accessed early in sensory stages of processing or later in decision stages. Because the earlier psychophysical findings of content-specific imagery-perception interaction consisted of perceptual facilitation, we expected the EP marker of these effects to be an enhancement of "processing negativity" (Näätänen, 1984). Greater processing negativity is generally obtained when the stimulus is more fully processed. So, the question is : Will we see content-specific processing negativity and if so, where in the brain and how early in the processing of the stimulus ?

2. MATERIALS AND METHODS

The experimental method was similar to that of the visual psychophysical experiments previously conducted (Farah, 1985). The subject's task had two main components : a perceptual component and an imagery component.

a) The perceptual component : Subjects viewed 20 msec presentations of either an H, a T, or a blank, followed by a 500 msec presentation of a vertically symmetrical, but otherwise random, pattern mask. Subjects were to decide if they had seen a letter or not, and push either the "letter" or "no letter" response button accordingly. Letters, blanks and masks occurred inside a 0.6 degree square frame, with a fixation point at the center. Thus the task was a simple detection task. Subjects did not identify the letter, they simply indicated whether or not they saw a letter.

b) The imagery component : Before each trial, digitally synthesized speech provided an imagery cue : to image an H, image a T, or not image anything. Each image cue occurred equally often with each stimulus (H, T, or no letter) and was thus completely non predictible.

This design resulted in three relevant conditions of stimulus presentation, with a matching image, a non-matching image, and no image, and two conditions of no stimulus presentation, with an image, and with no image. So, subjects heard an image cue, formed an image, initiated the detection trial by pushing a "ready" button, and stimulus presentation occurred 500 msec later. Subjects were told to initiate a trial only if they had projected a clear, vivid image of the cued letter into the square frame and were fixated on the fixation point. They were informed that the image cues were not predictive of the stimuli. Fifteen subjects participated in the experiment. Four subjects were eliminated from final data analysis because of large amounts of alpha rythm in their average EPs. Each subject performed a total of 360 trials.

EPs were recorded at 16 sites covering the whole scalp (Figure 1). EEG was amplified with a 16-channel ECEM electroencephalograph. The bandwidth of the filters was 0.23 to 35 Hz. Averaging was conducted on-line by a Solar 16/40 Bull minicomputer. The analysis time was 400 msec with a sampling rate of 1.56 msec. The data processing program provided an automatic equalization of the gain between channels. The baseline was corrected, separately on each channel, according to the EEG DC-level preceding the stimulus. Artefactual signals (due to movements or eye blinks) were automatically rejected.

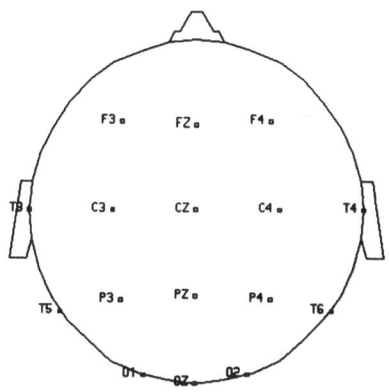

FIGURE 1. Electrode placement using the standard internatio-nal system (Jasper, 1958). The reference electrode is on the forehead (Fpz) and the ground electrode middle between Fz and Fpz.
F=frontal, T=temporal, C=cen-tral, P=parietal, O=occipital.

3. RESULTS

The most straightforward measure of the content-specific effect of imagery on perception, and the principal measure used in previous psychophysical studies on the effect of imagery on perception, is the difference in stimulus processing while holding a matching versus a non-matching mental image. The general effort of forming and holding an image (which interferes with stimulus processing) will be constant between the two conditions ; furthermore, the frequency of occurrence of each stimulus and each image is equal in the two conditions, so that differences in the detectability or imageability of the stimuli will not affect this measure.

Figure 2 shows the averaged EPs for all 11 subjects recorded at the 16 scalp locations. The traces are arranged roughly like the electrodes from the front (up) to the occiput (down). The first thing to notice is that there was a content-specific effect of imagery on the EPs. The traces are not exactly the same. The second thing to notice is that the difference emerges relatively early and at the posterior electrodes, in the form of increased negativity between roughly 150 and 300 msec. After 300 msec, the matching image condition causes increased positivity compared to the non-matching image condition. The waveforms from the no image condition, not shown here, either fall intermediate between the matching and non-matching image conditions or, at some latencies, show somewhat more negativity.

11 SUBJECTS   IMAGE = STIMULUS ——————   IMAGE ≠ STIMULUS ··············

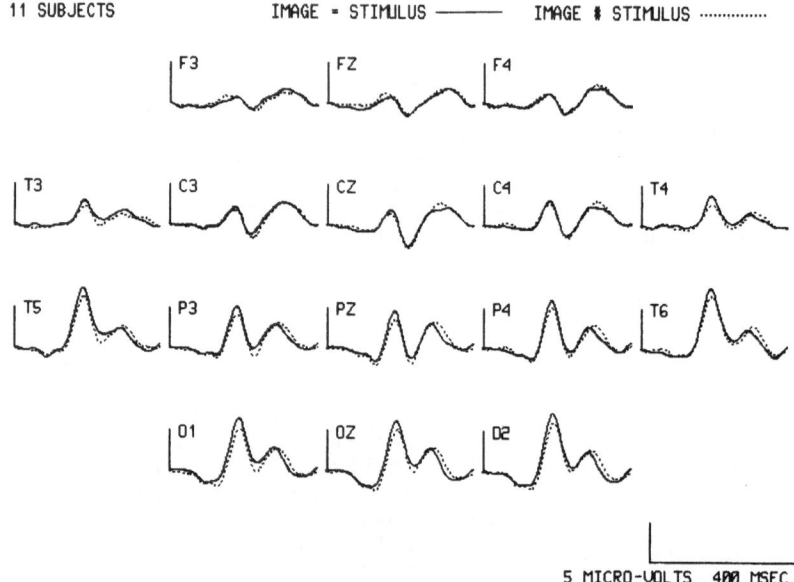

5 MICRO-VOLTS   400 MSEC

FIGURE 2. Grand mean responses from 11 subjects in the matching image condition (solid line) and the non-matching image condition (interrupted line). Negativity is up.

Let us first consider our prediction regarding early modality specific processing negativity. This was tested by a Hotelling multivariate test at the latency of the first negative peak at the three occipital electrodes and was significant at the 0.05 level. Individual t tests at each of the occipital electrodes at the same latency yielded significant levels of 0.01, 0.05 and 0.05 for left, center and right occipital, respectively. Inspection of the waveforms shows a later effect of imagery as well at the latency of a second positive peak, maximal in the left temporo-occipital region. Although a priori statistical tests are not strictly appropriate here, an a posteriori test did not reach the 0.05 level of significance. Further research to examine this late effect is planned. In the meantime, we present, in addition to the map of the (predicted) early effect (Figure 3), a map of the later effect (Figure 4). The map in Figure 4 also highlights an asymmetry in the effect of imagery, in favor of the left hemisphere. This is consistent with recent findings on the laterality of mental image generation, using a variety of behavioral measures with brain-damaged and normal subjects (Farah, 1984). By t test, the significance level of this asymmetry at the occipital electrodes was 0.01 at this latency.

These topographical maps (Giard, Péronnet, Pernier,

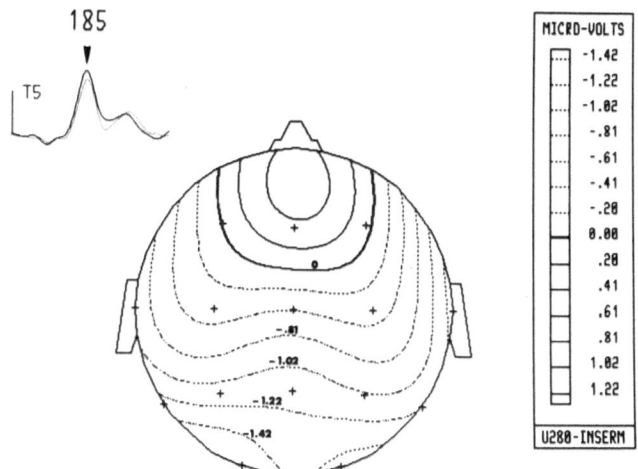

FIGURE 3. Topographical map of the difference between EPs in the matching image and the non-matching image conditions at the latency of the first negative peak of the evoked responses (185 msec).

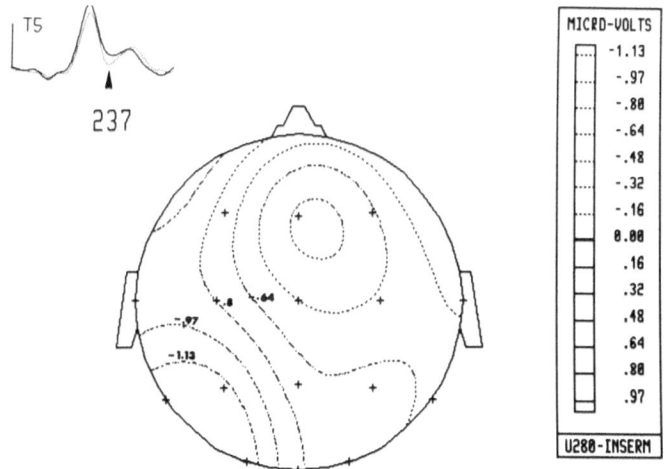

FIGURE 4. Topographical map of the difference between EPs in the matching image and the non-matching image conditions at the latency of the second positive peak of the evoked responses (237 msec).

Mauguière, & Bertrand, 1985) are constructed from the difference between the EPs in the matching and non-matching image
conditions, using the spline technique (Perrin, Pernier,
Bertrand, Giard, & Echallier, 1987) for interpolating between
electrodes.

Although further experiments within the imagery-perception interaction paradigm are needed to clarify the mechanism
through which images and percepts interact, the effects
reported here appear to involve EP components related to
visual pattern recognition and/or visual discrimination.

In summary, mental imagery causes changes in the evoked
potential to visual stimuli that are sensitive to the relative content of the image and the stimulus and distributed over
the occipital and occipito-temporal regions of the scalp.
This implies that mental imagery accesses visual representations in the visual system proper.

REFERENCES
1. Farah, M.J. (1984). The neurological basis of mental
   imagery : A componential analysis. Cognition, 18,
   245-272.
2. Farah, M.J. (1985). Psychophysical evidence for a shared
   representational medium for mental images and percepts.
   Journal of Experimental Psychology : General, 114,
   93-105.
3. Giard, M.H., Péronnet, F., Pernier, J., Mauguière, F., &
   Bertrand, O. (1985). Sequential colour mapping system of
   brain potentials. Computer Methods and Programs in
   Biomedicine, 20, 9-16.
4. Jasper, H.H. (1958). The ten-twenty electrode system of
   the international federation. Electroencephalography and
   Clinical Neurophysiology, 10, 371-375.
5. Näätänen, R. (1984). Processing negativity : An evoked
   potential reflexion of selective attention. Psychological Bulletin, 18, 245-272.
6. Perrin, F., Pernier, J., Bertrand, O., Giard, M.H., &
   Echallier, J.F. (1987). Mapping of scalp potentials by
   surface spline interpolation. Electroencephalography and
   Clinical Neurophysiology, 66, 75-81.
7. Segal, S.J., & Fusella, V. (1970). Influence of imaged
   pictures and sounds on detection of visual and auditory
   signals. Journal of Experimental Psychology, 83,
   458-464.

PATTERN OF REGIONAL CEREBRAL BLOOD FLOW RELATED TO VISUAL AND MOTOR IMAGERY: RESULTS OF EMISSION COMPUTERIZED TOMOGRAPHY

GEORG GOLDENBERG, IVO PODREKA, MARGARETE STEINER, ERHARD SUESS, LÜDER DEECKE

NEUROLOGISCHE UNIVERSITÄTSKLINIK WIEN, AUSTRIA

and KLAUS WILLMES

NEUROLOGISCHE ABTEILUNG DER RWTH AACHEN, F.R.G.

ABSTRACT
    Regional cerebral blood flow (rCBF) was investigated in episodic and semantic memory tasks which partially required the use of imagery. Visual imagery led to an increase of rCBF in the left inferior occipital lobe. Analysis of correlations between regions suggested the emergence of a functional system of bilateral occipital and medial inferior temporal regions in tasks that involved imagery. In the episodic memory tasks the system included lateral inferior temporal regions whereas in the semantic memory tasks the left inferior parietal lobe was included. Imagery had no influence on global asymmetry of cerebral blood flow.

1. INTRODUCTION

    Psychological considerations have led to two major hypotheses concerning the neurological basis of visual mental imagery. On the one hand, it has been said that "a subject is imaging whenever he employs the same cognitive processes that he would use in perceiving, but when the stimulus input that would normally give rise to such a perception is absent" (Neisser, cited by Eysenck, 1984). Logically, it seems likely that imagery activates the same areas of the brain that are activated by actual visual perception, namely visual cortical areas in the occipital lobe and its neighborhood. This hypothesis is corroborated by numerous case studies that describe a loss of visual imagery in conjunction with visuoperceptive impairment (see Farah, 1984 for a review).
    On the other hand, imagery has been understood as a nonverbal mode of information processing that is opposed to verbal processing (Paivio, 1979, 1986). Since verbal abilities are lateralized to the left hemisphere it has been concluded that imagery is a domain of the right hemisphere (e.g. Denis, 1979; Paivio, 1979; Ley, 1983). However, little empirical support has been found for this hypothesis (see Ehrlichman and Barrett, 1983 for a review), and recently even the opposite claim of a left hemisphere superiority for imagery has been made (Kosslyn et al., 1985; Farah 1986).
    We investigated changes in regional cerebral blood flow (rCBF) in verbal tasks which partially required employing of

363

M. Denis et al. (eds.), Cognitive and Neuropsychological Approaches to Mental Imagery, 363–373.

visual imagery. A first question was whether the use of imagery would lead to any consistent changes in blood flow patterns. Secondly we looked at whether any of the hypotheses mentioned above could be supported by our results.

Single Photon Emission Computerized Tomography (SPECT) offers the possibility to visualize the distribution of an isotope over the whole brain. The isotopes used were 123-I-isopropylamphetamine (IMP) in the first study, and Tc-99-Hexamethylpropylenamineoxime (HMPAO) in the second. For both isotopes the cerebral distribution is proportional to rCBF, but the steady state that allows measurement of local count rates is reached after about 2 minutes by HMPAO whereas IMP takes approximately 20 minutes to reach a steady distribution. In both cases, however, the cerebral distribution represents a summing up of rCBF patterns of the whole period during which the steady state was achieved. Acquisition of data was performed by a dual head rotating gamma camera (SIEMENS ZLC37), the spatial resolution is 14 mm FWHM for IMP and 12 mm FWHM for HMPAO. Regions of interest were delineated in 4 appropriate horizontal slices of 21.9mm (IMP) or 15.7mm (HMPAO). Relative local count rates were obtained by dividing the count rate of each region of interest by the mean count rate of all regions taken together.

2. IMAGERY IN EPISODIC MEMORY

The first set of experiments used IMP and was aimed to investigate rCBF changes induced by imagery in an episodic memory task.(An extensive description and discussion of this experiment is given in Goldenberg et al., 1987). We investigated a resting state and 4 stimulated conditions. In the resting state subjects were blindfolded. They had no protection against background noise but nobody talked in the room during the experiment. In the stimulation studies subjects listened via earphones to a list of words spoken at 5 second interval. Then, after a further interval of 30 seconds, they heard another word and had to flash a light held by the left hand if they thought that this word had been present in the preceding list.

Phonotactically correct meaningless words were derived by reversing and exchanging syllables and letters within real German words (e.g. "Riroff, Schramsol, Tressebust, Popnos, Gatilu "). 36 lists of 8 stimuli were given. Abstract nouns had a rating of no more than 3 on a 7 point scale of imageability of German nouns (Mitterndorfer, 1978). 24 lists of 12 nouns were given. Concrete nouns had been rated no less than 6 on the 7 point scale of imageability. Again, 24 lists of 12 nouns were given.

In memorizing the concrete words, subjects followed one of two different instructions: In the condition without explicit imagery subjects first memorized a pilot list of concrete nouns and were then asked how they had proceeded. One subject who had used an imagery strategy was excluded. The other subjects had either tried to silently rehearse the words or reported no particular strategy at all. They were instructed to carry on the same way as they had done with the pilot list. In the _imagery_ condition subjects were instructed not to rehearse the words but to try to visualize the objects named and to concentrate upon the mental images. They were told that consecutively created images might form a composite image and that this would be advantageous.

3. RESULTS

The numbers of correct responses were virtually identical with abstract nouns and with concrete nouns given without an imagery instruction. By contrast, the imagery instruction led to a significant improvement of performance. Variations of the mean relative count rates of individual regions across conditions were evaluated by one-factorial ANOVAs and subsequent multiple t-tests. Condition had significant effects on several regional count rates but no difference between any two stimulated conditions reached a statistical significance level. Thus, no specific effects of imagery could be proven by this form of statistical analysis. Visual inspection of the SPECT images, however, showed that some subjects in the imagery group had particularly high activities unilaterally in the left frontal and inferior occipital lobe (Fig. 1).

FIGURE 1: Top: Study of a subject who memorized concrete nouns without an imagery instruction. Bottom: Study of a subject who used imagery to memorize the concrete nouns list.

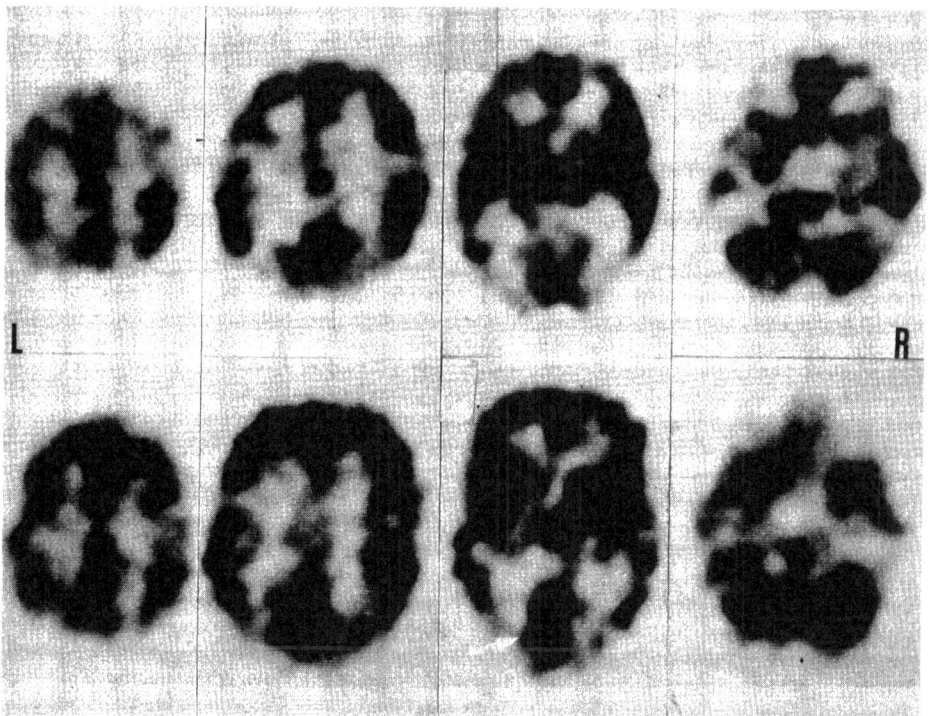

An index of hemispheric asymmetry was obtained by dividing the mean count rate of the left hemisphere by the mean
count rate of the right hemisphere. The concrete nouns conditions were at the opposite extremes of the total range of
hemispheric asymmetries: Whereas the imagery instruction led
to the largest leftward shift of activation of all the stimulated conditions, the same concrete nouns given without the
imagery instruction gave rise to a bias in favor of the right
hemisphere which was larger than that displayed by any of the
other conditions.

Smallest Space Analysis (SSA) (Lingoes, 1979) was applied to study the pattern of correlations between regions
within each condition. This procedure yields a spatial representation of the ordinal relations among correlation coefficients in such a way that the order among the correlations is
represented by the order among the distances between points
in a Euclidean space of as few dimensions as possible. Adequate fit was obtained for three dimensional representations
in each condition. Figure 2 shows projections upon the first
two dimensions which contain the main structural information
that will be interpreted.

There appeared to be a relation between the index of
hemispheric asymmetry and the SSA representations: In the
conditions with the highest asymmetry in favor of the right
hemisphere - rest and concrete nouns - SSA showed a rather
clearcut separation between left and right cortical regions
which was absent in the other conditions.

In SSA the presence of a continuous subspace indicates
that the variables contained in the subspace have closer
relations among themselves than to the other variables. After
stimulation with meaningless and abstract words continuous
subspaces could be identified around the regions of the
inferior temporal lobes. With the imagery instruction a continuous subspace could be defined around all inferior temporal and occipital regions of both hemispheres. For concrete
nouns without an imagery instruction such a subspace could be
identified as well but it included only those regions of the
right hemisphere which were represented within the representational space occupied by left cortical regions, namely the
hippocampal and the inferior occipital regions.

4. EVIDENCE FOR ACTIVATION OF VISUAL AREAS

Performance of all memory tasks led to the formation of
a continuous SSA subspace containing the hippocampal and
inferior temporal regions of both hemispheres. Most likely,
the relationship between the regions indicates that they form
a functional system related to those task demands that are
common to all conditions. When concrete nouns were being
memorized the subspace comprised occipital regions as well. A
straightforward explanation for the association between occipital and inferior temporal regions would be that the use of
visual imagery led to the inclusion of occipital visual areas
into a functional system related to basic task demands. The
finding of a particularly high blood flow in the left inferior occipital lobe of some subjects who were advised to use

FIGURE 2: Projections of 3-dimensional SSA representations
upon the first two dimensions. Empty symbols: Right; Black
Symbols: Left; SF = superior frontal; MF = middle frontal;
IF = inferior frontal; OF = orbitofrontal; C = central ;
SP = superior parietal; IP = inferior parietal; SO = supe-
rior occipital; IO = inferior occipital; ST = superior tem-
poral; IT = inferior temporal; H = Hippocampus; AB = ante-
rior basal ganglia; TH = Thalamus; CB = Cerebellum. In the
HMPAO study SF was divided in SM=superior medial frontal,
SF=superior lateral frontal, and AF=anterior frontal.

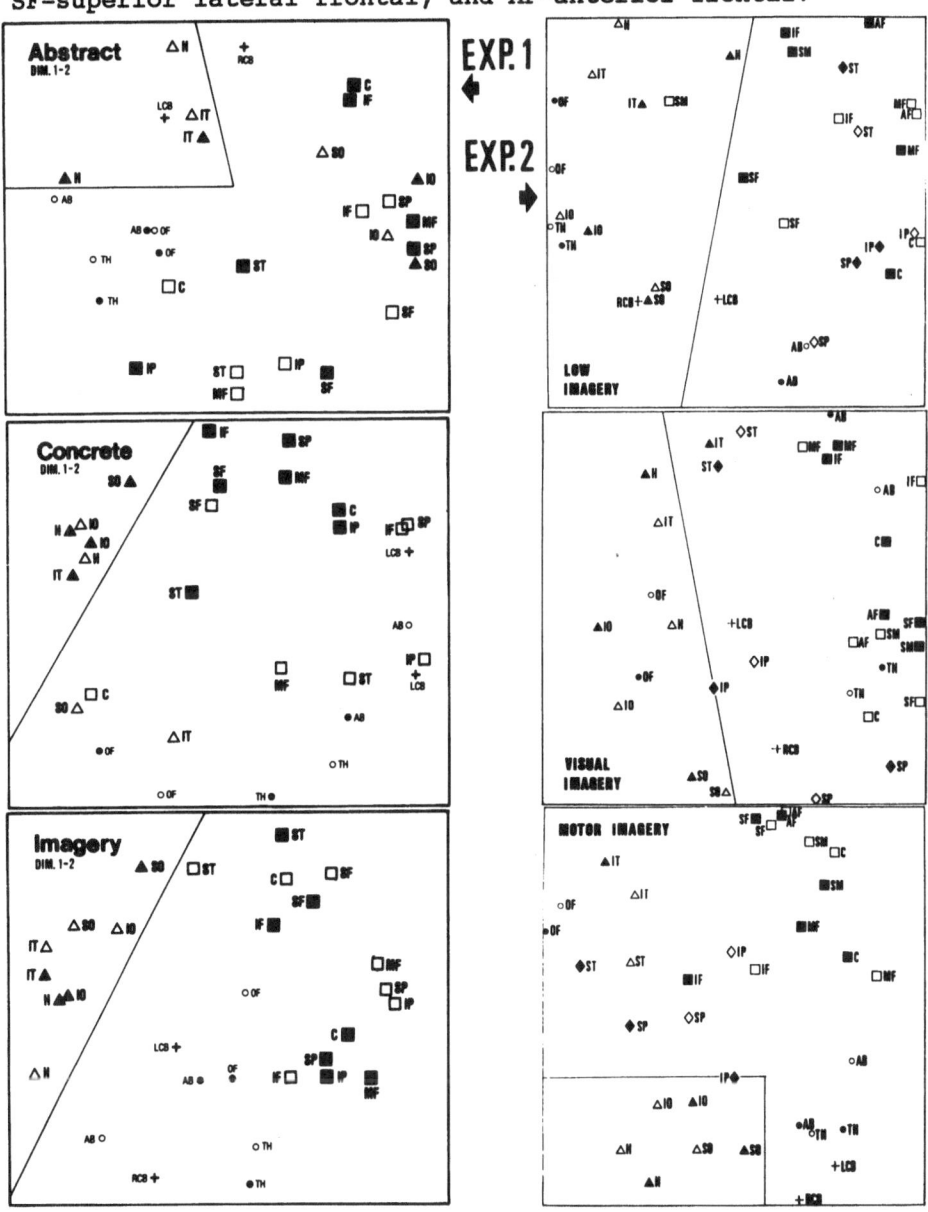

imagery points to a possible prominent role of that region in visual imagery (Basso et al., 1980; Farah, 1984).

5. HEMISPHERIC ASYMMETRY

Memorizing of concrete nouns without an imagery instruction gave rise to an asymmetry of mean count rates in favor of the right hemisphere, the numerical value of which was even higher than that of the resting state. At the same time SSA showed a separation between right and left hemispheric region. Only the right superior frontal, inferior occipital, and hippocampal regions were placed within the representation of the left hemisphere. This structure could indicate that only the left hemisphere together with a few right hemispheric regions was engaged in the solution of the task. Within the left hemispheric functional system a distinct subspace was occupied by regions supposed to be engaged in visual imagery. This physiological evidence of the employment of visual imagery contrasts with the results of the recognition task which showed no improvement compared to the memorizing of abstract words. Possibly, the gain in efficiency obtained by "dual coding" was used to release the remaining regions of the right hemisphere from participation in the task. The higher metabolic activity of the right hemisphere might thus stem from attention to background stimuli rather than from an involvement in task solution. On an introspective level the restriction of task dependent activity to only a part of the brain may have been experienced as the task being "easy".

Regardless of whether imagery was used intentionally or not, the imagery system was composed of regions of both hemispheres. The explicit instruction to use imagery led to a marked leftward shift of hemispheric activity but at the same time the functional system comprised more right hemispheric regions than without an imagery instruction. The difference in hemispheric asymmetries is thus to be attributed to different modes of interhemispheric collaboration. Probably, these modes are determined by the intentional control of visual imagery or the amount of attention paid to the mental visual images rather than by visual imagery per se.

6. IMAGERY IN SEMANTIC MEMORY

In the second set of experiments a semantic judgment task was introduced to evoke mental visual images.

Subjects were divided in two groups and within each group each subject took part in two experiments. Again, subjects were blindfolded. In the high imagery group subjects listened via earphones to a list of 50 "high imagery sentences" (Eddy and Glass, 1981) and had to judge whether the respective propositions were correct or not. Five seconds later they heard a beep and had to flash a light when they had judged the preceding sentence to be wrong. Order of conditions and hand of response were counterbalanced across subjects. In the visual imagery condition, all sentences required the imaging of visual percepts in order to be evaluated (e.g., " The green of pine trees is darker than that

of grass" = correct; "The letter W consists of three lines" =
wrong). In the motor imagery condition the evaluation of the
sentences required imaging of motor actions (e.g., " When you
turn a screwdriver the whole forearm rotates" = correct; "One
can elevate the arm above the head without moving the shoul-
der" = wrong).

The second group of experiments did not involve the use
of imagery: In the low imagery sentences condition the experimental setting was the same as in the high imagery
group,but subjects had to rate the correctness of "low imagery sentences" (e.g., " Columbus named the natives of America
Indians because he believed he was in India" = correct; " The
categorical imperative is an ancient grammatical form " =
wrong). In the "Yes-No" condition subjects heard either
"yes" or "no", followed after 5 seconds by a beep, and had
to flash the light only after "no". Again, hand of response
and order of conditions were balanced across subjects.

Table 1 shows the mean count rates for all regions.
Planned comparisons were carried out between the "Yes-No"
condition and low imagery sentences and between visual and
motor imagery (t-test for repeated measures), as well as
between low imagery and visual imagery sentences and between
low imagery and motor imagery sentences (t-test for independent measures). Their results are shown in the table. This
time, the activation of the left inferior occipital lobe
reached statistical significance at least for the comparison
between low imagery and visual imagery sentences. The numerical value of the left inferior occipital count rate was
somewhat lower with motor imagery than with visual imagery
(see Fig 3). In the left hippocampal area the activity was
significantly higher with visual than with motor imagery. In
contrast to the first experiment, count rates of frontal
regions were now generally higher in the low imagery conditions.

The index of global hemispheric asymmetry showed a statistically reliable leftward shift from the "Yes-No" condition to low imagery sentences, whereas there was no marked
difference between low and high imagery sentences. Obviously,
global hemispheric asymmetry is determined by the difficulty
of the task or by the requirement of semantic processing
rather than by the employment of imagery.

Interpretation of SSA-representations (see Fig 2) was
guided by the assumption that imagery should give rise to a
functional system combining visual areas of the inferior
temporal and occipital lobes. Since temporal visual association areas are located on the medial rather than the lateral
face of the inferior temporal lobe, we decided to look for a
"core-system" comprising inferior and superior occipital and
the hippocampal regions. Adequate subspaces could be defined
in all conditions, but in the "Yes-No" condition they en-
closed both anterior basal ganglia, the right thalamus and
both orbitofrontal regions, and with low imagery sentences
both thalami, the right cerebellum, the right superior medial
frontal region, both lateral inferior temporal regions and
both orbitofrontal regions were within the region. By con-

TABLE 1: MEAN LOCAL COUNT RATES

		YES-NO (Y)		LOW IMAGERY(L)		VISUAL IMAGERY(V)		MOTOR IMAGERY(M)		p .05*)
		Mean	SD	Mean	SD	Mean	SD	Mean	SD	
Sup.medio	L	100.6	5.4	100.0	4.7	100.3	4.8	100.8	4.6	
frontal	R	100.4	5.1	98.8	5.1	100.4	4.3	100.1	4.6	
Superior	L	90.6	3.0	91.1	2.1	89.8	3.1	91.5	3.4	
frontal	R	92.4	2.7	91.6	3.0	89.3	4.0	91.7	3.8	
Anterior	L	106.1	3.0	106.3	3.6	104.3	3.0	104.0	3.8	
frontal	R	106.6	3.5	107.5	2.8	104.7	3.3	104.8	5.0	L>V
Middle	L	97.9	2.5	98.9	2.4	99.1	4.0	99.4	4.8	
frontal	R	101.2	3.0	100.5	3.5	101.0	2.8	100.8	3.5	
Inferior	L	102.2	3.3	103.1	2.3	102.9	2.7	102.0	2.9	
frontal	R	107.0	3.5	106.0	2.3	105.2	3.7	105.8	2.8	
Orbito	L	100.9	8.5	100.3	7.4	102.5	5.2	99.3	5.3	
frontal	R	100.1	7.8	99.5	7.8	104.4	6.1	98.0	6.3	
Central	L	89.3	1.7	89.4	2.2	88.3	2.1	90.2	2.0	V<M
	R	92.1	3.0	91.3	3.0	90.5	2.5	92.5	3.6	V<M
Superior	L	95.3	2.7	95.4	2.8	94.8	3.3	95.9	2.8	
parietal	R	97.5	2.5	95.8	2.8	95.4	3.9	94.9	3.1	Y>L
Inferior	L	98.6	2.1	99.1	2.9	98.1	3.0	99.6	2.3	
parietal	R	100.0	3.1	98.8	4.4	96.5	3.4	98.7	2.3	
Superior	L	100.5	2.7	102.1	2.8	100.2	3.4	101.1	2.0	
temporal	R	106.1	2.3	105.3	3.7	103.4	2.7	103.4	1.9	
Inferior	L	89.4	4.4	91.8	6.4	93.3	3.9	91.7	3.6	
temporal	R	93.5	4.6	94.2	6.2	96.6	4.7	96.0	2.6	
Hippocamp	L	92.3	3.7	93.8	6.2	96.6	4.3	92.5	4.8	V>M
	R	90.0	5.7	92.4	4.8	95.1	4.9	92.2	4.8	
Superior	L	106.9	3.7	106.5	4.3	108.4	3.8	108.5	2.9	
occipital	R	109.7	3.5	106.9	4.8	109.8	2.9	109.9	3.2	Y>L
Inferior	L	105.1	3.4	104.8	3.2	109.5	6.4	107.4	4.3	L<V
occipital	R	106.0	4.6	106.1	3.9	107.2	6.5	105.7	4.9	
Basal	L	104.8	3.7	106.2	5.1	105.9	4.6	104.9	5.9	
ganglia	R	106.7	3.3	105.9	4.7	104.4	4.3	104.2	3.8	
Thalamus	L	94.3	5.9	94.0	5.4	98.5	3.7	97.7	3.9	L<V
	R	96.6	5.5	95.8	6.6	100.5	4.1	98.6	5.2	L<V
Cerebellum	L	102.9	4.1	103.9	4.1	105.9	4.1	105.3	6.0	
	R	104.7	4.6	105.3	4.3	106.8	3.4	106.7	4.8	
Left/Right		98.3	1.0	99.8	1.2	99.6	1.5	99.9	1.4	Y<L
Errors				9.5	4.9	4.5	2.3	6.0	3.1	L>V,L>M

trast, in the visual imagery condition only the orbitofrontal regions, the right inferior temporal region and the left inferior parietal region were included in addition to the "core-regions", and in the motor imagery condition the only additional region was the left inferior parietal one.

7. VISUAL AREAS ENGAGED IN IMAGERY

The significant activation of the left inferior occipital region with visual imagery sentences points to a prominent role of that structure in visual imagery. In addition, both thalami showed a significant increase of rCBF with visual imagery. There is evidence that the thalami are in-

FIGURE 3: Studies of one subject, judging visual imagery sentences (TOP) and motor imagery sentences (BOTTOM). Images are scaled to the maximum rather than to the mean local count rate. The maximum is in the left inferior occipital lobe in both cases, but since it is higher in the visual condition (119 vs 110 %), other regions look less activated in that condition.

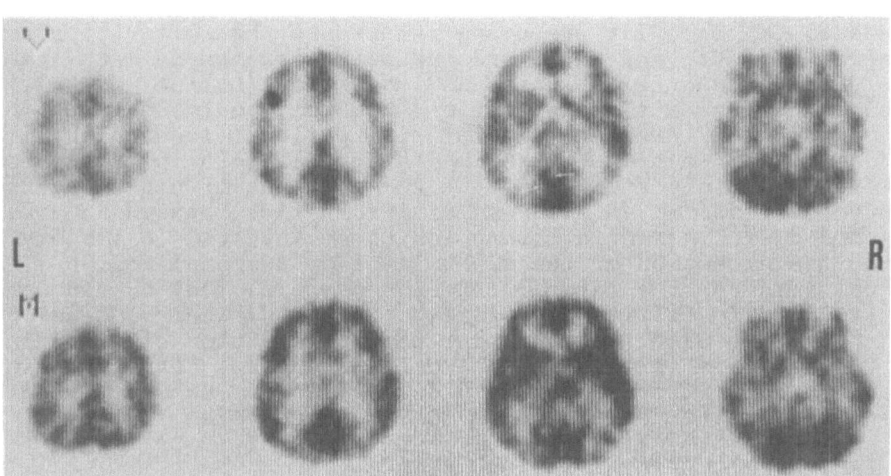

volved in the control of visually guided eye movements (Denny Brown et al., 1976; Ogren et al., 1984). Their activation by imagery might hence be attributed to concomitant eye movements. This sort of coactivation needs not necessarily lead to an increase in the strength of correlation between thalami and visual areas: We think that such an increase would be produced only by the constitution of a chain of information processing in which the amount of output of one processing unit determines the amount of processing done by the following unit. If eye movements are a motor epiphenomenon of imagery rather than a functional link in the information processing chain, then no strict correlation is to be expected between structures that control eye movements and those involved in processing the information contained in the visual images. The same might apply to the central regions which were more active with motor than with visual imagery. They may have controlled subliminal motor actions that accompanied motor imagery.

As far as correlational structures are concerned, however, the results of the second experiment were less clearcut than those of the first. To defend the hypothesis that a functional system of visual areas is specific to imagery one has to accept the inclusion of orbitofrontal regions into this system in the visual imagery condition. However, the number of unexpected regions located within the SSA representation of the system was considerably higher in both low imagery conditions. In contrast to the first experiment, the imagery system of the second experiment included the left inferior parietal region. The semantic judgement tasks frequently required the imaging of several objects or of movements rather than of single static objects. The difference may thus be attributed to different involvement of two visual systems, an inferior one being related to the recognition of single objects and a dorsal one being concerned with the analysis of spatial relation and movements (Levine et al., 1985). An alternative explanation, however, could be based on the assumption that the left inferior parietal lobe which is adjacent to Wernicke's area has a crucial role in semantic memory. One might speculate that the judgment of high imagery sentences required an exchange of information between an area concerned with semantic memory and those involved in imagery. With the exception of the right inferior temporal region in visual imagery, the lateral inferior temporal regions did not participate in the imagery system. Possibly, their inclusion in the first experiment was due to the formation of a chain of information processing between structures involved in imagery and structures involved in episodic memory rather than to a greater extension of the imagery system itself.

8. HEMISPHERIC SPECIALIZATION

Imagery per se had no influence on the global asymmetry of hemispheric blood flow, and the functional system related to imagery was composed of regions of both hemispheres. A distinct bias in favour of the left side was observed only with respect to regional blood flow of the inferior occipital lobe. It must be emphasized, however, that we investigated only verbal tasks. Further experiments exploring the use of visual imagery in visuospatial tasks will be necessary to decide whether this lateralization does indeed reflect a lateralization of a neurological correlate of visual imagery or whether it is to be attributed to an interaction between verbal processes and imagery (Paivio, 1986).

ACKNOWLEDGEMENTS

Parts of this research were supported by grant P6085 from the "Fonds zur Förderung der wissenschaftlichen Forschung"

REFERENCES

1. Basso A, Bisiach E, and Luzatti C. (1980) Loss of mental imagery: A case study. Neuropsychologia 18,435-442.
2. Denis M. (1979) Les images mentales. Presses universitaires de France: Paris.
3. Denny Brown D, and Fischer EG.(1976) The subcortical visual direction of behavior. Archives of Neurology 33,228-242.

4. Eddy JK, and Glass AL. (1981) Reading and listening to high and low imagery sentences. Journal of Verbal Learning and Verbal Behaviour 20,333-345.
5. Ehrlichman H, and Barrett J. (1983) Right hemisphere specialization for mental imagery: A review of the evidence. Brain and Cognition 2,55-76.
6. Eysenck MW. (1985) Imagery and visual working memory. A Handbook of Cognitive Psychology pp 173-195.
7. Farah M. (1984) The neurological basis of mental imagery: A componential analysis. Cognition 18,245-272.
8. Farah M. (1986) The laterality of mental image generation: A test with normal subjects. Neuropsychologia 24,541-552.
9. Goldenberg G, Podreka I, Steiner M, and Willmes K. (1987) Patterns of regional cerebral blood flow related to meaningfulness and imaginability of words - An emission computer tomography study. Neuropsychologia 25, 473-486.
10. Kosslyn SM, Holtzman JD, Farah MJ, and Gazzaniga MS. (1985) A computational analysis of mental image generation: Evidence from functional dissociations in split-brain patients. Journal Experimental Psychology: General 114,311-341.
11. Levine DN, Warach J, and Farah M. (1983) Two visual systems in mental imagery. Dissociation of "what" and "where" in imagery disorders due to bilateral posterior cerebral lesions. Neurology 35,1010-1018.
12. Ley RG. (1983) Cerebral laterality and imagery. in: Sheikh AA (ed): Imagery: current theory, research, and application. John Wiley and Sons, New York. 252-287.
13. Lingoes JC. (1979) The Guttman-Lingoes nonmetric program series. Mathesis Press: Ann Arbor.
14. Mitterndorfer F. (1978) Imagery und Konkretheits-Abstraktheitswerte für 1003 Hauptwörter. Ph. D. Thesis, Philosophische Fakultät der Universität Wien.
15. Ogren MP, Mateer CA, and Wyler AK. (1984) Alterations in visually related eye movements following left pulvinar damage in man. Neuropsychologia 22,187-196.
16. Paivio A. (1979) Imagery and Verbal Processes. Second Edition. Lawrence Erlbaum Associates Inc.: Hillsdale, N.J.
17. Paivio A. (1986) Mental representations: a dual coding approach. Oxford University Press, Oxford, New York.

MENTAL IMAGERY AND THE EFFECTS OF CLOSED HEAD INJURIES

JOHN T. E. RICHARDSON

DEPARTMENT OF HUMAN SCIENCES, BRUNEL UNIVERSITY,
UXBRIDGE, MIDDLESEX, U.K.

ABSTRACT
    Patients with minor closed head injuries show a selective deficit in the recall of concrete material, and this suggests an impairment in their use of imagery as a mnemonic code. However, under interactive imagery instructions both head-injured and control patients show superior performance on concrete material, and there is no sign of any difference between these two groups of subjects. The effects of minor closed head injuries upon memory may thus be interpreted as a functional deficit attributable to the patients' failure to employ the optional strategy of constructing interactive images. Training in the use of relevant strategies is likely to be beneficial to patients who are suffering from memory impairment following brain damage. However, there is also evidence that imagery instructions are helpful only to subjects from the higher social classes.

1. INTRODUCTION

    My research on mental imagery and human cognition has been carried out since 1971. It has covered a number of general themes: the relative importance of imaginal processes and linguistic factors in human memory; the relevance of mental imagery to the theoretical distinction between primary and secondary memory; the exploration of individual differences in the use of mental imagery; and the role of mental imagery in the retention of meaningful sentences. However, during this time I have had a special interest in the effects of brain damage upon cognitive function, and I have conducted several studies which link together these two strands in my work.

2. CLINICAL ASPECTS OF CLOSED HEAD INJURIES
2.1. Mechanics of closed head injuries

    A closed head injury is an injury to the head which does not expose the contents of the skull. Such injuries are a common outcome of industrial, domestic, and recreational accidents, and especially of accidents on the roads. Head injuries give rise to shearing forces which produce diffuse effects within the brain. The most common effect of these forces is an immediate loss or disturbance of consciousness known as concussion. The clinical significance of loss of consciousness is that it marks the dividing line between a trivial knock on the head and a more serious injury which may subsequently give rise to neurological complications.

M. Denis et al. (eds.), Cognitive and Neuropsychological Approaches to Mental Imagery, 375–380.
© 1988 by Martinus Nijhoff Publishers.

2.2. Memory loss and closed head injuries

On recovery of consciousness head-injured patients show a characteristic and major disruption of memory function, described as posttraumatic amnesia. The duration of the period of post-traumatic amnesia is typically used as an index of the severity of the head injury: severe head injuries give rise to a period of posttraumatic amnesia of longer than 24 hours, while minor head injuries give rise to a period of posttraumatic amnesia of 24 hours or less. However, even beyond the end of the period of posttraumatic amnesia, most head-injured patients demonstrate a measurable and persistent disturbance of memory function. For many years, I have been interested in analyzing this disturbance of cognitive function using techniques derived from experimental research on human memory. I have been especially concerned to compare the performance of head-injured patients on concrete and abstract material as a way of considering the relevance of imagery to the question of understanding the nature of their memory impairment. More recently I have also considered the effects of instructions to use mental imagery in learning such material. All of the patients that I have examined were hospitalized following serious accidents and were tested within a few days of their admission to hospital.

3. MEMORY FOR CONCRETE AND ABSTRACT MATERIAL
3.1. The effects of closed head injury

The first experimental investigation contrasted 40 cases of minor closed head injury with a control group of 40 orthopaedic patients (Richardson, 1979). The results are shown in Table 1. The head-injured patients were impaired in their recall of lists of concrete words, but not in their recall of lists of abstract words. The control patients demonstrated the usual pattern of better recall in the case of concrete words than in the case of abstract words. However, the head-injured patients showed no significant advantage in terms of their recall of concrete material. This pattern of results was replicated in a subsequent study (Richardson & Snape, 1984). I attributed the superior performance of the control subjects in the recall of concrete items to their use of mental imagery as an additional memory code in the case of concrete material. The failure of the head-injured patients to demonstrate any difference in performance between concrete and abstract items was taken to mean that mental imagery was not being employed by these subjects. I concluded that closed head injury gave rise to a

TABLE 1. Mean percentage correct in free recall of concrete and abstract words by head-injured patients and orthopaedic controls (Richardson, 1979).

	n	Concrete	Abstract
Control patients	40	32.1	23.1
Head-injured patients	40	26.9	23.6

TABLE 2. Mean percentage correct in free recall of concrete and abstract words by patients treated microneurosurgically for ruptured intracranial aneurysm and tested six weeks and six months after discharge.

	n	Concrete	Abstract
Control patients	18	39.5	30.4
Aneurysm patients: six weeks	57	30.0	21.4
Aneurysm patients: six months	29	31.9	23.2

specific impairment in the use of mental imagery as a form of elaborative encoding in long-term memory.

3.2. The effects of ruptured intracranial aneurysm

It is possible that the pattern of results obtained in these studies was merely an artefact of the particular experimental procedure employed. There is fortunately now evidence that this selective pattern of impairment is not obtained in the case of other conditions involving diffuse brain damage. In particular, Table 2 shows unpublished results which I obtained from the same procedure administered to patients at the Radcliffe Infirmary, Oxford, who had suffered subarachnoid haemorrhage as a result of ruptured intracranial aneurysm. They were tested six weeks and six months after their discharge from hospital following microneurosurgical treatment, and on both occasions they were significantly and roughly equally impaired on both concrete and abstract material. Elsewhere I described similar findings in the case of two patients with spontaneously arrested congenital hydrocephalus (Richardson, 1978). Nevertheless, a selective impairment has also been found in the case of patients with diabetes mellitus (Prescott, Richardson, & Gillespie, in preparation). Table 3 shows that the degree of metabolic control that these patients achieved did not show a significant relationship with recall performance, but that the duration of

TABLE 3. Mean percentage correct in free recall of concrete and abstract words by patients with well and poorly controlled diabetes mellitus of long and short duration (Prescott, Richardson, & Gillespie, in preparation).

	n	Concrete	Abstract
Good control	20	40.2	32.7
Poor control	20	37.7	31.0
Long duration	20	37.2	30.9
Short duration	20	40.7	32.9

their illness was significantly and selectively related to their recall of concrete lists.

3.3 Analysis of intrusion errors in free recall

An analysis of the errors produced by the patients in my original study produced further evidence consistent with the hypothesis that a closed head injury would give rise to a selective impairment in the imaginal encoding of verbal information (Richardson, 1984). Inspection of Table 4 shows that the control patients tended to produce intrusion errors of similar concreteness to the current list; that is, most intrusion errors produced in attempting to recall concrete lists came from previous concrete lists, and most intrusion errors produced in attempting to recall abstract lists came from previous abstract lists. However, the head-injured patients showed no sign of such an effect: the concreteness of their intrusion errors was quite unrelated to the concreteness of the list which they were attempting to recall. This suggested that the concreteness or image-evoking quality of verbal material was simply not a salient dimension of that material in the case of patients with closed head injuries.

TABLE 4. Numbers of intrusion errors produced in immediate free recall by head-injured patients and orthopaedic controls (Richardson, 1984).

Current list: Source list:	Concrete		Abstract	
	Concrete	Abstract	Concrete	Abstract
Control patients	58	20	28	58
Head-injured patients	37	46	31	45

4. THE EFFECTS OF IMAGERY MNEMONIC INSTRUCTIONS

The use of mental imagery has of course been known to be an effective technique for improving memory for over 2,500 years. Together with Chris Barry, I investigated the usefulness of imagery instructions in the case of patients with closed head injuries (Richardson & Barry, 1985). Table 5 shows that the main effects of such instructions were to enhance the patients' memory performance to the level obtained by orthopaedic control subjects, and to reinstate the superior recall of concrete material over that of abstract material. From a theoretical point of view, these results imply that closed head injuries do not affect the patients' ability to use mental imagery per se, but that they disrupt their ability to employ active learning strategies in an appropriate and spontaneous manner. In other words, the focus should be not upon the ability to remember, but upon the ability to manage one's memory. From a practical point of view, these results also suggest that training in the use of relevant strategies is likely to be beneficial to other patients suffering from memory impairment after brain damage, although evidence on this point is not very impressive (Richardson, Cermak, Blackford, & O'Connor, 1987).

TABLE 5. Mean percentage correct in free recall of concrete and abstract words by head-injured patients and orthopaedic controls under standard learning instructions and imagery mnemonic instructions (Richardson & Barry, 1985).

	n	Concrete	Abstract
Standard instructions			
Control patients	24	35.3	27.1
Head-injured patients	24	25.5	25.4
Imagery instructions			
Control patients	24	39.4	29.5
Head-injured patients	24	37.5	28.3

5. SOCIAL CLASS AND THE EFFICACY OF IMAGERY INSTRUCTIONS

Finally, one surprising outcome of the experiment which I carried out with Chris Barry was that the orthopaedic control subjects failed to show any significant improvement in their recall as a result of having been given instructions to use mental imagery. This raises the possibility that samples of subjects who are more typical of the general population might not demonstrate the substantial increases in memory performance which are normally obtained in laboratory research using college students. Although there are a great many respects in which college students might be different from the general population, the critical difference seems to be that students on courses of study in higher education come almost entirely from nonmanual or middle class families (Richardson, 1987). Table 6 shows indeed that enhanced performance under imagery mnemonic instructions is only achieved by subjects from the higher social classes. These results encourage a considerable degree of scepticism concerning the possibility of generalizing from experimental work based upon samples of college students.

TABLE 6. Mean percentage correct in free recall by head-injured patients and orthopaedic controls under standard learning instructions and imagery mnemonic instructions classified by social class (Richardson, 1987).

Social class	Controls		Head-injured	
	Standard	Imagery	Standard	Imagery
I and II	30.4	39.0	25.8	36.6
III(Nonmanual)	32.1	36.8	27.8	35.2
III(Manual)	31.4	31.3	24.3	33.7
IV and V	32.5	28.2	24.2	26.6

ACKNOWLEDGEMENTS
    I am grateful to the surgical and orthopaedic consultants of Ealing and Hillingdon Hospitals, and to the neurosurgical consultants of the Radcliffe Infirmary, Oxford, for their permission to examine patients under their care and for access to medical records.

REFERENCES

1. Prescott, H., Richardson, J. T. E., & Gillespie, C. R. (in preparation). The effects of chronicity and metabolic control on cognitive function in diabetes mellitus.
2. Richardson, J. T. E. (1978). Memory and intelligence following spontaneously arrested congenital hydrocephalus. British Journal of Social and Clinical Psychology, 17, 261-267.
3. Richardson, J. T. E. (1979). Mental imagery, human memory, and the effects of closed head injury. British Journal of Social and Clinical Psychology, 18, 319-327.
4. Richardson, J. T. E. (1984). The effects of closed head injury upon intrusions and confusions in free recall. Cortex, 20, 413-420.
5. Richardson, J. T. E. (1987). Social class limitations on the efficacy of imagery mnemonic instructions. British Journal of Psychology, 78, 67-79.
6. Richardson, J. T. E., & Barry, C. (1985). The effects of minor closed head injury upon human memory: Further evidence on the role of mental imagery. Cognitive Neuropsychology, 2, 149-168.
7. Richardson, J. T. E., Cermak, L. S., Blackford, S. P., & O'Connor, M. (1987). The efficacy of imagery mnemonics following brain damage. In M. A. McDaniel & M. Pressley (Eds.), Imagery and Related Mnemonic Processes, pp. 303-328. New York: Springer-Verlag.
8. Richardson, J. T. E., & Snape, W. (1984). The effects of closed head injury upon human memory: An experimental analysis. Cognitive Neuropsychology, 1, 217-231.

A COMPARISON OF FOUR MNEMONIC SYSTEMS WITH BRAIN DAMAGED AND NON BRAIN DAMAGED PEOPLE

BARBARA ANN WILSON

UNIVERSITY DEPARTMENT OF REHABILITATION, SOUTHAMPTON GENERAL HOSPITAL, SOUTHAMPTON, SO9 4XY, ENGLAND

ABSTRACT

Five lists of words were presented to brain damaged and control subjects for immediate and delayed recall. One list required no strategy, the others used either method of loci, visual imagery, first letter cueing or the story method. The no strategy list was always presented first but otherwise all allocation of words to lists and order of presentation was controlled. There were significant differences between groups, lists, immediate and delayed recall as well as an interaction effect between groups and lists. Reasons for these differences and implications for rehabilitation are discussed.

1. INTRODUCTION

Both verbal and visual mnemonics have been used to improve recall (for example, Lorayne, 1979; Wilson and Moffat, 1984). Bower (1972) argues that mnemonics work because they allow previously isolated items to become integrated. However, it is not clear (a) whether all mnemonics do this to the same extent, (b) how far individual differences are important, and (c) whether those people with organic memory impairment benefit from the same strategies as those without organic involvement.

A number of mnemonic systems exist and some of these are in fairly widespread clinical use (see, for example, Wilson, 1987). Perhaps the four most commonly used are: first letter cueing, method of loci, interactive visual imagery and the story method.

First letter cueing uses the initial letters of the material to be remembered to form a word or to construct a sentence. Thus many people in Britain remember the order of musical notation by learning that the notes in the four spaces of a stave spell F-A-C-E and the notes on the lines can construct the sentence Every Good Boy Deserves Fruit. Gruneberg (1973) reports that 53 per cent of undergraduates employ this method when they revise for finals.

In the Method of Loci, places are chosen to act as retrieval cues. Luria's (1968) famous mnemonist 'S' formed mental images of the items he wanted to remember and imagined each item placed at a certain point along a familiar street. When he wanted to recall the items he imagined himself walking down the street and 'retrieved' each item as he passed by.

Interactive visual imagery is described by Lorayne and Lucas (1974). An image is formed of the first item to be remembered. This is then linked in some way with an image of the second word to be remembered. The linking process should involve the two images interacting.

The story method is perhaps best exemplified by Crovitz's (1979) Airplane List in which he required subjects to remember 10 items in a list by embedding them into a story. Gianutsos and Gianutsos (1979) also used the story method to improve recall of brain injured people.

M. Denis et al. (eds.), Cognitive and Neuropsychological Approaches to Mental Imagery, 381–386.
© *1988 by Martinus Nijhoff Publishers.*

This paper reports an investigation carried out to see which (if any) of these four strategies led to the best recall of information for (a) memory impaired people whose condition had been caused by brain damage and (b) non-impaired controls.

2. SUBJECTS

Forty subjects took part in the study, 20 of whom were memory impaired, brain injured people. All were patients at a Rehabilitation Centre. Their mean age was 31 years, with a standard deviation of 13.8 years and a range of 15 - 39 years. Ten had sustained a severe head injury, 4 were stroke patients, 3 had suffered from encephalitis, 2 had been treated for a cerebral tumour and 1 was diagnosed as having Korsakoff's syndrome. All were in the impaired range on the Rivermead Behavioural Memory Test (Wilson, Cockburn and Baddeley, 1985) with a mean score of 3.6, a standard deviation of 2.4 and a range of 0 - 8. The maximum score on this test is 12 and scores below 10 are considered impaired.

The normal control group was recruited from staff at the rehabilitation centre, students from a local college, and other working adults. The mean age for the control group was 27 years (S.D. 11.9 years, range 17 - 53 years). Seven of this group were male.

3. METHOD

Five lists of 10 words were constructed. Each list was suitable for allocation in each one of the following conditions: no strategy, first letter mnemonics (in this case the initial letters of each word in each list spelled out a word), story method (the format used was similar to that described by Crovitz, 1979), method of loci (the locations were rooms and other places in the subject's home), interactive visual imagery (the format was similar to that described by Lorayne and Lucas, 1974).

Subjects were seen individually. For the no strategy condition they were told, "I am going to read a list of words to you and when I have finished I want you to tell me back as many as possible in any order." Each word was repeated twice during a five second interval to ensure equivalent exposure for each condition. Similar wording was used for the other conditions together with any specific procedural explanation.

In order to avoid adoption of one of the other mnemonics, all subjects were given the no strategy condition first. Following this, the order of strategies was counter-balanced across subjects. Allocation of lists to strategies was also counter-balanced with the exception noted above.

Twenty four hours later, without warning, subjects were asked to recall as many words as possible from each list. In addition, the brain damaged people were prompted when necessary with the previous word. If no words at all were recalled from a particular list the experimenter would supply the first word from that list. This prompting was necessary because so many brain damaged subjects were at 'floor level'. The number of correct words from each subject for each condition was recorded.

4. RESULTS

Analysis of variance indicated the following:
(i) there was no significant difference between the groups
($F = 269$; df: 1, 380; $p < .001$);
(ii) there was a significant difference between lists
($F = 15.25$; df: 4, 380; $p < .001$);

(iii) there was a significant difference between immediate and
      delayed recall
      (F = 349; df: 1, 380; p < .001);
(iv) there was a significant interaction between groups and lists
      (F = 3.75; df: 4, 380; p < .01).
The mean number of words correct for both groups under all conditions
can be seen in Figure 1.

FIGURE 1. THE MEAN SCORES OF BOTH GROUPS UNDER ALL CONDITIONS

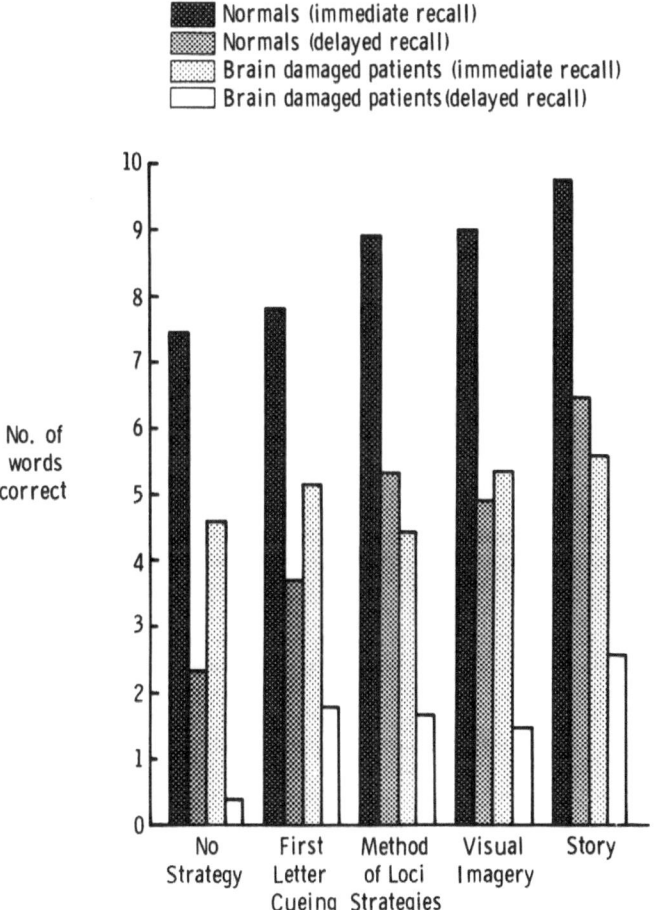

A series of Newman Keuls tests revealed that, for immediate recall,
the non brain damaged subjects showed no difference between first letter
cueing and no strategy, nor between visual imagery and method of loci. All
other comparisons were significantly different. The story method was the
most successful.

The tests indicated that the non brain damaged subjects scored in a similar pattern in the delayed condition, with the story method again producing the highest scores. It was very much more effective than either the no strategy or first letter cueing (p < .01). It was also more effective than method of loci or interactive visual imagery (p < .05).

As far as the brain damaged group was concerned, none of the strategies were significantly more effective than any other in the immediate recall condition. In the delayed recall condition, however, the story method again turned out to be the most effective, and, unlike the controls, first letter cueing was more effective than no strategy at all.

A forgetting score was also obtained (delayed recall as a percentage of immediate recall) for each subject. The purpose of this was to see whether those strategies which worked best in the delayed condition simply reflected a higher amount recalled in the immediate condition. There was no evidence that brain damaged subjects forgot more than controls as there was no interaction effect between group and time of recall in the original ANOVA.

For the non brain damaged, story (p < .01), visual imagery (p < .05), and method of loci (p < .05) all resulted in less forgetting than no strategy, although as much was forgotten in the first letter mnemonic strategy.

The brain damaged subjects showed a different pattern, with the first letter strategy being more effective than no strategy and, again, unlike the controls, they forgot as much using visual imagery as they did using no strategy. Despite the significant superiority of story, first letter and method of loci, the brain damaged people still retained little of the original material (see Figure 1).

5. DISCUSSION

It is not surprising that the brain damaged subjects scored less well than the controls as memory impairment was the criterion for selection into study. Nevertheless, they were able to benefit from some strategies in the delayed condition. The story method was particularly useful, and the most likely reason for this is that it requires dual coding as both visual and verbal techniques are in use during processing of the story. Others have found dual coding to be superior to single modality coding, for example, Paivio (1971). The same argument applies of course to the control subjects. It might also be the case that the story method is more effective because it provides, as Bower (1972) suggests, a more integrated system.

The two groups differed as far as the relative benefit they gained from first letter mnemonics, with the controls showing no benefit in comparison with the no strategy condition, and the brain damaged showing some benefit. This could be due partly to the fact that initial letters provide relatively ineffective cues when memory systems are functioning normally (at least as far as novel material is concerned). First letters are much more helpful when the material is already known to the subject and the problem results from ordering or sequencing difficulties (Harris, 1980). However, such cues may be better than nothing at all in an imperfect system. The discrepancy cue may also be due to the fact that the brain damaged people were so impaired in the delayed condition that it took very little to improve their performance, whereas the controls who remembered more from the no strategy list needed a relatively bigger increase for the difference to reach significance.

The brain damaged were equally good at interactive visual imagery and first letter mnemonics while the controls found interactive imagery easier. Such visual imagery is difficult for the organically memory impaired as they have problems retrieving one image to act as a cue for another. A previous study reported in Wilson (1987), using imagery with brain damaged people, demonstrated that, for those with severe memory impairment, experimenter drawn images were recalled better than mental images. Other studies (Wilson, 1987) suggest that imagery works better with memory impaired people when they are required to learn one thing at a time, and when material from real life is used rather than laboratory material. Hence, it is possible that the strategies would have been more useful if (a) experimenter drawn images had been used, (b) if learning had been broken down into smaller steps, and (c) if real locations and every-day situations had been selected.

6. IMPLICATIONS FOR REHABILITATION

A. Memory impaired people can use mnemonics to learn some new information. It is probably unrealistic, however, to expect them to apply and use mnemonics to cope with everyday memory demands.

B. Dual coding appears to be more effective than single coding. Thus, a combination of methods might be best for teaching new information to the severely impaired.

C. It is probably better to teach one step at a time.

D. Experimenter or therapist drawn images are likely to be remembered more easily than mental images.

E. Individual preferences and styles of patients should be taken into account by therapists.

F. Motivation and success are likely to be increased through avoiding experimental or laboratory material, and relying upon information that has relevance to the everyday lives of the memory impaired.

Footnote: Some of this material appears in Wilson (1987) with permission from Guilford Press.

REFERENCES
1. Bower G. H. (1972). A selective review of organizational factors in memory. In E. Tulving & W. Donaldson (Eds.) Organization of memory. New York: Academic Press.
2. Crovitz H. (1979). Memory retraining in brain damaged patients: The airplane list. Cortex, 15, 131–134.
3. Gianutsos R. & Gianutsos J. (1979). Rehabilitating the verbal recall of brain injured patients by mnemonic training: An experimental demonstration using single case methodology. Journal of Clinical Neuropsychology, 1, 117–135.
4. Gruneberg M. (1973). The role of memorization techniques in finals examination preparation – A study of psychology students. Educational Research, 15, 134–139.
5. Harris J.E. (1980). We have ways of helping you remember. Concord. The Journal of the British Association for Service to the Elderly, No. 17,
6. Lorayne H.(1979). How to develop a super power memory. Wellingborough: Thomas & Co.
7. Lorayne H. & Lucas J. (1974). The memory book. New York: Balantine Books.
8. Luria A. R. (1968). The mind of a mnemonist. New York: Basic Books.
9. Paivio A. (1971). Imagery and verbal processes. New York: Holt, Rinehart & Winston.
10. Wilson B. A. (1987). Rehabilitation of memory. New York: Guilford

Press.
11. Wilson B. A., Cockburn J. & Baddeley A. D. (1985). The Rivermead behavioural memory test manual. Reading, Berkshire: Thames Valley Test Co.
12. Wilson B.A., & Moffat N. (1984). Clinical management of memory problems. London: Croom Helm.

HEMINEGLECT AND MENTAL REPRESENTATION

EDOARDO BISIACH AND ANNA BERTI

ISTITUTO DI CLINICA NEUROLOGICA, UNIVERSITA DI MILANO, ITALY

ABSTRACT
Neuropsychological findings show that a spatially circumscribed
brain lesion may not only involve a spatially circumscribed
sensory loss, revealing the analog structure of relatively
peripheral sensory apparata; it may also involve a
circumscribed scotoma in representational space. From which we
may infer that mechanisms subserving representational activity
which function themselves as analogs, are present in the brain.

1. INTRODUCTION

Hemineglect is a disorder the most pronounced forms of which
appear, as a rule, as a consequence of focal lesions of the
right hemisphere. In simplistic terms it may be described as
failure to respond to stimuli located in the hemispace
contralateral to the lesion, that is in the left hemispace, and
to initiate activities in that hemispace. To give just one
example, in drawing a clock-dial the patient may omit details
from the left half or transpose them to the right.

During the last ten years, hemineglect has been
systematically investigated in our laboratory. Although we
were already convinced, on purely clinical grounds and in spite
of alternative proposals, of the necessity of a cognitive
explanation of the disorder -- i. e. of an explanation
extending beyond the level of afferent and efferent
transduction mechanisms -- we first attempted to find
persuasive evidence supporting this opinion. We then started
analyzing the cognitive framework of space representation
revealed by the disorder. Finally, and with some hesitation
in view of the complex and far-reaching implications, we
subsumed hemineglect to a more general syndrome of space
misrepresentation, outlined a model which could explain this
syndrome, and faced its most critical predictions.

What follows is intended to provide a general outline of our
activity.

2. HEMINEGLECT AND MENTAL REPRESENTATION: EVIDENCE FOR ANALOG MECHANISMS

Our first aim was fulfilled on finding that, in describing
their mental image of a familiar view from a given vantage
point, right brain-damaged patients with left hemineglect were
prone to ignoring items located in the left side of that view.
Neglected items were afterwards recalled when the patients
described the image of the same place from the opposite view-

M. Denis et al. (eds.), Cognitive and Neuropsychological Approaches to Mental Imagery, 387-391.

point, whereas, amazingly, right-side items reported a few moments before were subsequently omitted (Bisiach and Luzzatti, 1978; Bisiach, Capitani, Luzzatti and Perani, 1981).

A case of imagery neglect following right parietal infarction has recently been studied by Barbut and Gazzaniga (personal communication). Among other things, the patient was asked to imagine himself in New York facing towards California and to name the states which lay in between. On the third day after the onset of the illness, he only named ten, all on the right of the imaginary line of sight. On the 7th day the patient had much recovered; however he still omitted six states on the left and only three on the right.

Imaginal neglect may also affect verbal processes. Baxter and Warrington (1983) described a patient who misspelled the left half of words, both forwards and backwards. Similar results were obtained by Barbut and Gazzaniga with their patient.

Imaginal neglect may also appear when the visual working memory is loaded with perceptual rather than with long-term memory information. Indeed, a further experiment with left-neglect patients showed that same-different judgments to pairs of stimuli, the components of which were presented one after the other, failed in trials in which the stimuli differed in their left halves. This happened both when the stimuli were stationary and exposed to unconstrained vision, and when they were moved horizontally either to the left or to the right behind a stationary vertical slit so that each part could be perceived in central vision but their complete shape could only be reconstructed in short-term visual memory (Bisiach, Luzzatti and Perani, 1979). Our results were replicated by Ogden (1985) with different patterns.

We interpret all these data as evidence for an analog format of visual images in working memory (see Kosslyn, 1980), as well as for an actual confluence of perceptual and representational processes on some common mechanism (see Finke, 1985).

An objection, however, could be raised to the effect that the very appeal to a disordered analog exposes the non-cognitive nature of hemineglect. We endeavoured to counter this objection on the grounds of experimental data (Bisiach, Berti and Vallar, 1985). Patients with left hemineglect had to press a lit key of the same colour flashed by a diode. Diodes were located in both halves of egocentric space and flashed either a red or a green light. On each trial two keys of different colour (red on the left and green on the right, or vice versa) lit up simultaneously with the flashing of a diode and remained lit until one of them was pressed. There were therefore two uncrossed and two crossed S-R conditions. Only one aspect of the results will be illustrated here. Subjects were quite accurate whenever both stimuli and required responses were in the right, unaffected field. This shows that the elementary S-R algorithm was firmly established. However, more than 50% right stimuli requiring crossed (leftward) responses were followed by faulty reactions: the patient pressed a wrong key on the right, either the unlit key of the same colour flashed by the diode or the lit key of the wrong colour; on some occasions no response was given. This shows that the disorder underlying hemineglect is not confined to the left half of a cognitively incompetent analog, but involves the <u>unmonitored</u> failure of a logical rule, whatever format this rule might turn out to have.

3. THE STRUCTURE OF SPACE REPRESENTATION

In order to gain further insight into the structure of the putative analog subserving space representation we explored two different paths of inquiry.

One concerns the egocentric mapping of spatial relations among objects relative to a representational system which has, itself, a complex spatial articulation. Therefore, we investigated the out-of-sight tactual exploration of a display placed in different positions relative to the line of sight and to the trunk's sagittal midplane: (a) line of sight and display at 0 degrees with respect to the trunk's sagittal midplane; (b) line of sight at 0, display 60 degrees to the right; (c) line of sight and display 60 degrees to the right; (d) line of sight 60 degrees to the right, display at 0 degrees (Bisiach, Capitani and Porta, 1985). The results obtained in neglect patients suggest the existence of at least two frames of spatial reference: one of them retinotopic, the other related to the trunk's sagittal midplane.

The other relates to the parsing of space representation into processes nearer to the input and output side respectively. In order to disentangle these two aspects, which -- as first hypothesized by Watson and associates (1978) -- might be separately involved in hemineglect, we devised a modification of the time-honoured line-bisection task, in which, as a rule, left neglect patients set the subjective midpoint more or less to the right of the objective midpoint (Bisiach, Berti and Geminiani, ongoing research). In one condition of our experiment a pointer is directly placed by the patient's hand on the subjective midpoint of the line, as in the traditional task. In another condition, the pointer is indirectly displaced along the line by means of a pulley device, so that it moves contrarywise to the patient's hand. Purely "sensory" neglect would imply the same amount of rightward displacement of the subjective midpoint in either condition. Purely "motor" neglect would imply that in the second condition the subjective midpoint is set to the <u>left</u> of the objective midpoint, in a position symmetrical with respect to that of the subjective midpoint set in the first condition. The preliminary results of the investigation suggest that space representation might indeed be the resultant of complex interactions between processes developing at sensory and at pre-motor levels.

4. DYSCHIRIA

Following a lead implicit in a notable paper published by the Austrian neurologist Hermann Zingerle in 1913, we proposed to view hemineglect as an aspect of a more general syndrome of unilateral misrepresentation of egocentric space, for which we adopted the term "dyschiria" used by Zingerle himself. Besides neglect, this syndrome includes unawareness of disorders such

as left hemiplegia or left hemianopia as well as delusory
beliefs relative to the left half of personal and extrapersonal
space.

We outlined a model which could account for both aspects of
the syndrome, which are viewed as resulting from slightly
different dysfunctions of the same functional unit (Bisiach and
Berti, 1987).

To put it very briefly, the model is a spatial analog similar
to Baddeley's "scratch-pad" for the working memory system
(Baddeley and Hitch, 1974; Baddeley and Lieberman, 1980).
"Veridical" cell assemblies in this analog are bottom-up
recruited by input from a sensory transducer. Top-down
recruited cell assemblies subserve mental imagery; in normal
conditions their activity is damped down by spatially
corresponding sensory-driven cell assemblies, so that no belief
of reality is fixed to their representational content and the
output of the system is a relatively faithful rendering of
sensory input. Complete inactivation of one half of the analog
gives rise to hemineglect phenomena. Inactivation
circumscribed to sensory-driven cell assemblies, by freeing
internally driven activity from bottom-up inhibition, may
release uncontrolled mental representation and misbeliefs
relative to one half of space.

It is important to note that the cell-assembly medium of the
spatial analog may easily account for representational
structures such as those suggested, e. g., by Hinton (1979).
Indeed, this medium -- unlike media inspired by physical optics
-- predicts that meaningful blobs of information may be ignored
or misrepresented all of a piece, as actually happens in
dyschiria.

Our model predicts that the profound disorder of
consciousness underlying anosognosia -- i. e. unawareness or
explicit denial of an extremely severe impairment such as left
hemiplegia -- might be manipulated by the same physical
manoeuvres affecting hemineglect. Thus we started exploring
the effect of vestibular stimulation ipsilateral to the brain
lesion, which has been found to transitorily remove or reduce
hemineglect (Rubens, 1985). In two out of four patients with
intractable anosognosia so far studied, we obtained a remission
of the disorder: a mild remission in the first case and a
marked one in the second (Cappa, Sterzi, Bisiach and Vallar,
ongoing research). Should these findings be confirmed, their
theoretical significance could scarcely be overestimated.

REFERENCES

1. Baddeley AD, & Hitch GJ (1974). Working memory. In G Bower
   (Ed), Recent advances in learning and motivation (Vol.
   8, pp 67-89). New York: Academic Press.
2. Baddeley AD, & Lieberman K (1980). Spatial working memory.
   In RS Nickerson (Ed), Attention and performance VII (pp
   521-539). Hillsdale, NJ: Lawrence Erlbaum Associates.
3. Baxter DM, & Warrington EK (1983). Neglect dysgraphia.
   Journal of Neurology, Neurosurgery, and Psychiatry,
   48 ,141-144.

4. Bisiach E, & Berti A (1987). Dyschiria. An attempt at its systemic explanation. In M Jeannerod (Ed), Neurophysiological and neuropsychological aspects of spatial neglect. Amsterdam: North Holland.

5. Bisiach E, Berti A, & Vallar G (1985). Analogical and logical disorders underlying unilateral neglect of space. In MI Posner & OSM Marin (Eds), Attention and performance XI (pp 239-249). Hillsdale, NJ: Lawrence Erlbaum Associates.

6. Bisiach E, Capitani E, Luzzatti C, & Perani D (1981). Brain and conscious representation of outside reality. Neuropsychologia, 19, 543-551.

7. Bisiach E, Capitani E, & Porta E (1985). Two basic properties of space representation in the brain. Journal of Neurology, Neurosurgery, and Psychiatry, 48, 141-144.

8. Bisiach E, & Luzzatti C (1978). Unilateral neglect of representational space. Cortex, 14, 129-133.

9. Bisiach E, Luzzatti C, & Perani D (1979). Unilateral neglect, representational schema and consciousness. Brain, 102, 609-618.

10. Finke RA (1985). Theories relating mental imagery to perception. Psychological Bulletin, 98, 236-259.

11. Hinton G (1979). Some demonstrations on the effects of structural descriptions in mental imagery. Cognitive Science, 3, 231-250.

12. Kosslyn SM (1980). Image and mind. Cambridge, Mass.: Harvard University Press.

13. Ogden JA (1985). Contralesional neglect of constructed visual images in right and left brain-damaged patients. Neuropsychologia, 23, 273-277.

14. Rubens AD (1985). Caloric stimulation and unilateral visual neglect. Neurology, 35, 1019-1024.

15. Watson RT, Miller BD, & Heilman KM (1978). Nonsensory neglect. Annals of Neurology, 3, 505-508.

16. Zingerle H (1913). Uber Stoerungen der Wahrnehmung des eigenen Koerpers bei organischen Gehirnerkrankunken. Monatsschrift für Psychiatrie und Neurologie, 34, 13-36.

WEAKNESSES OF IMAGERY WITHOUT VISUAL EXPERIENCE: THE CASE OF THE TOTAL CONGENITAL BLIND USING IMAGINAL MNEMONICS

CESARE CORNOLDI and ROSSANA DE BENI

DEPARTMENT OF PSYCHOLOGY, UNIVERSITY OF PADOVA, ITALY

ABSTRACT

Since visual imagery is usually considered to be not only analogical but also founded on visual experience, blind people should perform poorly on visual imagery tasks. Instead, many experiments on blind performance in tasks thought to involve visual imagery processes have often shown that the blind do not behave differently from matched sighted subjects. In the present paper visual images are considered as representations maintaining some of the properties of visual objects and constructed from information from various sources. The limitations of these representations are explored in a series of experiments. Results show that, presumably because of the deprivation of visual experience, the blind have particular difficulty in constructing multiple interactive images.

1. INTRODUCTION

Experimental research on the imaginative memory of completely congenitally blind subjects has often failed to show differences between them and sighted control subjects (see, for example, Kerr, 1983; Jonides et al., 1975; Marmor, 1978).

The totally congenitally blind person has never had visual experience. The above results are often thus interpreted as meaning that the absence of visual perception implies the absence of mental images. The conclusion is that in memory tasks apparently demanding the use of visual imagery, it is either not required or that although it may be for some (sighted) subjects, it is not necessarily so for everyone, considering that blind persons may not need to use visual imagery (Zimler & Keenan, 1983). The alternative interpretation is that using specific cognitive behaviours as indicators of the presence of mental images, blind subjects evidently do have mental images which are comparable to those of seeing people (Kerr, 1983). This interpretation assumes that a mental image does not require visual experience for its creation. However, it may be specified in two ways: believing that mental images specifically connected to the various senses do exist, and believing that mental images are the result of a synthesis of information

393

M. Denis et al. (eds.), Cognitive and Neuropsychological Approaches to Mental Imagery, 393–401.
© 1988 by Martinus Nijhoff Publishers.

coming from various sources and characterized by special functional analogic modalities with respect to the functioning of
perceptual activities. As regards the former interpretation,
attempts have been made to distinguish stimuli according to the
type of image they are capable of eliciting. This has been done
mainly by referring to visual and auditory images, by observing
how blind people, compared to sighted individuals, evidence
better performance with stimuli with high auditory image values
(Paivio & Okovita, 1971).

It should also be recalled that few stimuli are experienced
by means of a single sense and that in the representations we
adopt in our cognitive activities, we probably use information
from long-term memory, originally obtained from various sources
(Sholl & Easton, 1986). It therefore becomes important to examine which type of information is specific to visual experience
and is so important that it is essential to our representations, thus differentiating between the cognitive activities of
blind and sighted individuals.

In this work, visual images are considered as representations which retain some of the properties of visible objects
and are constructed on the basis of information from various
sources. It is therefore assumed that although congenitally
blind subjects do have images, they are specifically limited
due to the absence of visual experience. These hypotheses are
explored by examining the capacity of sighted and blind subjects to use imagery in situations linked to memory techniques.

Results presented at the First International Imagery Conference of Queenstown (De Beni & Cornoldi, 1985) showed that even
the blind are able to use "loci" memory techniques when asked
to memorize a list of isolated words. Instead, when the test
material is composed of a list of triplets of words, blind subjects' performance is greatly inferior not only to that of
sighted subjects who use this technique but also to that of
sighted subjects who do not. These results show that the blind
cannot form images starting from a spatial reference point involving several elements which have to be imagined inter-
actively. Our most recent (still unpublished) results, in which
the same task is given with improved procedure, confirm the
above results.

This work is an extension of this type of investigation,
with reference to two other situations classically involved in
the art of memory, i.e., the use of bizarre images and the
chaining strategy (see Higbee, 1977). These two situations
allow for a better distinction of certain aspects involved in
the above tasks.

The difficulty in memorizing pairs or triplets of words by
forming multiple progressive images may be due to the fact that
when the material is chosen randomly, the images subjects are

asked to construct may be only rarely encountered in everyday life and are frequently strange or bizarre. Blind subjects' difficulty may therefore be causal, not so much because of image construction but of the character of the images themselves, i.e., the difficulty of going beyond ordinary stereotyped representations. For this reason we chose a memorization task composed of bizarre sentences already used by various authors and originally proposed by Merry & Graham (1978), in which subjects are asked to imagine and then recall a list of six sentences describing bizarre situations and six describing respectively common concrete or abstract situations. If blind subjects have difficulty with bizarre images, their performance should be very poor on bizarre sentences and, in the case of total incapacity to form images, should descend to the low levels of abstract sentences. Alternatively, if performance is not far removed from that of sighted subjects, it may be concluded that the blind do not find it particularly difficult to imagine bizarre situations and we should instead find differences on the chaining task.

In the mnemonic strategy of chaining, which may also be called the link system, subjects memorize a list of words forming multiple interactive images: i.e., first they form an image involving the first two elements of the series and then a separate image involving the second and third elements, and so on. Difficulty in using the strategy generally leads to poor performance. Moreover, the person using the technique generally remembers better by maintaining pairing on the interactive images formed by having the previously used image available first, followed by the image of the next item. Lastly, if performance is not perfectly accurate, it is expected to be better on the first part of the list than on the second. This is because retrieval starts from the first item (whose image is recalled in relation to its interaction with the second item), and proceeds in sequence to the last item. In principle, when using the chaining technique, if one element in the chain is lost, it should be impossible to continue retrieval.

2. METHOD

2.1. Subjects:

25 totally congenitally blind people, 14 male and 11 female, aged between 14 and 45 (mean age 27;3). They had either attended junior high school (3 subjects), senior high school (20), or university (2).

The control group was composed of 25 sighted subjects, matched for sex, age, education and social level to the blind group.

2.2. Recall task with common and bizarre sentences

2.2.1. Material: 18 sentences (6 common, 6 bizarre, 6 abstract) composed of subject noun, verb, object noun. The common sentences described typical situations regarding animate or inanimate objects (e.g., "The boss is reading the newspaper"; "The packet contains cigarettes"). The bizarre sentences contained the same words but in different combinations, so that the action or typical characteristic was attributed to an absurd subject (e.g., "The monkey is reading the newspaper"; "The clothes-hanger contains cigarettes"). The abstract sentences described situations which are very difficult to imagine (e.g., "Promise induces hope"). The sentences were all taken from a pool used by PraBaldi, De Beni, Cornoldi & Cavedon (1985) and used to form four different lists, one randomly assigned to each subject. The words used to form the sentences were imaginable and commonly used even by blind people.

2.2.2. Procedure: Subjects were tested individually, basically following Merry & Graham's (1978) procedure. All subjects were instructed to form an image as soon as they heard each sentence and to rate the image verbally on one of the following classifications: "ordinary" - the sort of thing you might easily meet in the real world; "bizarre" - unlikely, ridiculous, the sort of thing you would not normally meet even though you can form an image of it in your mind; "don't know" - unable to decide whether the image is ordinary or unlikely, but can form an image; "can't image" or "abstract" - very difficult or impossible to form an image at all. The subjects were helped in the identification of the four categories by prior presentation and discussion of some examples.

When subjects had clearly understood these distinctions, the test was begun. Subjects were asked not so much to memorize as to form good images whenever possible and to classify them. The sentences were presented at 10-second intervals. Following this presentation subjects were given an interpolated task: the experimenter read a newspaper article slowly and subjects were asked to say "yes" after every word containing the letter E. An oral recall test then followed.

2.3. Chaining test

2.3.1. Material: 18 words of high imagery value and commonly used in Italian, chosen so as to have both high imagery value and be well-known to blind subjects too. The words were: curtain, book, funeral, ice-cream, salt, tree, gun, lemon, car, handkerchief, concert, laugh, tie, shower, chain, glasses, rain, and sound. They were taken from the list used by De Beni & Cornoldi (1985).

2.3.2. Procedure: Subjects were tested individually. They were first shown and then taught the chaining technique, following the illustrations and examples in Forno's (1980) memory technique manual, which have been proved suitable for rapid and effective teaching of the technique. When subjects were clearly able to use it, the test itself began. The experimenter read out the 18 words at 10-second intervals and then gave an interpolated task (identical to that used for the recall task with common and bizarre sentences), reading a newspaper article slowly. About half the subjects did the chaining test first and then the recall test, and the other half vice versa.

3. RESULTS

3.1. Ratings and recall of common, bizarre and abstract sentences

Previous research with this material had shown that our sentence classification was shared by most normal seeing adult subjects. In this case, it was interesting to see whether the blind subjects found it equally easy to classify or not. We thus calculated how many sentences were classified in each of the three categories as we had defined them and how many were not, because subjects either gave different classifications or did not know in which category to put them. Fig. 1 shows that the number of cases in which sentences were classified as expected is slightly higher for seeing subjects; discrepancies mainly deal with the bizarre and abstract ones. A 2 x 3 ANOVA (groups x type of sentence) for mixed design showed only one significant effect related to type of sentence ($F(2,96) = 21.33$; $p < .001$). Common sentences appeared to be correctly evaluated in the great majority of cases, while for many of the bizarre and abstract sentences some subjects (mainly the blind ones) differed, generally because they were unsure and refused to assign a category to a sentence.

Therefore, as regards memory performance, we decided to evaluate memory in relation not to subjects' classification but to the sentence category we had established. An initial evaluation of recall was carried out by considering the number of sentences of each type entirely recalled by both groups of subjects (Fig. 2). A 2 x 3 ANOVA (groups x type of sentence) for mixed design showed one significant effect for type of sentence ($F(2,96) = 36.56$; $p < .001$) (F values on the other main factor and interaction were less than 1).

Considering that the grammatical parts of the sentences could have been recalled differently according to group and type of material, the numbers of totally recalled subject nouns, verbs, and object nouns were evaluated separately, as shown in Fig. 3. A 2 x 3 x 3 ANOVA (groups x type of sentence x part of sentence) was then calculated for mixed design, and showed the following significant effects:

398

- type of sentence: F(2,96) = 39.30; p < .001 (Ms = 157.87; er = 4.01);
- part of sentence: F(2,96) = 14.38; p < .001 (Ms = 2.38; er = .17).

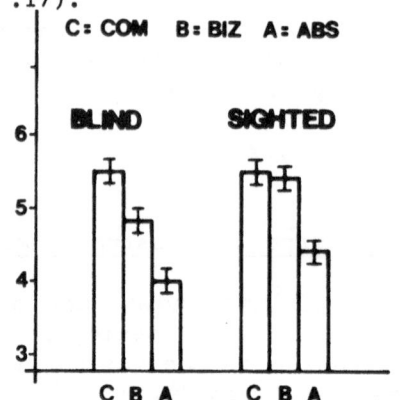

FIGURE 1. Mean number of correct classifications made by 2 groups of subjects (blind and sighted) on 3 kinds of sentences (common, bizarre, abstract).

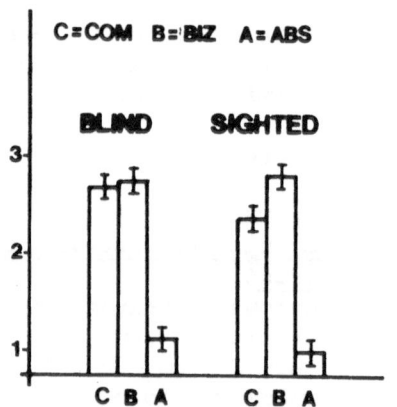

FIGURE 2. Mean number of complete sentences of 3 kinds (common, bizarre, abstract) recalled by blind and sighted subjects.

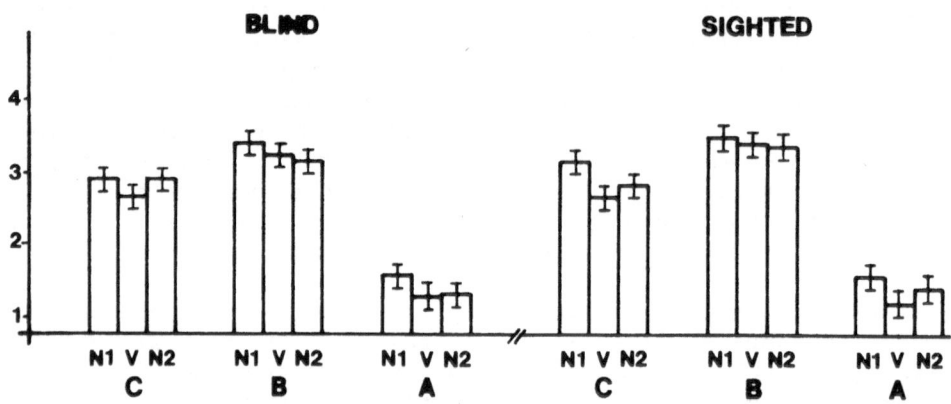

FIGURE 3. Mean number of part of sentences (N1 = subject noun, V = verb, N2 = object noun) recalled by sighted and blind subjects.

As Fig. 3 shows, the effect associated with type of sentence is related to poorer recall of words contained in abstract sentences and to better recall of words in common and bizarre sentences. As regards parts of speech, subject nouns are better recalled than other parts. In particular, this difference tends to vary according to type of sentence: the interaction type of sentence x part of speech yields F(4,192) = 2.37; p = .053.

3.2. Chaining test

We first considered the total number of words recalled by the two groups, divided according to whether the word fell in the first or second part of the list. A 2 x 2 ANOVA (groups x part of list) for mixed designs showed that both effects were significant: for groups (F(1,48) = 4.86; p = .02) and for part of list (F(1,48) = 12.18; p = .001). Interaction was not significant (F < 1). Fig. 4 shows that blind subjects recalled fewer words and that the first part of the list was generally recalled better than the second.

In this type of analysis we considered the total number of words recalled, independently of whether they were recalled in sequence or whether they somehow showed that they had been recalled by the chaining principle. For this reason, we decided to distinguish two methods of recalling the items: "chained" in which the strategy had probably been used, and "scattered" in which it had presumably not been used. A word was considered as recalled in a "chained" way if it was recalled after the word immediately preceding it in the order of presentation. We hypothesized in this case that it had been recalled thanks to chaining with the preceding word. If the first word of the list was remembered first, it was considered as having been recalled according to the chaining strategy.

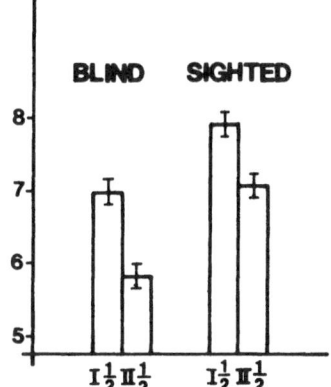

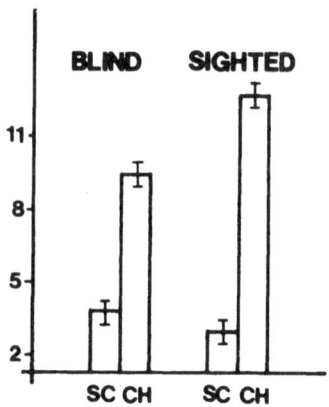

FIGURE 4. Mean number of words of first and second halves of list recalled by blind and sighted subjects.

FIGURE 5. Mean number of chained recall words and scattered recall words remembered by blind and sighted subjects.

For an overall analysis of these data, we decided to consider the "chained" and "scattered" recall modalities as two levels of a variable. A 2 x 2 ANOVA (groups x recall modalities) for mixed designs showed that all effects were significant: for groups (F(1,48) = 4.75; p = .03), recall modality

$(F(1,48) = 52.39, p < .001)$, and interaction $(F(1,48) = 3.7; p = .05)$. As Fig. 5 shows, the number of "chained recall" words is clearly higher than "scattered recall" ones, but this difference is greater for the sighted group, showing that they use chaining to a greater extent.

On the other hand, blind subjects do show partial improvement with the chaining technique. This conclusion was reached by considering the performance of a group of ten adult sighted subjects (a control group of blind subjects could not be found), who were tested with the same words in the same way but who did not use the chaining technique. They recalled a significantly lower number of words $(x = 7.4)$.

4. CONCLUSIONS

Our results show that even congenitally blind subjects can perform quite well in memory technique situations requiring the use of mental images. Their performance on imagining bizarre situations and recalling them is much better than on abstract situations, more or less like that of sighted subjects. Blind subjects are also able to improve their performance by using the chaining memory technique, but they are at a disadvantage when compared with sighted subjects. In this latter case, it is thus assumed that mental images are used, but that they are limited because of image weakening due to the element differentiating them from sighted subjects, i.e., the absence of visual experience. If we relate this difficulty to that emerging from our previous research, we see that both on chaining and on the triplet tasks, subjects were asked to form interactive images which were both progressive and multiple. In both cases, three aspects represented by the request to form an interactive image were implicit: the multiplicity and progressivity of this image first dealt with the interaction of one element with a second, and then with the interaction of one of the elements (in the chaining task) or of both elements (in the triplet task) with a third. Instead, with respect to previous investigations on memory techniques for loci, no reference to a mental place was required in the present test. We may therefore conclude that this was not the only critical element for blind subjects, although their much poorer performance in previous research indicates that the place reference may also be a problem for them.

REFERENCES

1. Cornoldi C., Calore D. & Pra Baldi A. (1979). Imagery ratings and recall in congenitally blind subjects. Perceptual and Motor Skills, 48, 627-629.

2. De Beni R. & Cornoldi C. (1985). The effects of imaginal mnemonics on congenitally total blind and on normal subjects. In D.F. Marks and D.G. Russell (Eds.) Imagery 1, Human Performance Associates, Dunedin, New Zealand.

3. Forno G. (1980). Sviluppare la memoria è facile e divertente. Universale MEB, Torino.

4. Higbee K.L. (1977). Your memory. How it works and how to improve it. Prentice-Hall, Englewood Cliffs, New Jersey.

5. Kerr N.H. (1983). The role of vision in "visual imagery" experiments: evidence from congenitally blind. Journal of Experimental Psychology: General 2, 265-267.

6. Jonides J., Kahn R. & Rozin P. (1975). Imagery instructions improve memory in blind subjects. Bulletin of the Psychonomic Society, 5, 424-426.

7. Marmor G.S. (1978). Age at onset of blindness and the development of the semantics of color names. Journal of Experimental Child Psychology, 25, 267-278.

8. Merry R. & Graham N.C. (1978). Imagery bizarreness in children's recall of sentences. British Journal of Psychology, 69, 315-321.

9. Paivio A. & Okovita H.W. (1971). Word imagery modalities and associative learning in blind and sighted subjects. Journal of Verbal Learning and Verbal Behavior, 10, 506-510.

10. Pra Baldi A., De Beni R., Cornoldi C. & Cavedon A. (1985). Some conditions for the occurrence of the bizarreness effect in free recall. British Journal of Psychology, 76, 427-436.

11. Sholl M.J. & Easton R.D. (1986). Effect of referent object familiarity on verbal learning in the sighted and the blind. Journal of Experimental Psychology: Learning, Memory and Cognition, 12, 2, 190-200.

12. Zimler J. & Keenan J.M. (1983). Imagery in the congenitally blind: how visual are visual images? Journal of Experimental Psychology: Learning, Memory and Cognition, 2, 269-282.

4.3. DISCUSSION OF PART 4

THE FUNCTIONAL ROLE OF IMAGERY IN COGNITION ?

MARC MARSCHARK

THE UNIVERSITY OF NORTH CAROLINA AT GREENSBORO
GREENSBORO, NORTH CAROLINA, USA

ABSTRACT
The role of imagery in learning, memory, and cognition can be clarified if the storage of information is distinguished from the use of that information following retrieval. Empirical findings from studies in several domains represented at this conference indicate a functional role for imagery in human cognition, but neither previous data nor any of the new findings require the conclusion that images serve as analog representations in long-term memory. Rather, the results from most studies are consistent with the notion that concreteness and imagery effects result from differential processing of distinctive and relational information for high- and low-imagery materials and contexts.

1. INTRODUCTION

If one surveys recent literature on mental imagery, most investigators seem to fit into one of three orientations. The two primary (and traditional) orientations include those who deny a functional role for imagery per se in cognition (Anderson, 1978 ; Pylyshyn, 1980) and those who ascribe the analog, perception-like quality of images with an essential role in learning, memory, and performance in several domains (e.g., Helstrup, this volume ; Kosslyn et al., 1979 ; Paivio, 1986). These two positions can be described as opposing parties in the "analog versus propositional debate", although the argument has been made elsewhere that the two argue on different, and not mutually exclusive levels (Marschark et al., 1987).

The third orientation in imagery research has been suggested periodically over the last 10 years (Marschark & Paivio, 1977 ; Nelson et al., 1977 ; Snodgrass, 1984), but until recently was never fleshed out in any way that led to a priori predictions directly challenging the more traditional views of imagery. From this perspective, mental imagery may be involved in "on-line" processes such as language comprehension, mental manipulation, and verbal learning, much as described by Baddeley and his colleagues in their "visuo-spatial sketchpad" (Baddeley, this volume ; Logie et al., this volume) but analog representation in long-term memory is denied (Marschark et al., 1987). Descriptions of imaginal and verbal systems in such views therefore tend to include some amodal memory that preserves both perceptual and non-percep-

M. Denis et al. (eds.), Cognitive and Neuropsychological Approaches to Mental Imagery, 405–417.
© *1988 by Martinus Nijhoff Publishers.*

tual information in similar forms. For convenience, this position will be referred to as the "imagery as process" view, so as to emphasize that imagery is assumed to play its role during processing rather than in memory.

The problem, heretofore, with the imagery as process view, is that most of its support has been in the form of negative evidence. That is, the data that have compelled this approach derive from findings that are inconsistent with representational imagery theories, such as Paivio's (1971, 1986, this volume) dual coding model. The theoretical mechanism by which imagery might facilitate learning and memory for verbal materials while not actually being the form of memorial representation meanwhile has remained absent if not elusive. (It is worthwhile noting here that tasks such as mental rotation and mental scanning provide evidence of on-line analog processes but are mute with respect to the form of long-term memory representations. See Marschark et al., 1987, for the distinction in symbolic comparisons.)

Recently, however, my colleagues and I have developed a theory of mental imagery, based on the imagery as process view, that provides a description of its functional role in learning and memory (Hunt & Marschark, 1987 ; Marschark, 1985; Marschark & Hunt, 1987 ; Marschark et al., 1987). The goals throughout this research have been consistent with those espoused by John Richardson in his concluding comments at the European Workshop on Imagery in Cognition (EWIC). Richardson asked for a theory of imagery rich enough to generate predictions not only in new (laboratory-specific) methodologies, but also in more traditional paradigms. Challenging existing theories in this way and using existing data when available enable researchers to satisfy another of Richardson's requests : avoiding the proliferation of "arbitrary frameworks" by being willing to discredit and abandon personal views of imagery in the search for some "higher truth". In this spirit, the present chapter will provide some speculation and extrapolation from my preferred account of imagery effects in considering some of the data presented at the EWIC and some other new findings using those "traditional paradigms".

2. CONCRETENESS EFFECTS IN MEMORY FOR LANGUAGE : THE RESULT OF PROCESSING DISTINCTIVE AND RELATIONAL INFORMATION

2.1. A theoretical framework for imagery in verbal learning

This interpretation of concreteness effects in memory draws on several existing theories of memory and thus shares several characteristics with them. Consistent with the general framework proposed by Einstein and Hunt (1980) and Hunt and Marschark (1987), for example, recall of any given verbal unit is assumed to depend upon initial encoding of distinctive attributes of that unit as well as relations between it and other units in the immediate context. In retrieval, relational or shared information delineates a search set from which the target may be drawn and distinctive information then discriminates the target from other potential targets within the delineated set.

This framework was first applied to the role of imagery in memory for sentences and prose by Marschark (1985) and has been elaborated by Marschark and Hunt (1987) to account for related effects in paired-associate learning. At all three levels, the presence or absence of concreteness effects lies in the greater distinctiveness of encoded concrete items in memory relative to abstract items because of the availability of item-specific perceptual information. (Concrete and abstract materials can be assumed to involve the encoding of comparable item-specific semantic information). Depending on one's theoretical preference, this "extra" information can be seen as resulting in a "dual coding" (cf. Paivio, 1971, 1986) of perceptual and semantic information, although not in analog or verbal forms (Marschark et al., 1987), or of a more distinctive encoding for concrete words and sentences (Hunt & Marschark, 1987 ; Kieras, 1978 ; Schwanenflugel & Shoben, 1983).

2.2. Concreteness effects in paired-associate learning

In paired-associate learning (PAL), processing of individual word information is subordinated to the relational processing of stimuli and responses, which produces pair-specific information. Presentation of a stimulus word in recall serves as a relational cue to pair-specific information (i.e., delineating the set from which the response is to be drawn). The greater distinctiveness of concrete encodings then has its influence, producing the concreteness effect. Interestingly, this interpretation leads to the prediction that concreteness effects in PAL should be relatively easy to eliminate. One means of accomplishing this would be to block the effects of relational information at the time of recall so that no retrieval set would be delineated and the effects of encoded distinctive information could not come to bear. Alternatively, relational processing at encoding could be disrupted so that higher-order distinctive representations are not formed in the first place (see Hunt & Marschark, 1987, for further discussion). As long as the procedures are such that both imaginal and verbal representations are likely to be generated, a dual coding position would predict concreteness effects in virtually all of these situations.

Marschark and Hunt (1987) recently used the above and other manipulations in six PAL experiments and obtained the predicted results. In two experiments, for example, the relational role of retrieval cues was eliminated by having a free recall task follow the usual PAL task for half of the subjects. Those subjects who received standard cued recall tests showed robust concreteness effects whereas those who received free recall tests showed none. In another experiment, subjects rated either the ease of integrating stimulus and response elements into a single wholistic unit or rated the imageability of the individual items, still presented in pair format. Obviously, the lack of any relational processing in the imagery rating conditions would be expected to atte-

nuate or eliminate the formation of any pair-specific encodings, and, in fact, neither cued or free recall led to
concreteness effects under those orienting instructions.
Concreteness effects were obtained with integration rating
instructions.

2.3. Concreteness effects in memory for sentences

For over a decade, there has been a theoretical puzzle
concerning the role of imagery in memory for concrete and
abstract sentences. Concrete sentences in lists are typically
remembered better than abstract sentences, but both appear to
be stored in some holistic or integrated fashion (Brewer,
1975 ; Franks & Bransford, 1972 ; Marschark & Paivio, 1977).
Although the former finding is consistent with the dual
coding model, the basis for explaining that result is
directly contradicted by the latter finding, and both have
been demonstrated within the same experiment. Both findings,
however, are consistent with the present theoretical view.

Like PAL, the acquisition of concrete and abstract sentences in lists involves the subordination of word-specific
processing to a higher-order relational processing, here, the
derivation of sentence meaning. This process should be the
same for concrete and abstract sentences (cf. Kieras, 1978),
yielding the finding of similar integrated storage. At the
same time, however, comprehension of concrete sentences can
lead to the on-line construction of meaning-preserving images
and encoding of relevant perceptual information, thus providing additional sources of item-specific information not
matched by abstract sentences. This added distinctive information produces the typical overall superior recall of concrete sentences relative to abstract sentences that is found
even when indices of integration do not reveal differences
(Marschark & Paivio, 1977).

2.4. Concreteness effects in memory for prose

At the level of multi-sentence prose, the preceding
levels of processing still occur in the interpretation of
component propositions. At least for incidental memory,
however, recall should be more a function of relational
processing between propositions and the theme of the passage
(i.e., macrolevel relationships) than item-specific processing of units (microlevel information) within the passage
(Kintsch & van Dijk, 1978). Concreteness effects, which are
the result of item-specific encoding, thus should be attenuated if not eliminated in prose learning. Although this prediction may seem counterintuitive and is clearly contraindi-
cated by the dual coding model (e.g., Paivio, 1971 ; Yuille &
Paivio, 1969), it has been supported in several studies
(e.g., Bunn, 1986 ; Marschark, 1978, 1985) in which concreteness has been a between-subjects variable. When concreteness is a within-subjects variable, the situation is more
complex because mixed material sets can affect distinctiveness (see Hunt & Marschark, 1987, for discussion), and
results from such studies have been inconsistent (see
Marschark et al., 1987).

2.5. Summary

The locus of concreteness effects in memory for verbal materials has been described here in terms of the processing of shared and distinctive information. This theoretical view is consistent with a variety of findings previously taken as support for dual coding, insofar as both verbal and perceptual information may be involved in comprehending high-imagery sentences and in learning lists of concrete words. But going beyond previous accounts of imagery, this view also can provide explanations for several findings that appear contradictory to the thesis that concrete and abstract materials differ in the form of their storage in long-term memory. Although this does not rule out a role for imagery in list learning or text comprehension, it is clear that the complex processes involved in comprehension and memory for language go beyond mechanisms supplied by a theory based on the availability of modality-specific mental representations. The task now is to determine the viability of the theory in other domains.

Several domains of imagery research presented at EWIC provided fertile ground for evaluating my theoretical viewpoint. Although not all provide a basis for distinguishing representational theories of imagery from the imagery as process view, there are data in several areas that are more consistent with the latter than the former. In other cases, there are at least potential sources of evidence that would allow such a distinction. Given the structure of the conference and the chapters by Desrochers and McDaniel in this volume, my speculations here are confined to research concerning motor programs and memory, individual differences, emotion and memory, and neurophysiological bases of imagery. Given this considerable task and the fact that these areas are outside of the original (and previously tested) scope of the theory, my comments necessarily will be brief and speculative.

3. INDIVIDUAL DIFFERENCES, EMOTION, AND IMAGERY

There can be little doubt that there are individual differences in both the fluency and vividness of mental imagery (e.g., Aylwin, this volume ; Conway, this volume ; Denis, 1987 ; Ernest, 1983, 1987 ; Katz, 1983), and that, Pylyshyn's (1980) arguments notwithstanding, these images play a functional role in our behavior in a variety of domains, including emotion, mental comparisons, perception, language comprehension, and motor performance (e.g., Acosta et al., this volume ; Bunn, 1986 ; Cocude, this volume ; Conway, this volume ; Cornoldi & De Beni, this volume ; Helstrup, this volume ; see also Paivio, 1986a, for a review). McDaniel (this volume) has reviewed some of the relevant literature and described its contribution to imagery research at-large, and so that need not be reconsidered here. It is important to re-emphasize, however, just how little we know about individual differences in imagery skill, precision, and use. Consistent relationships between self-reports of imagery use and assessments of imagery abilities through the use of standardized tests are relatively hard to find (e.g., Katz, 1983), and neither of these are as strongly related to behavioral indices of imagery as one might suppose (or desire).

Even more important for the present purposes is the fact that what we do know about individual differences in the speed, vividness, and spontaneous use of imagery generally relates to imagery as a process and says remarkably little about imagery as a long-term representational modality. Task dependence is a hallmark of imagery use and, for that matter, of verbal and nonverbal strategies in general (Bischof, this volume ; Cocude, this volume ; Denis, 1987 ; Katz, 1983 ; Paivio, 1986). Although "high-imagers" appear to construct images more quickly (Ernest & Paivio, 1971) and surpass "low-imagers" in various tasks involving picture recognition and mental comparison (Paivio, 1986, Chapters 6 and 9), the finding that imagery ability is not related to recognition thresholds (Ernest, 1983) or speed of retrieval of magnitude information (Marschark et al., 1987), suggests a disassociation between the form of memorial information and its use after retrieval.

Symbolic comparisons represent a paradigm case for this argument. In a variety of experiments, Paivio (1975, 1978) has shown that "high-imagers" make mental judgments on perceptual dimensions faster than "low-imagers", whereas "high-verbalizers" are faster in making judgments on linguistic dimensions. My own research on bipolar comparative judgments (some of it with Paivio, e.g., Marschark & Paivio, 1981), however, has indicated that the retrieval of magnitude information in such tasks can be empirically distinguished from a subsequent comparison stage in which that information is used (e.g., Marschark, 1983 ; see also Duncan & McFarland, 1980). Further, what little evidence is available indicates imagery ability to be related to the speed of comparisons but not the speed of retrieval (see Marschark et al., 1987, for details). This result is consistent with Cocude's (this volume) demonstration of a distinction between image generation and image maintenance with regard to individual differences, and consistent findings of imagery-like effects in some aspects of spatial processing in subjects who lack histories of visual experience (Cornoldi & De Beni, this volume ; see Ernest, 1987, for a review).

Considerably more work needs to be done in determining exactly what it means to be a "high-imager", as well as what it means to be a "high-verbalizer" in comparable situations. Nonetheless, it seems likely that the distinctions involved relate more to the strategic and spontaneous use of different strategies and the resolution of something like Baddeley's visuo-spatial sketchpad than the extent to which the world is preserved in memory in some analog form. There may be empirically verifiable differences in the extent to which individuals encode and remember perceptual information from stimulus arrays, but demonstrations thereof need to distinguish such behavior from the on-line use of imagery per se.

4. IMAGERY AND MOTOR SKILL

Although study of the role of mental imagery in motor performance and the effectiveness of mental (motor) rehearsal has increased considerably over the last 20 years, the area still appears to be in its infancy. As in the research described in the preceding section, the empirical results from investigations of imagery and motor skill have been variable with regard to domain specificity, the effects of instructional manipulations, and individual differences. Paivio (1985), however, recently offered a framework for research in this area, following his observation of the inconsistent effects of mental practice in various sports. He suggested that both general (e.g., affective and physiological) and specific (e.g., goal-oriented) motivational factors in mental practice need to be considered in concert with cognitive factors (also at both levels). This approach seems likely to clarify a variety of issues and contradictory findings in the area, and readers interested in background information are directed to his 1985 paper and another by Denis (1985).

Of interest here are the attempts of several investigators, including Engelkamp (this volume) and Perrig (this volume), to distinguish motor codes from "imaginal" codes in memory. Acknowledging that one goal of this paper was to integrate several new areas of research into the framework described in Section 2, this is one area in which a good theoretical fit was remarkably straightforward, and perhaps conceptually simpler than the alternatives presented at EWIC.

Perrig (this volume), for example, attempts to differentiate motor and imaginal codes on the basis of his consistent finding that motor ("enaction") coding leads to better memory than imaginal coding. While Denis (1985) had suggested that imagery might enhance the memorability of kinesthetic information through the elaboration of the memorial code, Perrig suggested that kinesthetic (motor) coding might improve memorability through the restriction of the potential retrieval set from which a to-be-recalled item would be drawn. This latter interpretation should sound familiar, insofar as it fits precisely the earlier description of item-specific processing as the basis of concreteness effects in memory for verbal materials. That is, motor encoding may improve recall by creating a more distinctive representation in memory (influenced by the egocentric nature of encoding as well as the restricted set size), effectively producing a "smaller underlying set", in Perrig's terms. In this view, Perrig's results no more require postulation of a separate motor code in memory than concreteness effects require postulation of a long-term imaginal code. Our two views, in fact, are highly compatible, and testing them head-to-head may lead to some interesting new findings.

Engelkamp (this volume) and Engelkamp and Zimmer (1985) have attempted to distinguish a "motor sub-system" in memory from the "visual sub-system" (i.e., visual imagery) and to describe its functional role in verbal processing. In particular, Engelkamp (this volume) argues that the motor sub-system might be responsible for differences in organization of the subjective lexicons for concrete and abstract words. On one hand, one can imagine Paivio arguing that any effects of "motor imagery" on differential memory for concrete and abstract verbal materials are already incorporated in dual coding theory. The onus would then be on Engelkamp and his colleagues to demonstrate functional differences between the two theoretical views (see Engelkamp & Zimmer, 1985). Alternatively, the effects of their "motor sub-system" on encoding and memory could be described, as above, in terms of the enhanced distinctiveness of concrete and/or motor-related concepts in particular encoding contexts, thus precluding any necessity for yet another memory code. Engelkamp's theoretical view, like Perrig's, thus appears to differ from my own view in much the same way as does Paivio's (1971, 1985, 1986). The question in Engelkamp's and Perrig's cases is whether the postulation of a separate mental code, in addition to verbal and "imaginal" codes, is necessary, or whether a more general principle such as differences in relational and distinctive processing of motoric information can account for his novel findings as well as those indicating the influence of verbal and imaginal processing. Only empirical tests will allow a definitive answer, but thorough consideration of the evidence for imaginal memory codes (Marschark et al., 1987) would appear to favor the processing approach.

5. IMAGERY AND THE BRAIN

The neuropsychological bases and correlates of imagery, of course, cannot be fully understood independently of individual differences, task domains, and the various modalities of mental imagery, a complex relationship outside of the scope of the present chapter. This discussion thus is intended to highlight several general but important issues, while deferring more precise comment to other authors in this volume.

We have known for some time that the right hemisphere typically plays a major role in spatial processing (but see Bryden, 1979 ; Ernest, 1983, for evidence of alternative possibilities) and several investigators have explicitly described neurophysiological commonalities in visual imagery and perception (e.g., Farah, 1985 ; see Finke & Shepard, 1985, for a review) and the roles of the right and left hemispheres in imaginal and verbal processing, respectively (e.g., Ernest, 1983 ; see Paivio, 1986, for a review). These commonalities are components in the theoretical views of imagery by Paivio (1986), Brooks (1968), Hebb (1968), and others.

With regard to the commonalities between imagery and perception, Péronnet et al.'s (this volume) research using visually evoked potential recordings supported Farah's (1985) earlier findings indicating that imagery and perception have some common underlying structures and obtained further evidence indicating that imagery activates the visual system relatively early in an image-object comparison task. Bisiach and Berti's (this volume) evidence that unilateral neglect in visual processing extends to imaginal processing is also consistent with an hypothesized intimate relationship between visual perception and visual imagery and the work with PET scan technology by Goldenberg et al. (this volume) has now clearly demonstrated cortical localization during and after imaginal processing.

Such results are impressive and support our intuitions and behavioral data indicating that high- and low-imagery materials may be processed in qualitatively different manners (see also Marschark, 1979, for differences in perceptual encoding strategies). Nevertheless, these results do not speak to the issue of whether images play any role in long-term memory. The indication of neurological differences in processing concrete and abstract material is, at some level, necessary for both representational and process views of imagery. They provide sufficient grounds for accepting the process view of imagery, but do not rule out a process-plus-representation difference in memory for the two material types.

Some potentially more definitive evidence is offered in examining data from brain damaged patients of the sort described by John Richardson (this volume) and in some of his previously published research (e.g., Richardson, 1979, 1984 ; Richardson & Barry, 1985). Two findings are of interest here. In an evaluation of a group of 40 individuals with closed-head brain injuries, Richardson (1979) found an impairment in free recall of concrete word lists but not abstract lists (i.e., subjects did not demonstrate concreteness effects). Interpreting his results in terms of Paivio's (1971) dual coding theory, Richardson assumed that his subjects had imagery-specific deficiencies : they either failed to construct images, failed to store their images, were prone to forget their images, or simply could not retrieve them. In subsequent research, Richardson and Barry (1985) found that brain-injured subjects did obtain concreteness effects when instructed to use imagery and they thus concluded that the lack of observed effects reflected a deficiency in spontaneous encoding of verbal material into an imaginal form (cf. Baddeley & Warrington, 1973).

In encouraging individuals to use imagery, however, Richardson and Barry (1985), and essentially all other researchers and therapists who have done work in this area, instructed them to "make up mental images which related together the things described by the words in each list" (p. 16). Thus, an alternative interpretation of their results is that both control and brain-injured subjects spontaneously generated images (and resultant item-specific encodings) for the words, but the brain-injured subjects failed to spontaneously link those encodings relationally. In recall, the lack of such relational information would have eliminated the effects of item distinctiveness : the concreteness effect.

Although speculative, there is some evidence that appears to support the relational-distinctiveness interpretation over the dual coding interpretation of Richardson's results. One source of evidence comes from Professor Herb Crovitz's research with brain-injured patients (including university students and faculty). Part of Crovitz's standard evaluation following an individual's head injury is presenting a sentence like "John took a shower before Mary bought the cake" and then asking "When did Mary buy the cake ?" After 5-6 seconds, the usual answer is "Before John took a shower". Not for another 7-8 seconds do subjects offer something like "No, that can't be right !" (personal communication, November, 1986). Although such disruptions in relational processing are common, Crovitz does not observe deficits in the formation of item-specific images. Baddeley and Warrington (1973) similarly found concreteness related deficits in amnesics who claimed to be able to form visual images, thus indicating a post-image construction problem.

Another source of evidence that appears to support my case comes from a study by Richardson (1984). In brief, he found that when control subjects made intrusion errors in recall of concrete or abstract lists, those errors were consistent with the concreteness of the to-be-recalled words (e.g., concrete words intruding into other concrete lists). Brain-injured subjects did not produce similar homogeneity in their intrusions. Although Richardson suggested that this finding may have indicated a disruption in "the normal encoding of the image-evoking quality of the stimulus material" (p. 158), a failure in relational processing is just as viable an explanation (see also Wilson, this volume).

The alternative interpretations of both of Richardson's findings could be evaluated in a task in which brain-injured subjects learned categorized and control word lists under rote, item-specific imagery, verbal relational, or relational imagery instructions. An imagery encoding deficit would be reflected in a) item-specific imagery and imagery-relational instructions producing better performance than rote and relational instructions and b) heterogeneous intrusions under rote and relational instructions. A relational encoding deficit would be reflected in a) relational and imagery-relational instructions producing better performance than rote and item-specific instructions and b) homogeneity in recall of categorized relative to control lists, regardless of instructional condition. Research along these lines is now being initiated in my laboratory.

6. CONCLUSIONS

Most of the papers presented at EWIC reinforced existing evidence for modality-specific processing of information and its effects on performance in several domains. As should be evident by now, however, I do not believe that any of that research or any previous findings compel us to assume that modality-specific analogs are retained in long-term memory. Certainly modality-relevant information is retained, but that is a very different matter. Analog representations (visual, olfactory, motor, etc.) entail multiple memory codes ; processing differences can be accounted for in terms of the sensory apparatus and on-line processes. The latter does not eliminate the need to understand how perceptual information is represented in the short term (see, e.g., Baddeley, this volume), both on the encoding end and the retrieval or redintegration end, but it does solve a variety of empirical puzzles and diffuse the always impending threat of infinite numbers of codes, interlinguae, and analog-versus-propositional arguments.

On the basis of my own research on symbolic comparisons, language comprehension, and memory for verbal materials, the most viable account of both imagery and concreteness effects appears to lie in the differential processing of relational and item-specific information under different instructional conditions, with different materials, and among individuals in differing physiological states or with different cognitive skills and preferences. This view does not deter me from imagery research, but rather encourages my further search for the "higher truths" of imagery and cognition.

REFERENCES

1. Anderson, J.R. (1978). Arguments concerning representations for mental imagery. Psychological Review, 85, 249-277.
2. Brewer, W. (1975). Memory for ideas : Synonym substitution. Memory and Cognition, 3, 458-464.
3. Brooks, L.R. (1968). Spatial and verbal components of the act of recall. Canadian Journal of Psychology, 22, 349-368.
4. Bryden, M.P. (1979). Evidence for sex-related differences in cerebral organization. In M.A. Wittig & A.C. Peterson (Eds.), Sex-related differences in cognitive functioning: Developmental issues. New York : Academic Press.
5. Bunn, C. (1986). Individual differences in spatial-imagery ability and memory for concrete and abstract prose. Unpublished honors thesis, Trent University, Peterborough, Ontario, Canada.
6. Denis, M. (1985). Visual imagery and the use of mental practice in the development of motor skills. Canadian Journal of Applied Sport Sciences, 10, 4S-16S.
7. Denis, M. (1987). Individual imagery differences and prose processing. In M.A. McDaniel & M. Pressley (Eds.), Imagery and related mnemonic processes : Theories, individual differences and applications. New York : Springer/Verlag.
8. Duncan, E.M. & McFarland, C.E., Jr. (1980). Isolating the effects of symbolic distance and semantic congruity in comparative judgments : An additive-factors analysis. Memory and Cognition, 8, 612-622.
9. Einstein, G.O. & Hunt, R.R. (1980). Levels of processing and organization : Additive effects of individual item and relational processing. Journal of Experimental Psychology : Human Learning and Memory, 6, 588-598.

10. Engelkamp, J. & Zimmer, H.D. (1985). Motor programs and their relation to semantic memory. The German Journal of Psychology, 9, 239-254.
11. Ernest, C. (1983). Spatial-imagery ability, sex differences, and hemispheric functioning. In J.C. Yuille (Ed.), Imagery, memory, and cognition : Essays in honor of Allan Paivio. Hillsdale, N.J. : Lawrence Erlbaum.
12. Ernest, C. (1987). Imagery and the blind : A review. In M.A. McDaniel & M. Pressley (Eds.), Imagery and related mnemonic processes : Theories, individual differences, and applications. New York : Springer/Verlag.
13. Ernest, C. & Paivio, A. (1971). Imagery and sex differences in incidental recall. British Journal of Psychology, 62, 67-72.
14. Farah, M.J. (1985). Psychophysical evidence for a shared representational medium for mental images and percepts. Journal of Experimental Psychology : General, 114, 91-103.
15. Finke, R.A. & Shepard, R.N. (1985). Visual functions of mental imagery. In L. Kaufman and J. Thomas (Eds.), Handbook of perception and performance. New York : Wiley.
16. Franks, J.J. & Bransford, J.D. (1972). The acquisition of abstract ideas. Journal of Verbal Learning and Verbal Behavior, 11, 311-315.
17. Hebb, D.O. (1968). Concerning imagery. Psychological Review, 75, 466-477.
18. Hunt, R.R. & Marschark, M. (1987). Yet another picture of imagery : The role of shared and distinctive information. In M.A. McDaniel & M. Pressley (Eds.), Imagery and related mnemonic processes : Theories, individual differences, and applications. New York : Springer/Verlag.
19. Katz, A. (1983). What does it mean to be a high imager ? In J.C. Yuille (Ed.), Imagery, memory, and cognition : Essays in honor of Allan Paivio. Hillsdale, N.J. : Lawrence Erlbaum.
20. Kieras, D. (1978). Beyond pictures and words : Alternative information processing models for imagery effects in verbal memory. Psychological Bulletin, 85, 532-554.
21. Kintsch, W. & van Dijk, T.A. (1978). Toward a model of text comprehension and production. Psychological Review, 85, 532-554.
22. Kosslyn, S.M., Pinker, S., Smith, G.E., & Shwartz, S.P. (1979). On the demystification of mental imagery. The Behavioral and Brain Sciences, 2, 535-581.
23. Marschark, M. (1978). Prose processing : A chronometric study of the effects of imageability. Unpublished doctoral dissertation, University of Western Ontario, London, Ontario, Canada.
24. Marschark, M. (1979). The syntax and semantics of comprehension. In G. Prideaux (Ed.), Perspectives in experimental linguistics. Amsterdam : John Benjamins B.V.
25. Marschark, M. (1983). Semantic congruity in symbolic comparisons : Salience, expectancy, and associative priming. Memory and Cognition, 11, 192-199.

26. Marschark, M. (1985). Imagery and organization in the recall of prose. Journal of Memory and Language, 24, 734-745.
27. Marschark, M., & Hunt, R.R. (1987). Imagery effects in paired associate learning : Now you see 'em, now you don't. In preparation.
28. Marschark, M. & Paivio, A. (1977). Integrative processing of concrete and abstract sentences. Journal of Verbal Learning and Verbal Behavior, 16, 217-231.
29. Marschark, M. & Paivio, A. (1981). Congruity and the perceptual comparison task. Journal of Experimental Psychology : Human Perception and Performance, 7, 290-308.
30. Marschark, M., Richman, C.L., Yuille, J.C., & Hunt, R.R. (1987). The role of imagery in memory : On shared and distinctive information. Psychological Bulletin, 102, 28-41.
31. Nelson, D.L., Reed, V.S., & McEvoy, C.L. (1977). Learning to order pictures and words : A model of sensory and semantic coding. Journal of Experimental Psychology : Human Learning and Memory, 3, 485-497.
32. Paivio, A. (1971). Imagery and verbal processes. New York: Holt, Rinehart, and Winston.
33. Paivio, A. (1975). Perceptual comparisons through the mind's eye. Memory and Cognition, 3, 635-647.
34. Paivio, A. (1978). Comparisons of mental clocks. Journal of Experimental Psychology : Human Perception and Performance, 4, 61-71.
35. Paivio, A. (1985). Cognitive and motivational functions of imagery in human performance. Canadian Journal of Applied Sport Sciences, 10, 22S-28S.
36. Paivio, A. (1986). Mental representations : A dual coding approach. Oxford : Oxford University Press.
37. Pylyshyn, Z.W. (1980). Computation and cognition : Issues in the foundations of cognitive science. The Behavioral and Brain Sciences, 3, 111-169.
38. Richardson, J.T.E. (1979). Mental imagery, human memory, and the effects of closed head injury. British Journal of Social and Clinical Psychology, 18, 319-327.
39. Richardson, J.T.E. (1984). The effects of closed head injury upon intrusions and confusions in free recall. Cortex, 20, 413-420.
40. Richardson, J.T.E. & Barry, C. (1985). The effects of minor closed head injury upon human memory : Further evidence of the role of mental imagery. Cognitive Neuropsychology, 2, 149-168.
41. Schwanenflugel, P. & Shoben, E.J. (1983). Differential context effects in the comprehension of abstract and concrete prose. Journal of Experimental Psychology : Learning, Memory, and Cognition, 9, 82-102.
42. Snodgrass, J.G. (1984). Concepts and their surface representations. Journal of Verbal Learning and Verbal Behavior, 23, 3-23.
43. Yuille, J.C. & Paivio, A. (1969). Abstractness and the recall of connected discourse. Journal of Experimental Psychology, 82, 467-471.

PART 5

CONCLUDING REMARKS

EUROPEAN CONTRIBUTIONS TO RESEARCH ON IMAGERY AND COGNITION

JOHN T. E. RICHARDSON
DEPARTMENT OF HUMAN SCIENCES, BRUNEL UNIVERSITY,
UXBRIDGE, MIDDLESEX, U.K.

MICHEL DENIS
CENTRE D'ETUDES DE PSYCHOLOGIE COGNITIVE,
UNIVERSITE DE PARIS-SUD, ORSAY, FRANCE

JOHANNES ENGELKAMP
DEPARTMENT OF PSYCHOLOGY, UNIVERSITY OF THE SAARLAND,
D-6600 SAARBRUECKEN, F.R.G.

1. THE EUROPEAN WORKSHOP ON IMAGERY AND COGNITION

In this volume, we have reported selected contributions to the European Workshop on Imagery and Cognition, whose objectives were as follows: to extend existing efforts aimed at enhancing scientific exchange among European cognitive psychologists and neuropsychologists involved in imagery research; to provide a setting where researchers could mutually inform each other of their recent as well as future lines of research; to provide an opportunity for initiating collaboration in the field of imagery; and to discuss possible new forms of scientific interaction among European imagery researchers. As the members of the scientific committee responsible for the scientific content and organization of the Workshop, we ourselves can hardly claim to be neutral evaluators. Nevertheless, we are confident in concluding that all of these objectives were admirably fulfilled. We were perhaps even a little embarrassed at the amount of interest which the Workshop attracted, and the large number of participants meant that the proceedings were occasionally more formal (and polite) than we had originally intended. On the other hand, the participants were most cooperative in submitting themselves to the rather gruelling schedule. To be sure, the wealth of material contained in this volume testifies to the tremendous potential for European collaboration in the area of imagery and cognition in the immediate future.

2. CURRENT DEVELOPMENTS IN IMAGERY RESEARCH

Some of the topics examined during the Workshop have been raised since the earliest days of imagery research. For instance, a central issue is that of the relationship between imagery and perception and the question of the commonality of the psychological structures and processes implicated in imaging and perceiving. The paper by Allan Paivio discusses some of the other "basic puzzles" that have preoccupied the scientific investigation of mental imagery. Although such problems may be old ones, many of the papers presented here are

421

M. Denis et al. (eds.), Cognitive and Neuropsychological Approaches to Mental Imagery, 421–428.
© 1988 by Martinus Nijhoff Publishers.

based upon new conceptualizations and methodologies that
confront and challenge older approaches. Be that as it may,
several of the topics which were examined in the Workshop would
simply not have been addressed at a similar event five or ten
years earlier. Furthermore, what is striking is that in each
case European scientists have made significant contributions
to recent developments in research on imagery and cognition.
We would point to three major examples of this trend.

One persistent issue in imagery research has been that of
defining the relationship between imagery and linguistic
representations. However, work on this topic has until
recently been restricted to language processing at the sentence
or even the word level. It is only in the last few years that
the first few steps have been taken to study the role of mental
imagery in the realm of text processing. Such a task requires
the careful elaboration of theoretical presuppositions and
hypotheses not only with respect to the cognitive processes
which are involved, but also with regard to the nature and
organization of the representational structures that are
assumed to be activated by such processes.

A formally similar yet totally new development is the
discussion of the relationship between imagery and action (or
motor activity in general). In principle, images and actions
seem to involve different processes. Not only are they
different insofar as the former are private mental events
whereas the latter are directed outwards and are publicly
observable, but they also produce clearly different effects
upon performance. On the other hand, the two kinds of
processes are not totally independent of each other. Recent
research has clearly demonstrated the importance of mental
imagery in the acquisition of certain motor skills and in the
internal representation of actions and behaviour. This
research illustrates the potential relevance of imagery
research to a wider range of human activities than has
previously been considered.

A third area of interest is that of brain research, which
is reflected here in a variety of approaches and methodologies.
There are two principal lines of inquiry which can be
distinguished: one group of researchers aims to identify the
neurophysiological manifestations and neuroanatomical basis of
imagery processes in intact subjects, while the other group is
concerned with evaluating the performance of patients with
brain damage in order to enhance our understanding of mental
imagery. In both cases, however, it would appear that genuine
scientific progress is likely to be contingent upon the
development and testing of detailed theoretical specifications
of the cognitive processes assumed to be involved.

3. FRAMEWORKS, MODELS, AND METHODS

Despite these undoubtedly important contributions of
European research on mental imagery, several considerations are
likely to weaken the impact which such research is likely to
make upon the wider international scene. The first point is
that much of the work that was presented at the European
Workshop was empirically driven, rather than theoretically
driven. This is not to say that there was any paucity of

theoretical frameworks on offer; indeed, if anything there were too many frameworks which seemed quite arbitrary and lacking in firm epistemological grounding, and which appeared to have been developed purely to handle fairly isolated empirical phenomena being studied in particular laboratories. Conversely, there were far too few really well articulated models of the role of mental imagery in human cognition which transcended local interests and findings, and which directly motivated specific empirical predictions across a wide range of experimental situations. Because of the relatively weak conceptual link between theoretical frameworks and empirical data, the relevant researchers showed relatively little inclination to discard models which had not been experimentally confirmed. It was therefore quite unclear what arguments or evidence would in fact lead them to revise or reject their speculations.

At the same time, the papers contained in this volume provide evidence of a further increase in the number of different procedures which have been devised to study mental imagery and its role in human cognition. This is especially true of those presentations concerned with the investigation of stimulus attributes, where the general approach is typically to set them up in competition with one another, to see which has the greatest capacity for predicting performance in some criterion task. Nevertheless, each is based upon a specific experimental situation itself, and our understanding of the theoretical basis of that situation is often extremely vague. Instead, we need an integrative model which identifies the processes involved in each such situation and which relates the various procedures concerned within a single unified account.

4. CONVERGENCE IN CONTEMPORARY THEORIZING

In short, current European research on mental imagery appears to lack a theoretical framework which is epistemologically firmly grounded, genuinely integrative in its approach, and heuristically powerful. Nevertheless, the contributions to this volume indicate that there are converging elements of thinking amongst imagery researchers in both Europe and North America which offer some basis for theoretical consensus. This would include the following principles:

(1) There are different forms of human information processing and these can give rise to qualitatively different effects upon performance.

(2) Information processing can be classified according to its modality; in particular, a plausible distinction is that between imaginal and verbal processing.

(3) The type of information processing which is used in any particular task depends upon optional control processes; these are influenced by particular characteristics of the stimulus material and of the task situation and also by the subject's cognitive preferences or "style", but they are not wholly determined by these factors.

(4) Imaginal and verbal information processing are directly amenable to conscious introspection; that is, conscious thought is manifested in the form of verbal, imaginal, or other modality-specific processes.

Although some might disagree, it seems plausible that

modality-specific information processing should be associated with distinct systems, and thus that images should be generated in a system different from that responsible for the generation of verbal responses. The various slave systems proposed within Baddeley's (1986) theory of working memory can be interpreted as one model for this distinction, but it is unclear whether the theory can handle all that is currently known about the generation and manipulation of mental images. Within research on human learning and memory more generally, if it is true that information processing is modality-specific, then the question arises whether the various operations of encoding and retrieval should also be characterized as modality-specific. Again, this seems to be intuitively reasonable, but basically remains a matter of theoretical predilection.

5. ALTERNATIVE METHODS OF INQUIRY

In our collective role as the Scientific Committee responsible for the European Workshop on Imagery and Cognition, we agreed that the event should be restricted to topics on imagery in experimental cognitive-oriented work. However, there was certainly no explicit requirement that our contributions should come solely from within the behaviourist tradition. Indeed, John Yuille (1986), one of the foremost researchers in imagery research during the last 20 years, has delivered a scathing attack on the value of a purely experimental approach to the study of human cognition (though in fact most of his empirical evidence for the limitations of this sort of approach was itself obtained from formal laboratory experiments). It can be argued that current work on imagery and cognition does not pay enough attention to the potential value of nonexperimental forms of investigation. Approaches of a qualitative, phenomenological, or even anthropological nature have proved valuable in cognate fields of inquiry such as text processing (see, e.g., Marton, Hounsell, & Entwistle, 1984), and they might well have something to contribute to the development of understanding in the present context as well. It might also be added that perspectives of this sort represent a distinctively European contribution to research on human cognition.

6. THE FUNCTIONS OF MENTAL IMAGERY

One aspect of Yuille's (1986) criticism of laboratory-based research on human cognition is that it tells us very little about the "natural history" of cognitive faculties. In particular, it reveals little or nothing about the real-life functions of mental imagery. Certainly, many contributors to this volume have merely considered the role of imagery within artificial experimental situations and have not discussed whether their findings might generalize to everyday life, though there are one or two obvious exceptions to this. Moreover, those researchers who have addressed the question of the functions of mental imagery tend to characterize it as a set of fairly simple, quasiperceptual processes, and they seem to assume that more sophisticated intellectual skills depend upon more abstract, propositional representations and the inferential power of systems of production rules.

Certainly, imagery does not appear to contribute to many forms of high-level communication that we engage in from day to day. One might assume that the broadcast media would be more likely to engage nonverbal processing than written media, but as Charles Pulteney (1986) recently pointed out, the majority of the discourses that are transmitted on radio and television are actually oral recitations of written texts. Michael Eysenck and David Warren Piper (1987) report that the economist J. K. Galbraith introduced a series of television programmes on economic theory by displaying the wondrous range of visual aids with which he had been provided, but qualified this by remarking, "And if all this fails, I can always just explain it to you; after all, a word is worth a thousand pictures".

Nevertheless, there do seem to be occasions when mental imagery supports equally powerful and impressive feats of intellect. For instance, the recognition of familiar faces appears to be achieved by means of visual cues and without the use of propositional descriptions (Richardson, 1980, pp. 64-65). Perhaps rather more impressive is the ability to recognize that a photograph shows someone as a child whom we have known only as an adult. To take quite a different example, in classical times mathematicians in China and India used to place considerable value upon geometrical figures which simply showed the necessity of mathematical theorems, and the concept of deductive proof was largely unknown.

7. OTHER TOPICS TO BE EXPLORED

There are many other questions which still need to be addressed in work on mental imagery. We shall merely identify two topics where we feel that European cognitive psychologists can make important contributions to future research. One of these is the "externalization" or communication of mental imagery. By this we mean the exploration of those communicative processes (including discourse elaboration, drawing, and also other forms of artistic expression) whereby an individual who has a particular mental image is able to convey the information contained in that image to another person, and to induce that person to form a similar mental image in order that efficient computations can be performed upon it. This is clearly of great practical importance to the teaching and application of the techniques of art and design.

Another topic which has been consistently neglected in imagery research is the whole area of human development. The conspicuously small number of investigations that have taken a developmental perspective are isolated and overwhelmed by the major currents in contemporary work on mental imagery. What is needed above all is an integrated developmental approach to imagery which takes into account the results of modern cognitive research including information-processing accounts and computational theories. Unfortunately, since Piaget, research on mental imagery has been somewhat hesitant to approach the question of the ontogenetic construction of the system which enables individuals to form and manipulate mental images. This question is certainly one which should receive increasing attention in the future.

8. STRUCTURES FOR FUTURE EUROPEAN COLLABORATION

It is certainly our hope that the scientific interchange made possible by the Workshop should continue in the future. Each of us made a number of acquaintances who might well prove invaluable in the development of our own ideas and research in the imagery field. Nevertheless, it was also our intention that the Workshop should be a unique event in that field, that it should give rise to new and different forms of collaboration, and that it should not itself become a regular scientific meeting. We were grateful to many of the participants for their kind suggestions that we should organize further activities along the same lines, but we were perhaps more pleased (and certainly a little relieved) when they themselves started to discuss spontaneous initiatives for future collaboration. We also considered it to be important to point out that existing national or international societies already contained structures for encouraging such collaboration.

REFERENCES

1. Baddeley, A. D. (1986). Working Memory. Oxford: Oxford University Press.
2. Eysenck, M. W., & Warren Piper, D. (1987). "A word is worth a thousand pictures." In J. T. E. Richardson, M. W. Eysenck, & D. Warren Piper (Eds.), Student Learning: Research in Education and Cognitive Psychology, pp. 208-220. Guildford: SRHE & Open University Press.
3. Marton, F., Hounsell, D., & Entwistle, N. (1984). The Experience of Learning. Edinburgh: Scottish Academic Press.
4. Pulteney, C. (1986). Word blindness. The Times Higher Education Supplement, 19 September, p. 17.
5. Richardson, J. T. E. (1980). Mental Imagery and Human Memory. London: Macmillan.
6. Yuille, J. C. (1986). The futility of a purely experimental psychology of cognition: Imagery as a case study. In D. F. Marks (Ed.), Theories of Image Formation, pp. 197-224. New York: Brandon House.